'The skill of this book is that it understands self-harm so broadly, sweeping within its remit a range of other forms of injur~ ~~~~~~~~~ bloodletting, castration and flagellation . . . She is a diligent and exte~ ~~~~~ ~~~ ~~~ ~~~~~~~~~ ~~~ ~~~ amassed sources and the sensitivity beh~ ~~~ ~~~~~~~ ~~~ ~~~~ ~~ ~~~ discover and understand in the history ~

'The book is deeply important, both for ~~~~~~~ ~~~~~~ ~~~~~~~~~ to self-harm and for the broader critique it offers of diagnosis and medicalization. Chaney sends a message I think more people in the field need to hear.' – *PsycCritique*

'A valuable contribution . . . Chaney insightfully highlights the gender biases that have pervaded the discourse from the start: the way self-harmers were caricatured in gendered terms as deceitful and devious; the habit among some researchers of excluding men or older women from sample groups (on grounds of being "atypical") in order to reinforce the assumption that the typical cutter was a young woman; and the tendency of practitioners to overlook sexual abuse – marginalized under the euphemistic purview of "family troubles" if mentioned at all – as a possible causative factor when considering a patient's motives for self-harming . . . Chaney's emphasis on the importance of communities and mutual support groups is especially apposite in the wake of last year's closures of a number of state-funded Crisis Recovery Unit centres across the UK, in the name of fiscal austerity.' – *TLS*

'It's an exquisitely original take, and one evinced by Chaney with an attractive intensity and wavering levels of confidence. Discursive, meticulously politically correct and, at times, metallic in tone, she attacks the shifting borders of psychiatry and its baleful gender bias.' – *The Australia*

'There is a lot of careful detail here, balanced against a set of "bigger pictures" – trends in medicine, politics and culture, with particular attention to gender differences. I enjoyed the eclecticism and fast pace; it is worth noting also the careful scholarship and respectful tone . . . by assembling a set of competing definitions, Chaney shows that the field of self-harm is contested and therefore contestable, not least by those who (like the author) have experienced medical treatment that they found alienating, or cruel.' – *Social History of Medicine*

'In *Psyche on the Skin*, Chaney traces the illuminating and disturbing history of self-mutilation and other forms of self-harm . . . This work offers a fascinating look at a set of topics often as taboo to talk about as the acts themselves. It is strongly recommended for professionals likely to encounter individuals who have engaged in such acts.' – *Choice*

'Self-harm is a crucially important topic for understanding psychology and culture in general and, often, religion in particular. For that reason, Sarah Chaney's *Psyche on the Skin* is a welcome contribution.' – *Anthropology Review*

'*Psyche on the Skin* is a historical analysis of the global psychological issue of self-harm. My concern when choosing this book to review was that it might end up being a self-indulgent account of the author's own experience of self-harm. This book however offers an interesting and detailed account of different kinds of self-harm throughout the ages, beginning with the religious practice of castration and historical practice of therapeutic blood-letting.' – *Nursing Times*

'Well-written, clearly organized, and entirely intriguing . . . *Psyche on the Skin* is a fascinating and impressive piece of social history and analysis. Equally illustrative and didactic, it is a compelling argument against a universal model of self harm. It is also a model for how to approach other categories that have been caught up in the maw of psychiatric reductionism, certainly eating disorders, but perhaps even mood disorders like depression. For those skeptical or concerned over present day ideas about mental health and illness, including practitioners, mental health service users, social historians and philosophers of psychiatry, this is a valuable contribution.' – *Metapsychology*

'The author demonstrates the dubious utility of trying to contain such a range of behaviours, with so many antecedents, within a single diagnostic construct. It reminded me of one of my most important tasks as a psychiatrist. To, without preconceptions, help the patient in front of me to construct a narrative, articulate their predicament and use this understanding to enable change. Which, the author tells us, is what she has achieved by writing this book and, in doing so, I think she has succeeded in helping the reader to reflect on his or her assumptions about self-harm.' – *British Journal of Psychiatry*

'Eloquent, awe-inspiring, and sassy. This book will captivate anyone curious about the body and pain.' – Joanna Bourke, author of *The Story of Pain: From Prayer to Painkillers*

'A remarkable account from the pen of a young and brilliant scholar of the history and meaning of self-harm. Insightful and immensely readable.' – Sander L. Gilman, Professor of Psychiatry at Emory University and author of *Making the Body Beautiful: A Cultural History of Aesthetic Surgery*

PSYCHE ON THE SKIN

PSYCHE ON THE SKIN

A HISTORY OF SELF-HARM

SARAH CHANEY

reaktion books ltd

With love to Gail, Holly, Tara, Shaz, Kate, Nat and all the forum folks old and new. I could never have got this far without you.

Published by REAKTION BOOKS LTD
Unit 32, Waterside
44–48 Wharf Road
London N1 7UX, UK
www.reaktionbooks.co.uk

First published 2017
First published in paperback 2019
Copyright © Sarah Chaney 2017

Printed and bound in Great Britain by CPI Group (UK) Ltd, Croydon CR0 4YY

A catalogue record for this book is available from the British Library

ISBN 978 1 78914 148 1

CONTENTS

INTRODUCTION

When I was in my early twenties, I determined to begin life anew. Filled with nervous optimism, I decided it was time to erase the visible evidence of my past. I had read about a scheme run by Samaritans. They offered free make-up matched to your skin tone, and advice on covering scars. The only catch? You had to be referred by your GP. I was living in my fourth home, and fourth London borough, in four years. The concept of a regular GP was alien to me. I got an appointment with the first doctor available. I'd never met him before – I don't even know if he was from my local practice or a locum, just passing through. Hesitantly, I explained what I needed from him. He stared at me in condescending disbelief. 'Why should I refer you?' he said scathingly. 'You'll only go and do it again!' In a decade or so of varied experience of primary care and mental health services, this is by no means the only occasion I have encountered hostility like this. Certainly, I have also experienced the reverse. I'll never forget the doctor who caught me up in his enthusiasm as he drew circles on a piece of paper to try and explain my mental state, or the accident and emergency nurse who talked kindly while she bandaged up a deep wound, even though it was past 1 a.m. and there was a two-hour wait for stitches. These experiences stand out, however, because they have been relatively unusual.

What is it about self-inflicted injury that invites knee-jerk assumptions? And, more importantly, where do such assumptions come from? It might seem easy to dismiss these personal anecdotes as isolated experiences of poor patient care, or a simple failure in human understanding. Yet my opening example illustrates attitudes that have been written into psychiatric and medical explanations of self-inflicted injury over the past century or more. Hostility towards self-injury in a medical setting has often been founded on the assumption that self-harm is intended to manipulate others – a firm refusal by a physician to be 'duped' by a deceitful patient.[1] Yet a historical approach to self-harm indicates that this is by no means the obvious or only way of viewing self-inflicted injury. Indeed, it was not until the turn of the twentieth century that this assertion was first made, bound up with wider concerns over the economic effect of so-called 'malingering' on health care and society.[2] The other implication of the words cited above is that it might be 'pointless' to refer someone who presents with self-injury to other services, even at the patient's request. This assumption is historically more recent than the idea of self-harm as manipulative, founded largely in the connections formed between self-injury and borderline personality disorder from the 1960s onwards. This notion has been retained in the modern concept of self-injury as an 'addictive' behaviour, that once indulged in might be 'triggered' by external circumstances and can never be truly recovered from.

My personal reflections also provide an important context for this book. The history of self-harm is not simply about the past, but offers a source of insight into modern medicine and cultural ideals. If we dismiss as a one-off instance the circumstances that might lead a busy GP to refuse point-blank to refer a patient to a charity service, we miss an opportunity to improve medical services. If we assume that it is just a 'bad' psychiatrist who might reject anything else a patient tells them as unworthy of attention once they have admitted to self-harm, then we may fail to acknowledge our own prejudices and assumptions. Self-harm, it could be suggested, confounds the medical profession because it contradicts the efforts of practitioners to 'fix' or heal a patient. Yet this simplifies a complicated moralization of self-injury, involving a variety of value judgements often made in comparison to other forms of behaviour.[3] In contrast to this, in recent decades personal accounts have gained increasing recognition in mental health research, as a range of organizations and individuals have become engaged in mental health service user or survivor research on a national and international scale. User groups may highlight different ideas, challenging accepted psychiatric wisdom and hierarchies of evidence. Responding to self-harm in particular, peer-led advocacy and self-help groups, such as the Bristol Crisis Service for Women and Survivors Speak Out, coordinated publications and conferences from the 1980s onwards.[4] Personal accounts of self-injurious behaviour can be powerful and evocative, indicating the vast breadth and scope of the ways in which people make sense of their lives.[5] Sometimes they may engage directly with medical diagnoses, emphasizing or critiquing particular elements; sometimes they are explicitly anti-psychiatry or offer alternative user-led definitions of self-injury.[6]

Despite this background, however, in 2013 the fifth edition of the American Psychiatric Association's *Diagnostic and Statistical Manual of Mental Disorders* (DSM-5) incorporated non-suicidal self-injury (NSSI) as a category for the first time, as one of a number of 'conditions for further study'.[7] Some medical experts assume that it will become a discrete diagnosis the next time the volume is revised.[8] The inclusion of self-injury in the DSM may seem surprising, given that those advocating for it have often been those who take a broad trans-cultural and historical approach to the topic.[9] One reason for this is the importance of the DSM within the insurance model of health care operating in the United States: without a formal diagnosis, insurance companies will not pay for medical treatment. In the United Kingdom, and other countries with a state health care system, this may not be the case: those who self-injure can pass through general practice, accident and emergency and even some parts of the mental health service without being formally given a psychiatric diagnosis.[10] Enshrining NSSI as a specific syndrome runs the risk of imposing one specific cultural model of 'harm' across entire populations. The DSM definition, for example, states that it does not include 'socially sanctioned' behaviours; however, it is largely left to individual psychiatrists to decide what is or is not socially sanctioned. Body piercing and tattooing are listed as examples,

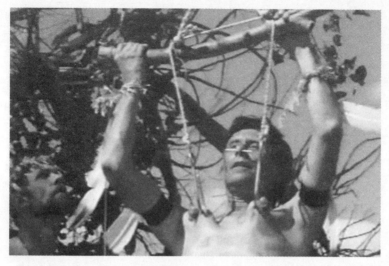

Fakir Musafar (b. 1930), founder of the Modern Primitives movement, shown suspended from flesh hooks during a ritual.

certainly; but what of other forms of body modification, acts defined as sexually masochistic or extreme performance art?[11] Both the second and third editions of Armando Favazza's *Bodies Under Siege* included an epilogue by Fakir Musafar, founder of the Modern Primitives movement, in which he described the spiritual value of branding, extreme waist reduction, the insertion of weighted flesh hooks and full body suspension.[12] How many psychiatrists taking up the new category of NSSI, one wonders, would accept Musafar's descriptions as culturally sanctioned and therefore not pathological?

Medical definitions have often been assumed to be neutral and objective in a way that personal experience is not. Yet, as this book shows, psychiatric definitions cannot be viewed outside the lives and experiences of medical practitioners. The political and cultural ideals we all hold impact the way our research is interpreted, whether we admit to this or not: a psychiatrist is no different in this respect from a mental health service user. Awareness of this is an important first step. Understanding our limitations improves our ability to critique. History itself is not a neutral set of ideas through which we understand the past, but an opportunity to reflect on our current experiences and practices. Viewing self-injury historically benefits practitioners and service users, taking us beyond a narrow model based either on personal experiences or medical theories. That does not mean we should ignore either of these things: indeed, they may well be the impetus that drives us to critique in the first place. Would I have been interested in exploring psychiatric models of self-harm if I had not wanted to understand my experiences of the medical profession better? If I had not wondered about those stereotypes and bitterly felt those assumptions? Perhaps I would, but the two things are impossible to disentangle. And if I pretend I can isolate either, I am only supporting the notion that objectivity might somehow be possible.

Rewriting psychiatry: countering the myth of objectivity

When I began my research, I held a number of preconceptions based on the work of other historians. I assumed that the emergence of a category of 'self-mutilation' in Victorian psychiatry was part of a drive towards classification within mental health care at the time, based on a pessimistic and determinist biological model of mental illness.[13] I was surprised to find that, of the small group of practitioners writing on self-mutilation in the Victorian era, many argued against this view. Instead, they read self-harm as evidence that mental health and illness were part of a continuum. They used the behaviour as justification for a psychological rather than a bio-logically determined model of mental illness, and even an argument for the value of diversity in evolution, as opposed to the so-called 'survival of the fittest'.[14] As we shall see in the chapters that follow, this did not mean that they were immune to the cultural stereotypes and moral concerns of their era: far from it. However, to interpret their ideas as evidence that self-harm is, and always has been, a universal category (supporting its inclusion in the *DSM*) is to utterly ignore this very important context. While it is certainly possible to find material in Victorian texts that supports modern ideas, there are just as many examples that contradict the psychiatry of today. To cherry-pick those elements that chime with contemporary assumptions is simply using history to justify our current concerns, setting them up as absolute truth.[15] If we learn but one thing from late Victorian psychiatry, it is the uncertainty of definition, which 'is after all but the summing up of the knowledge of to-day; it is not an absolute reflex of nature'.[16] Medical diagnoses – especially but not only in psychiatry – shift across time and culture. They change as new medical evidence is investigated, but also as cultural attitudes and ideas alter.[17] To assume that today's ideas are 'true' in a way that yesterday's were not is to suggest that modern science is omniscient.

In this book I explore psychiatric models of self-harm, but I do not begin with them. In this way I hope to avoid some of the artificial distinctions that a focus on descriptions of self-inflicted injury as pathology can impose. While, in the main, I don't cover body modification, ritual mutilation or performance art, I do not consider that there is an obvious distinction between the self-harming behaviour described in a psychiatric context and wider instances of self-inflicted bodily harm.[18] To that end, I begin with a 'pre-history' of self-harm, before it was first viewed in a psychiatric context in the late nineteenth century. Through this approach, I question the notion that self-mutilation can be thought of as a constant, universal human behaviour with a particular set of meanings. I explore three distinct eras and practices of self-injury, each of which differs in at least one significant way from modern definitions. The pagan and early Christian practice of religious castration had a very specific set of social and political – as well as spiritual – meanings. Importantly, maleness was not viewed as intrinsically linked to sex organs, as came to be the case in later years. The flagellant processions of the Middle Ages, meanwhile, reshaped earlier religious mortification into a very public group practice. As a group activity, often viewed in positive terms, religious flagellation in the Middle Ages has no connection to the modern assumption that self-harm is a personal, private activity. Finally, self-inflicted injury has an important connection to historical medical practice through the concept of bloodletting. In nineteenth-century definitions of self-mutilation,

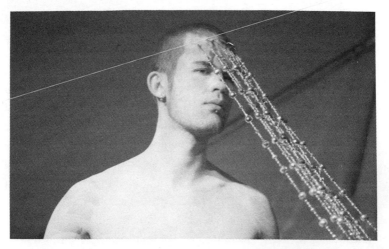

Dominic Johnson, *Transmission*, performed at 'Revisions of Excess', curated by Ron Athey and Lee Adams for Fierce Festival, Birmingham, 2007.

self-cutting was barely mentioned: today, it has become the archetype of self-harm.[19] Yet for Victorian doctors and patients, self-cutting was much closer to self-treatment than other forms of self-injury, for bloodletting had been an established medical practice for over two thousand years.

The modern concept of self-harm as a specific category of abnormal individual behaviour emerged in the second half of the nineteenth century, when 'self-mutilation' was defined within asylum psychiatry. I explain how this occurred in the context of the new asylum system and psychiatric profession in western Europe. While it has often been assumed that Victorian writers made no distinction between suicidal and non-suicidal self-injury, this was not the case. Psychiatrists in this era frequently argued that self-mutilation was not carried out for suicidal reasons, although they differed in their method of applying alternative meaning to such acts. While people had certainly harmed themselves in a variety of ways prior to this period, the late nineteenth century was the first time that diverse acts – from skin-picking to amputation – became regarded as equivalent behaviours. Combining them under the umbrella term 'self-mutilation' prompted the idea that some form of universal meaning might similarly be discoverable. Self-harm became viewed as an act that had meaning beyond the physical nature of any wounds inflicted, an act that revealed something of the character of an individual and, in addition, an act that might help to explain the relationship between individual and society.

The remainder of the book explores five distinct models or methods of understanding self-inflicted injury within psychiatry, from the 1880s to the present day. It is not a straightforward chronology. I argue that as self-harm is not a coherent or constant category, it follows that there can be no linear progress in 'understanding' it. I do not cover all instances or examples of self-mutilation, but instead explore particular models that have been put forward in different eras, indicating how these drew on a wide variety of contemporary medical, social and political ideas. While there has certainly been overlap between ways of viewing self-injury, authors of new models have often selectively interpreted past research in order to shoe-horn it into prevailing theories. Some notions, such as those outlined at the outset of this introduction, came to be imbued with a kind of independent 'truth', and continued to be put forward long after the cultural ideas they had grown out of were superseded.

The two late Victorian models outlined form an interesting comparison in relation to this tendency. The first, 'sexual self-mutilation', is likely to prove quite alien to modern readers. Self-castration became a significant concern in the 1880s – out of all proportion to reported incidence of acts of genital mutilation. Diverging sharply from a classical approach, late Victorian commentators viewed castration as linked to sexual desire. Sexuality was newly described as of great social and political importance, in the psychological development of the individual (usually male) as well as for the wider development of civilization. Conversely, the 'motiveless malingerer' described in the second model may, on the surface, appear much more familiar to modern readers. Studies in the century following have tended to claim that self-harm is more frequent among women than men and, in particular, among young, middle-class, educated women.[20] This was often the profile assumed by doctors treating so-called 'hysterical' women for self-inflicted injuries in the late nineteenth and early twentieth centuries. Yet this surface similarity should not blind us to the differences between hysterical 'malingering' and twenty-first-century self-harm. Turn-of-the-century male practitioners, from psychiatrists to dermatologists, shaped their explanations through a pre-existing understanding of gendered attributes. Hysterics – and often, by extension, *all* women – were thought to be inherently manipulative. Indeed, physicians' assumptions about their patients' personalities were often the only thing that united these disparate cases of female self-harm.

Modern researchers often date investigation into self-inflicted injury as beginning with Karl Menninger's *Man Against Himself* in 1938.[21] Menninger, an American Freudian psychoanalyst, regarded self-mutilation as an unconscious mechanism for avoiding suicide, by the concentration of a 'suicidal impulse' on one part of the body as a substitute for the whole.[22] Although Freud himself had shown little interest in self-injury, other psychoanalysts interpreted self-harm as proof of his theories. In particular, I explore the association of the psychology of self-harm with psychosexual trauma and the Freudian death instinct. This largely took place in psychoanalytic circles in the United States and, far from being universal, both explanations were specific to the contexts in which they were developed. *Man Against Himself*, in particular, emerged from Menninger's attempt to understand the apparently destructive nature of human psychology as world war loomed on the horizon for a second time.

Psychoanalytic ideas were adopted as background to the 1960s concept of 'delicate self-cutting'. Nonetheless, this characterization of self-mutilation altered significantly, as psychiatrists began to focus on one particular form of injury: that of cutting or scratching the skin. 'Self-cutting' had not been emphasized in any of the previous models, although today it is frequently assumed to be the paradigm for self-harm.[23] This shift in the types of behaviour associated with the term is an important argument against a universal model of self-harm. The articles on delicate cutting, moreover, reinforced stereotypes of gendered attributes, through generalizations made about a small number of inpatients in private hospitals in the northeastern United States. These assumptions were subsequently applied to *all* populations engaging in self-injurious behaviour and were used to generate a universal model, associated in the third edition of the *Diagnostic and Statistical Manual* of the American Psychiatric Association (*DSM-III*, 1980) with borderline personality disorder.

In the twenty-first century, however, the explanations applied to self-injury have changed once again. I explore the role of the World Wide Web and a new concept of self-harm based in modern notions of trauma. In particular, I look at the emergence of the 'trigger warning', in relation to psychological and cultural concepts of contagion. While the trigger is cited across a variety of psychiatric and medical fields, it is particularly problematic in relation to self-inflicted injury. On the one hand, the modern concept of self-harm usually describes the behaviour as a private, personal act related to individual inner turmoil; on the other, the trigger is embedded in a neurobiological model of conditioning, based on reflex responses.

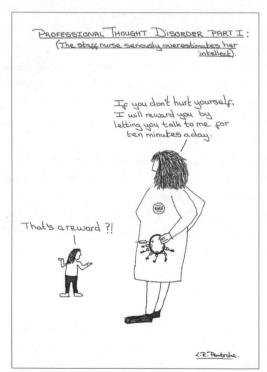

Cartoon by Louise Roxanne Pembroke, from 'Self-harm: Perspectives from Personal Experience', produced by Survivors Speak Out, one of the first organizations to hold a user-led conference on self-harm, in 1989.

Where does one begin and the other end? When we view self-harm from a historical perspective, modern notions can be as confused and confusing as Victorian ideas of self-mutilation.

This book is a medical history, in that I explore historical views of self-injury as a medical category, usually a psychiatric one. Although I do not take modern definitions as a given from which earlier models depart, I do refer interchangeably to self-harm, self-injury and self-mutilation (although not all these terms were used throughout the historical eras I describe).[24] I use all three primarily to refer to self-inflicted acts resulting in tissue damage of some kind, although sometimes the way definitions are shaped in a particular era means that I touch on other behaviours, in particular overdosing and food refusal. Focusing on self-injury in a medical context can risk reinforcing it as a medical (pathological) category. However, it is this use of history that I critique throughout: the assumption that modern definitions are simply new descriptive terms for acts that were previously defined differently. All the models of self-harm, self-injury or self-mutilation outlined here were specific to the times and places in which they came into being, associated with social, political, religious, moral and cultural ideals as well as medical theories. By examining the attribution of meaning to self-inflicted injury from a historical perspective, it becomes clear that self-mutilation emerged from a variety of contemporary concerns and frameworks for understanding human identity. Understanding the ways in which medical categories of self-mutilation were created can enable us to ask similar questions about self-harm today. Finally, while my approach sheds doubt on the existence of self-harm as a universal medical category, I do not intend to bring into question the need of many people who injure themselves to seek medical support: whether to repair tissue damage or in response to associated mental distress or trauma. However, recognizing the assumptions inherent in definitions of self-injury, and reflecting on the ways in which these came into being, *can* help to improve the services available: in general practice, accident and emergency and, of course, mental health care.

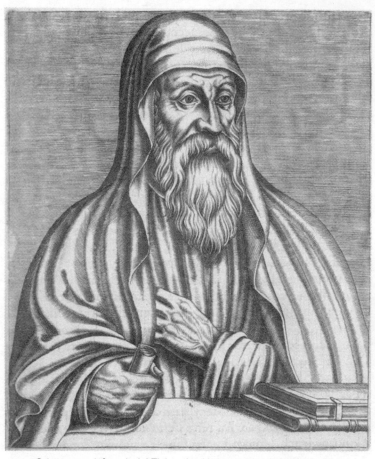

Origen, portrait from André Thévet, *Les Vrais portraits et vies des hommes illustres* (1673).

ONE

THE PRE-HISTORY OF SELF-HARM
From Ancient Castration to
Medicinal Bloodletting

In around 206 CE, so it is said, the Christian teacher Origen – at that time a young man of about twenty – had himself castrated. Origen lived and worked in Alexandria. A few years before his castration, his father Leonides was executed by the Augustal prefect, and thus became a Christian martyr. According to his chroniclers, the only reason the teenage Origen was not martyred alongside his father was because his mother hid his clothes so that he couldn't leave the house. Not long after his father's death, Origen became a spiritual guide and religious teacher. He taught in Alexandria until 234, before ending his life in virtual exile in Caesarea, on the coast of Palestine, where he continued to teach until his death around 253–4, the year after he suffered torture in the local prison.

Already a well-known theologian at the time of his castration, the young Origen reportedly tried to keep the act quiet, discreetly visiting a doctor for the purpose, although, ultimately, 'however much he might wish it, he could not possibly conceal such an act.'[1] Just over a century later, Church chronicler Eusebius considered Origen's act evidence of 'a mind youthful and immature', although he nonetheless praised the teacher's decision as indicative of his 'faith and self-mastery'.[2] The castration, Eusebius felt, had been carried out largely in order to avoid scandal: Origen taught women as well as men, and there was strong potential for unbelievers to accuse him of misusing his privileged position to develop sexual relationships. While this may sound flippant, the accusation that Christianity was synonymous with sexual promiscuity was widespread among pagan critics, and even between different Christian groups.[3]

Yet is this how Origen himself would have regarded the act of castration: as a purely practical measure in order to avoid gossip? Eusebius concluded that Origen had taken 'an absurdly literal' view of Matthew 19:12.[4] This gospel claimed to quote Jesus' words declaring the value of eunuchism:

> For there are some eunuchs, which were so born from their mother's womb: and there are some eunuchs, which were made eunuchs of men: and there be eunuchs, which have made themselves eunuchs for the kingdom of heaven's sake.[5]

This statement has been claimed as allegorical by many theologians both before and after Eusebius: for them, eunuchism referred to a state of mind and style of behaviour, rather than a bodily practice. However, the same text has also been used as justification by Christian sects practising voluntary castration, such as the Russian Skoptsy who are discussed at greater length in Chapter Three. Thus it was perfectly possible to interpret this passage literally, and many of the early Christian teachers, such as Augustine and Clement of Alexandria, who *did* claim this passage to be allegorical, attacked similar readings of other parts of the Bible as heretical.[6] Indeed, the Vulgate – the fourth-century CE Latin version of the Bible, edited by St Jerome – explicitly used the verb *castraverunt* (from *castro*, to castrate) to describe those who had 'made themselves eunuchs'.

Although some later writers claimed that Eusebius misinterpreted Origen's words, and that he was never castrated at all, it was certainly widely believed at the time that the teacher *had* undergone a physical alteration. Indeed, it would not be particularly surprising if he had. There is a great deal of evidence that voluntary castration was widespread in the second and third centuries, in both pagan and Christian religions, and for spiritual and commercial reasons. We must be hesitant, particularly in the absence of any record of eunuchs' own voices, in viewing these acts through the eyes of later commentators – or, indeed, applying a Western twenty-first-century lens directly to these practices: in particular a hetero- or gender-normative framework that assumes a two-sex model of humanity.[7] Eunuchs in antiquity were part of a complex political and religious framework that did not emphasize the same claims about the individual body and its connection with a self or psyche – or, indeed, sexuality – as modern psychology has done. Nonetheless, exploring the complex meaning of self-castration in antiquity (whether self-performed or as a voluntary operation, for contemporaries made little distinction between the two) has resonance for modern understandings of sex and gender. In particular, it highlights the fluidity of definitions of sex, gender and sexuality, and reminds us that there are a multitude of possibilities besides the rigid binary of male/female that was commonly accepted in the nineteenth century and for much of the twentieth.

In this chapter, I explore several specific ways of understanding the body in relation to self-inflicted injury throughout history. All of these differ significantly from those that emerged in modern Western psychiatry (from around 1850). While there are many other examples of self-inflicted injury I could have outlined, I have chosen three particular models that span the period from the first century BCE to about 1850, when psychiatric interpretations of self-injury first emerged. In all of these instances, at least one element of the practice differs considerably from later psychiatric models, above and beyond the religious and ritual context from which most of the acts outlined emerged. First, I look at voluntary castration in antiquity, both as a pagan ritual (carried out by the priests of Cybele) and in early Christian thought. I show that, although there may be some similarities in certain aspects, the meaning of castration in this period (including its perceived effects on the individual) differed significantly from the modern trope of gender dysphoria and/or concepts such as genderqueer.[8] All these tropes *begin* from the notion of binary gender as a normative category. When we look at other eras or cultures, we cannot assume that their ideas of gender emerged from the same norms. Self-castration in antiquity, as distinguished from the involuntary castration of slaves for commercial reasons, generally had a spiritual or ritual element. The religious meaning of eunuchism nonetheless merged with wider knowledge of eunuchs as a specific social and political grouping, and commentators often made little distinction between those who became eunuchs through a self-performed operation, through voluntary surgery or by coercion. This attitude differs significantly from modern understandings of self-harm, which makes voluntary eunuchism an important starting point. Following this, I move on to another practice which is at odds with current psychiatric models: self-flagellation in the Middle Ages. Here, I focus on the processionary flagellants of the thirteenth and fourteenth centuries. This practice of self-wounding was a new aspect of worship in the medieval era and, in the thirteenth century, was transformed from a private act of penance to a heavily symbolic group ritual, with significant social and political impact. Both the positive – even celebratory – view of flagellation by contemporaries, and the way in which it became a very *public* practice, differ completely from the modern concept of self-harm as a private, individual experience. Finally, I look at something very different from religious or spiritual self-mutilation: the medicinal practice of bloodletting. I focus primarily on the popularity of bleeding in the sixteenth and seventeenth centuries, despite major changes in anatomical and physiological knowledge in this era. Bloodletting remained an extremely popular practice, even into the early 1900s, and the widespread understanding of bleeding as therapeutic may explain the absence of many examples of self-inflicted cutting prior to the twentieth century.

From pagan castration to genderless Christianity,
C. 100 BCE–300 CE

Early eunuchs appear to have been found primarily in the Middle East, and the idea of eunuchs as 'Eastern' became an enduring association in later European texts. Eastern tended to denote an exotic 'otherness' for European writers and, after the Middle Ages, eunuchs were associated in Western popular thought with the imperial eunuchs of the later Ottoman

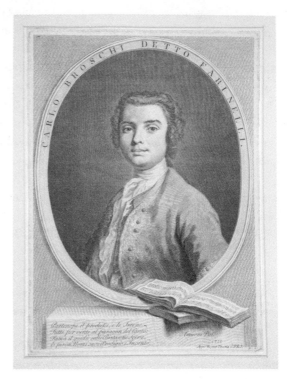

Empire (1453–1909) and the Qing dynasty in China (1644–1912). This connection was strong despite the existence of the practice across many parts of the Greek and Roman empires in antiquity, as well as later European traditions, such as the singers known as castrati. In what was primarily an Italian phenomenon, the singers were castrated as boys, in order to prevent their voices breaking. Some achieved great fame in the early days of opera in the seventeenth and eighteenth centuries and toured Europe to great acclaim. The most famous castrato was Farinelli (Carlo Broschi, 1705–1782), a favourite of the Spanish royal court. Although the castrati received less attention after 1800, castrated males continued to feature in church choirs until the early twentieth century. In 1902, Pope Leo XIII attempted to end the practice of castration by banning any new eunuchs from joining the Sistine Chapel choir.[9]

Carlo Broschi detto Farinelli by Jacopo Amigoni, 1735.

This commercial eunuchism – although it retained certain religious associations, through the 'angelic' voices of the castrati – was very different from voluntary castration in antiquity, on which I focus in this section. Both Greek and Roman historians attributed the origins of deliberate castration to the royal courts of Assyria and later Persia, and it seems that many eunuchs through history have been associated with royalty.[10] Stone reliefs depicting these eunuchs date back to at least the ninth century BCE. The popular assumption holds that eunuchs were useful specifically because their sterility made them ideal guardians for imperial harems. However, in practice they undertook a wide variety of administrative, military and personal duties in palaces and even private homes. Eunuchs were often slaves – both Roman and Islamic cultures held that citizens of their empires should not be castrated – and thus a foreign supply was required. Reasons for castration were varied. It might be inflicted as a punishment or to preserve a youthful singing voice or to create a 'guardian of the bed'.[11] Eunuchs were particularly expensive slaves, due to their relative scarcity, and thus became a status symbol for the elite, especially as personal attendants for men and women. Here, however, I want to focus on religious eunuchs. Religious emasculation was more often elective than in the case of slaves (although the castration of boys before puberty certainly occurred, a practice which would not be considered voluntary from a modern perspective) and thus more comparable with 'self-harm' than the commercial practice. The background is important, however, in that there was significant overlap between the positions held by religious eunuchs and those in the royal court. The Galli, the priests of Cybele, held a unique position in society, such that they often wore royal garments.[12]

The priests of Cybele practised a well-known form of self-castration, and the meaning of their ritual practice is an interesting contrast to the example of Origen. Self-castration in the Cult of Cybele was accounted for by the myth of Attis, although there has been some debate as to whether the myth inspired the practice or was adopted to account for a procedure already in use. Victorian writers certainly tended to assume the latter, probably

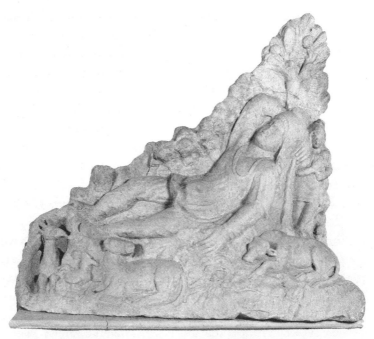

Relief from an Attideum in Ostia, showing Attis after castrating himself. According to Alvar, the original colouring may have shown blood pouring from the wound.

inspired by the description in the anthropologist James Frazer's *The Golden Bough* (1890). Frazer was adamant that 'the story of the self-mutilation of Attis is clearly an attempt to account for the self-mutilation of his priests',[13] an assumption incorporated into the definition of self-mutilation written by the psychiatrist James Adam in 1892. The association of self-castration with the Cult of Cybele was firmly enshrined by the Victorian era, generally set in an Oriental context. As Adam put it, 'this elementary principle of Eastern religion has deeply influenced the whole history of man, but it had made no progress in Europe till after the introduction of Christianity.'[14] Adam viewed the worship of Cybele as a clear bridge between Eastern practices and early Christian castration, such as that of Origen.

The myth of Cybele and Attis originated in a Phrygian (Turkish) version, which was the source of several classical variants of the story, such as those told by the Roman poets Catullus and Ovid.[15] Cybele, the Mother Goddess, has been identified with a large number of other goddesses appearing in Greek, Egyptian and Syrian texts.[16] Most versions of the story cast Attis as a young Phrygian herdsman (in some he is the son of a demi-god, in others not). When Attis decided to marry, the goddess Cybele took a terrible revenge on him for reneging on his promise to remain faithful to her alone. At Attis' wedding, she filled all the men present with a mad-dening sexual desire: Attis castrated himself with a flint and bled to death beneath a pine tree, which became his symbol as a god. Other men present cut off their testicles, although none suffered the same fate as Attis. The miserable bride, meanwhile, cut off her own breasts. Subsequently, Cybele decided she had been too harsh and begged Zeus, the father of the gods, to restore Attis to life. Zeus decreed that the herdsman's body would never decay, and although he remained in his tomb, Attis' hair continued to grow, and his little finger to twitch.[17] The poet Gaius Valerius Catullus (c. 84–54 BCE) dramatically described Attis' castration: 'straying from reason, he cut away with sharp flint the burden of manhood.'[18] Following this act, Catullus referred to Attis as 'she', and used the feminine form 'Gallae' to describe the priests. Like Attis, they were a 'slice of my former self, an unmanned man'.[19] Catullus focused on Attis' transformation, rather than his death. Following castration, Attis was both feminized *and* genderless (unmanned), indicating the dual role of the eunuch in late antiquity. In domestic circles, a eunuch was permitted to move in both male and female spheres: associating with the female side of the household, but also enter-ing public spaces usually forbidden to women. The castrated male was thus not quite considered a man, but neither was he entirely feminized.[20]

Cybele's priests, the Galli, occupied a similarly ambiguous status. They held a privileged position in Phrygia (although in Greece or Rome they were more likely to be associated with slave-eunuchs). However, they also existed outside society. They wore women's clothing: a colourful tunic and a veil covering long hair, alongside prominent ornaments – necklaces, rings and earrings – and often make-up.[21] Lucian reported that the Galli at Hier-apolis carried out women's work, as well as dressing in female clothing.[22]

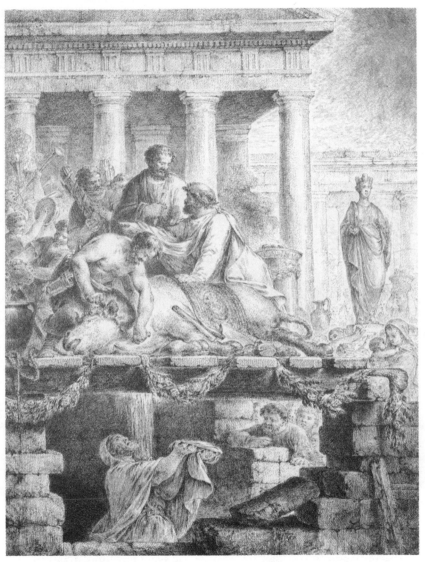

A tauroborium ceremony, indicating the importance placed on blood in the cult of Cybele. The priests of Cybele are being baptized with the blood of a sacrificial bull, which is lying on a stage in the centre. Christian Bernhard Rode, 1774-5.

It is impossible to know, in retrospect, how many of the devotees were actually castrated, although it is often assumed today that gelding was a requirement for initiation into the priesthood.[23] Contemporary social accounts suggested that initiates emasculated themselves during the spring festival. They were supposed to follow the example of Attis, castrating themselves while in a frenzy, using a pointed sherd or flint. The likelihood of this practice was later called into question due to the dangerous nature of such a procedure – although the Victorian accounts of self-performed operations with rudimentary instruments described in Chapter Three might attest to its being possible, albeit risky. It seems likely, however, that the Galli used a variety of methods, including ligature, crushing of the testicles and surgical removal, as well as self-ablation.[24] This would accord with other contemporary practices. According to one source, the Roman emperor Elagabalus (*c.* 203–222 CE) tied up his testicles while celebrating the rites of Cybele, and others may well have followed this example.[25]

But what did the practice signify? The priests themselves appear to have regarded the act of castration as a sign of their exclusive devotion to the Great Mother – unlike Attis, they would be physically incapable of breaking their promise to be faithful. But what did this faith mean? It did not, as we might assume, mean that the Galli renounced all sexual contact. Indeed, although sources are often euphemistic, there is some evidence that worship of Cybele included sacred prostitution: ritual sexual activity by both female and male (eunuch) devotees.[26] It was well known in antiquity that eunuchs (especially those castrated after puberty) could experience sexual desire and were often capable of achieving an erection.[27] Eunuchs could be paired sexually with either men or women. However, in the later Roman period it appears that the eunuch was most often assumed to be the passive recipient of anal intercourse with another man.

While people in antiquity did not recognize a clear division between homosexuality and heterosexuality as states of being, homosexual practices became increasingly frowned upon in the later empire, and new legislation attempted to prohibit such acts.[28] A law of 342 CE appeared to ban marriage between a man and a eunuch, while in 390 the death penalty was extended to apply to all men who had sex with eunuchs (and not just those who married them).[29] The Galli, by most accounts, were sexually active with both men and women. Their 'faithfulness', then, did not equate to modern assumptions concerning sexual or emotional monogamy. We should remember that the cult was inextricably linked with fertility: Cybele, the Great Mother, was a nature goddess, and the major rituals of the cult occurred at the outbreak of spring, which was associated with new life. The 'Day of Blood', the centre of the festival in April, celebrated this birth of the new as the Galli lacerated themselves in public.[30] However, although the spilled blood symbolized fertility and new growth, the fact that the Galli were castrated meant they would retain the pneuma (or life-force) thought to be contained in their seed. This ensured the Galli retained their spiritual integrity, and thus were faithful to Cybele alone.[31]

This retention of their vital spirit set the Galli apart from other mortals, just as their adoption of a very specific way of life set them apart from the wider social order. The Galli were able to act 'as mediators between the "otherness" and the "norm": able to foretell the future or heal the sick, they still remain[ed] separated from the social group'.[32] Like other priests, the Galli had an intimate connection with the gods, which endowed them with powers not possessed by other mortals. They existed *between* the mortal world and the divine realm, and their physical castration and stylized clothing were direct evidence of this special status, of being beyond or more than human. This point is further supported if we accept the claims of Stephen of Byzantium that it was Gallus, not Attis, who was the model for the priests. In one version of the myth, Gallus was the father of Attis' tragic bride. During the frenzy at the wedding party, Gallus too castrated himself: unlike Attis, he survived the act and thus did not become a mythical figure. Existing 'between mythical and ritual time', Gallus could be represented by the Galli, who were both men and not men at one and the same time.[33]

Given the link described by many writers between the eunuch priests of Cybele and sacred prostitution, as well as wider Greek and Roman understanding of the sexual life of eunuchs, Eusebius' assertion that Origen castrated himself in order to be seen as pure seems surprising. Yet the complicated division between allegorical and literal readings of sacred texts meant that early Christian writers often made such apparently contradictory claims. One of the first teachers to suggest that castration was desired by some Christians in order to cure them of earthly desires was Justin (c. 100–165 CE) who, in his *First Apology*, recorded an example of 'one of ours' (that is, a Christian) who had submitted a petition to the governor in Alexandria, 'praying him to permit a physician to remove his testicles, for the physicians there said that they were forbidden to do this without the permission of the governor'.[34] Yet, although Justin presented this example as evidence of the purity of conviction in the Christian faith, he elsewhere described the practices within the Cult of Cybele (including intentional castration) as a sign of immorality. As other authors had done, he explained that the self-castration of the cult was evidence of the priests' homosexual practices, for 'some openly emasculate themselves to become catamites'.[35] Catamite was the Roman term used to describe a young man who engaged in a relationship with an older man; usually, this assumed that the youth was the passive recipient of anal intercourse. In the same text, Justin condemned castration as a sexual act and paradoxically supported (if not advocated) its preservation of purity.

Biblical writings also showed conflicted attitudes towards castration. While eunuchs might be welcomed into the 'kingdom of heaven' and castration viewed as a positive act, it could also be interpreted as a pagan ritual and denounced as evidence of the barbarity of pagan myths. Some later writers have claimed that classical myths, such as that of Cybele and Attis, had a profound effect on Christian thought, and indeed the violent imagery of much of the Old Testament is comparable to the brutal bloodbath at Attis' wedding. Victorian medical writers certainly assumed such a connection. In his definition of self-mutilation, James Adam moved seamlessly from discussing the worship of Cybele to describing the castration of Origen, 'whose Christianity had a strong Oriental tinge', according to the later writer.[36] Conversely, modern historians have suggested that Christian leaders in the centuries following Origen's death actively promoted the idea of metaphorical eunuchism in order to encourage conversion to

Christianity, suggesting the assumption that castration meant a *physical* procedure remained widespread.[37]

Yet there were other reasons for this shift in thinking. Writers in the fourth and fifth centuries actively distanced themselves from some aspects of early Christian thought, as well as the pagan rituals represented by self-castration. Origen's teachings incorporated a very specific understanding of the body, and his physical castration was a telling example of his views. Some of the theologian's contemporaries saw the body as a spiritual obstacle, a temporary prison for an immortal soul. Origen, however, viewed the human body as a necessity, to ensure that the spirit was appropriately nurtured over time, increasing its desire to become one with God in death. The physical body, for Origen, was not a limiting corporeal form that prevented a true spiritual union with God, but a frontier that could be traversed. Yet the body was also something that changed throughout its existence. This being the case, none of its specific, time-bound characteristics while on earth could be regarded as essential to human nature. Sexual maturity, for example, did not last throughout even the fleeting existence of a mortal form and thus could not be part of the essence of the spirit. Instead,

> the body was poised on the edge of a transformation so enormous as to make all present notions of identity tied to sexual differences, and all social roles based upon marriage, procreation, and childbirth, seem as fragile as dust dancing in a sunbeam.[38]

In this way, Origen's teachings supported 'the genderless ideal' of early Christianity.[39] Certain early Christian teachers promoted a society in which all were equal, and some communities allowed the full participation of women in religious activities. A century and a half after his death, at the end of the fourth century, the discrediting of Origen's teachings was, at least in part, a reaction against this genderless ideal, which male writers denounced as heretical.[40] The later Judaeo-Christian tradition adhered to much more rigid notions of sex and gender than before, with 'little tolerance for intermediate categories and gender ambiguities' that remained permissible in other cultures, such as the Byzantine Empire.[41] At the same time, a literal interpretation of Matthew 19:12 was also condemned. By insisting that Christian lessons were metaphorical, rather than literal, writers from the fourth century onwards distanced themselves from the pagan traditions with which their religion had previously been associated. In later centuries, however, specific sects did return to this practice: the Skoptsy, for example, promoted not just physical alteration but also elements of the communal way of life adopted by early Christians.[42]

Attitudes towards castration in pagan and early Christian thought offer us an understanding of self-harm that diverges markedly from modern Western notions. It cannot be understood outside the religious, social and political context of the era. One element that particularly deviates from modern ideas of self-harm as intentionally inflicted by an individual is the lack of clarification in most cases as to whether castration was literally self-performed or carried out by a surgeon or other assistant. For ancient writers, whether or not an act was self-inflicted was of far less importance than the social role of the eunuch. While this social role was often clearly defined as 'not-male', it did not necessarily directly equate to performing a female role. The multiple meanings of castration in the later Roman Empire and in early Christianity – in particular the 'genderless ideal' of some Christian teachers – remind us that notions of sex, gender and sexuality are fluid cultural constructs. The Galli were eunuchs, but were often described in terms of their sexual acts and desires; early Christian castrates viewed themselves as without sex or gender at all. Neither of these interpretations fits into the rigid two-sex model that later medical, religious and popular thought deemed the proper way to interpret sex and gender, and they suggest potential for a much broader interpretation of human existence. Indeed, in Western science this model became widespread only in the 1700s, replacing a 'one-sex' view of humanity, in which the female sex organs were assumed to be an 'inverted' version of the male.[43] Understanding the species through a male/female binary is neither 'natural' (if we think of gendered characteristics, as Origen did, as a temporary part of corporeal existence), nor socially and culturally stable. The castration of the Galli, while remarked upon and part of the social awareness of everyday citizens, was less publicly visible than other aspects of the rituals of Cybele. The Day of Blood, during which the Galli practised self-laceration in the streets, was one of the most public of the sect's rituals, and more frequently described.[44] To explore the public performance of self-mutilation in more depth, however, I will now move away from pagan ritual and the Cult of Cybele to look at another religious form of self-injury: the processionary Christian flagellants of the Middle Ages.

Whipping up a storm: flagellant processions in Europe, c. 1260–1450

In 1446, Gertrud Becke confessed to an inquisition at Nordhausen (in what is now central Germany) that she had whipped herself daily since the age of fourteen. Most of the five men and eight women who were arrested in the same investigation similarly declared that they whipped themselves regularly, usually on Fridays. By this means, the prisoners declared that all sin in the world would be forgiven; they claimed that baptism by blood had replaced baptism by water. Indeed, the Nordhausen subjects reportedly regarded the single ritual of flagellation as an appropriate replacement for almost every other religious rite. Gertrud claimed that her mother had taught her to 'believe in flagellation instead of all the sacraments': a teaching that was reinforced by a network of people around her, all regarded as heretics by the established Church.[45] It was small wonder that such acts were prosecuted as heresy, for Becke and her fellows openly proclaimed themselves to be in opposition to the established Church. Their practice of flagellation, they declared, was the only true means of worship. Indeed, that Easter, after attending an ordinary church service, Becke and her husband had whipped one another in penance after a grandmother told the couple that such services were 'idolatrous and sheer insanity'.

The Nordhausen Inquisition was one of a number of investigations into the practice of flagellation in the later Middle Ages. As with the case of Gertrud Becke, most of these concerned heresy, rather than the practice of whipping per se, and followed the Pope's ban on flagellant processions in 1349. This edict did not forbid all religious mortification: rather, the major concern here was flagellation as a *public* practice, which appeared to have political and transgressive elements that individual penance did not. The painful and physically damaging practice of self-flagellation was not regarded as a problem in and of itself. Indeed, it is relatively recently that pain itself has come to be viewed primarily as a negative experience. Even in the early 1800s, philosophical models of human psychology saw an important role in pain as a motivator. As the utilitarian philosopher Jeremy Bentham (1748–1832) put it:

Nature has placed mankind under the governance of two sovereign masters, pain and pleasure. It is for them alone to point out what we ought to do, as well as to determine what we shall do.[46]

In the centuries prior to Bentham, pain was considered to have a multitude of uses, many of them positive. The experience of pain might be classed alongside redemption (particularly in a religious context), or considered a gift to remind an individual of the correct path to follow. In the medical realm, pain was a natural indicator that something was wrong with the body or mind; in the absence of diagnostic tests, it might even be the *only* sign a patient or physician had to work with. In medical texts, pain held positive connotations well into the Enlightenment, being regarded as a 'natural' process, which suggested that cure could in some cases be achieved only *through* the experience of pain.[47]

Attitudes to religious flagellation were intrinsically bound up in this changing understanding of pain and pleasure. As pain became increasingly viewed as something to be avoided or cured, and not an experience having value, understandings of flagellation shifted dramatically. For an eighteenth-century audience, flagellation became suspiciously sexualized: the pursuit of pain could no longer be understood unless it was simultaneously a route to pleasure. This idea increased in popularity during the nineteenth century, when the experience of pain began to be seen as fundamentally pathological. Following the work of sexologists, such as Richard von Krafft-Ebing, flagellation became firmly associated in the popular mind with sexual deviance through the masochistic and sadistic desires outlined in his *Psychopathia Sexualis* (1886). Religious flagellation came to be viewed primarily as a perversion, resulting from the absence of opportunity for so-called 'natural' sexual contact: the 'greatest evil' for those 'unable to find satisfaction in a natural manner, mostly tends in cloisters to self-pollution and to homosexual vice'.[48]

It is only by moving beyond these modern notions of pain and pleasure that we can hope to understand the ritual of group flagellation in the Middle Ages. As with castration, many Victorian writers assumed self-flagellation had its roots in pagan ritual. Jacques Boileau's history in 1888, for example, considered that voluntary flagellation was widespread in ancient times, and generally intended to appease the gods, although he also found examples of philosophers suggesting that flagellation served to correct their thoughts and focus their minds.[49] Boileau did not find many examples of early Christian mortification, and modern historians have also attested to a gap between the pagan and early Christian rituals already described and medieval flagellation. Although other types of asceticism existed in the intervening period (including fasting and the denial of comforts), this form of mortification – both as a public and private ritual – became popular in Christianity only in the Middle Ages. This popularity emerged from an increased emphasis in religious ideology on the sufferings of Jesus Christ, which elevated the mystical role of blood and pain in Christian thought. The first recorded example of this form of religious flagellation was in the life of St Pardulf, who died in 737 CE. However, it was not until the teachings of Peter Damian (*c.* 1007–1072/3) that flogging became widely regarded as a pious act. Damian's teachings transformed flagellation from a punishment (inflicted to promote monastic discipline) to an ascetic act, which held important spiritual meaning. The longer tradition of monastic beatings, however, enabled Damian to claim that flagellation as a religious practice had a legitimate history. However, there were two elements that were quite new in Damian's promotion of

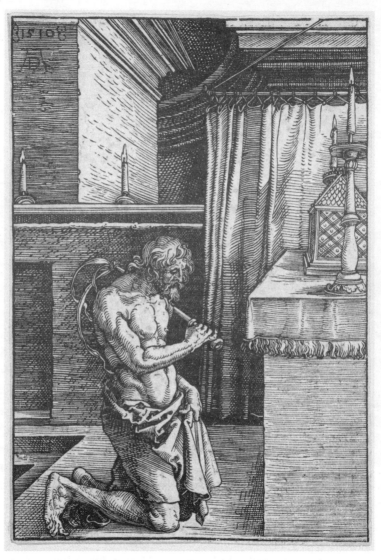

A penitent whips himself in private devotion in a German woodcut
by Albrecht Dürer, 1510.

mortification. First, it was self-inflicted; previously whipping would have been carried out by another monk. This shift meant flagellation could easily be carried out in private as part of individual devotional practice. Second, flagellation was transformed from an act of punishment or penance into a central element of spiritual life, becoming a literal embodiment of the sufferings of Christ: 'an actual inscription of the message of the Gospel in the ascetic's body'.[50]

There was a strong performative element to religious flagellation, as practised by Damian. Flagellation re-enacted the suffering of Christ, but it was also intended to reflect the experiences of the early Christian martyrs. While Christians no longer needed to physically prove their devotion by submitting to the violence of others, since the 'time of battle' was over, they *could* show their faith by inflicting hardships upon themselves. As Damian put it,

> when I freely scourge myself with my own hands in the sight of God, I demonstrate the same genuine and devout desire as if the executioner were here in all his fury.[51]

Moreover, inflicting the blows himself, Damian argued, was greater proof of faith, for it made him 'author of this ordeal'. The body, for Damian, was an instrument on which his faith could be made physically visible; he even compared the skin of the body to that of a tambourine, suggesting that both instruments might be 'played' in order to praise God. Damian's ideas did not receive universal acceptance, although for a long time it was assumed that they encouraged the widespread practice of self-flagellation. However, it was Peter Damian's description of flagellation as a performance that appears to have been a major impetus in the foundation of the flagellant movement of the later Middle Ages.

The processionary flagellants were a lay movement, and not a clerical one. Beginning in around 1260 in Italy, these groups travelled from town to town, participating in a group ritual of flagellation at each location. The first account of these processions was by St Justina of Padua, who claimed that the flagellants had appeared in Bologna. The ceremonies spread through Italy and then to Greece, Poland and Germany. In 1349, Albert of Strasbourg suggested that the resurgence of the practice was in direct response to the plague that devastated Europe in that period.[52] The processions were generally a temporary pursuit. Individual penitents would join a group for a period of days that corresponded with the number of years Jesus lived on earth: thirty-three and a half. Most groups consisted of about fifty to sixty members, who all lived by a prescribed set of rules. According to one commentator,

> they never spoke to women and refused to sleep upon feather beds. They wore crosses upon their coats and hats, behind and before, and had their scourges hanging at their waist.[53]

As they arrived at each new town, the group would perform a highly stylized ritual of flagellation in a public space. The church bells would be rung to attract the inhabitants, and a ceremony carried out that included prayers, songs, chanting and, of course, a ritual flogging. The movement spread rapidly across Europe during 1260–61 and – just as suddenly – disappeared. Individual penitents returned to their daily lives, nonetheless taking an oath to continue to practise private flagellation. In the years 1348–9, another mass phenomenon emerged, which again spread rapidly across the continent before dispersing.[54]

The interpretation of the flagellants' practices was strongly reminiscent of earlier concepts of private scourging. The flagellants used the body as an instrument of penance and devotion, to expiate sin and to praise God. The pain inflicted by scourging was not simply a punishment but a transformative practice, turning the bodies of the penitents into instruments of prayer. As a movement, however, the flagellants were considered dangerously heretical. According to contemporaries, all classes and types of people participated – in 1349, at least, this included women as well as men, contradicting official teachings. Communities apparently welcomed the flagellants. Conversions were common, and even those who did not participate turned out in

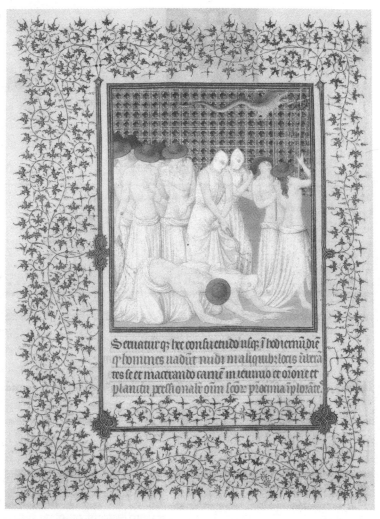

Flagellant procession in the *Belles Heures* of Jean de France, duc de Berry (1405-8/9).
Those standing on the left of the group are flagellating themselves, while the prostrated
flagellants are being whipped by their fellows.

throngs to witness the performance. This popularity suggested to Church authorities that the movement was subversive in nature. The flagellant processions were a challenge to the hierarchy of the Church itself, refuting established practices, as Gertrud Becke had the sacraments. Indeed, by turning the written word (which required the educated interpretation of a priest) into a public performance, understandable by all, flagellants reduced the power of the Church, whether they did so intentionally or not. Some movements were explicitly anti-clerical, as were networks of later flagellators, like Gertrud and her associates. Others were not, but were interpreted in this way when they performed their rituals in a public space. Hence the late medieval bans on flagellation prohibited not self-flagellation as a practice, but flagellation as a group activity: it was this that held social and political importance for contemporaries.[55]

The power and threat implicit in the late medieval flagellant movement, alongside a very positive interpretation of self-mortification as transformative (an association that remained strong in religion until at least the early 1800s, and in some cases beyond), meant that flagellation in the Middle Ages was understood from a very different perspective to later assumptions. Unlike the modern belief that self-harm is an isolated, individual, private act, flagellants performed their rituals as a group, a process that cemented their social identity. Hugh of Reutlingen, writing in 1349, declared that 'seldom does one see such a great number of people as in these processions of flagellants.'[56] It was not just the practices of the flagellants that were unusual, then, but their ability to bring large numbers of people together. For leaders of the established Church, this was a dangerous element in a lay movement. Thus, while private mortification continued to be seen as a pious act, group flagellation was banned in the late medieval period, although groups of flagellants, like Gertrud Becke and her friends, continued to meet in secret. It was not the expression of religious devotion through the body that challenged the authorities, but the social nature of the practice. Individual forms of asceticism, such as fasting, remained an important way of expressing religious ideals, especially for women.[57]

A flagellant resting
on a stone, undated.

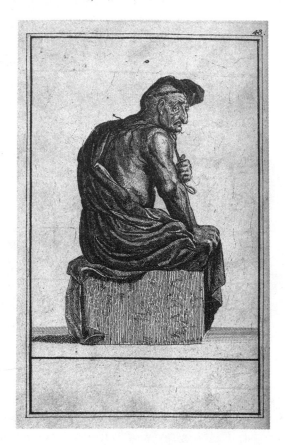

'A very large and copious bleeding':
bloodletting as a healing practice

In 1860, the 38-year-old housewife Elizabeth T. was admitted to the Bethlem
Royal Hospital, the first time she had experienced any form of mental
illness. Diagnosed with acute melancholia, Elizabeth had sought her own
treatment prior to her admission to hospital. Her admission record
described how she had 'latterly some indications of a wish to injure herself
. . . to draw blood which she fancies would relieve her'. On one occasion,
she had rushed into a chemist's shop and asked to be cupped immediately,

'as the only means to relieve the distress of her head'. When admitted, she had wounds on her right temple and left hand, both of which were self-inflicted with a pair of scissors.[58] Elizabeth was adamant that her self-mutilation was a form of therapeutic bloodletting. Indeed, her ideas were not too distant from medical practice of the time. Although most physicians had reduced their reliance on therapeutic bloodletting by the mid-nineteenth century, it was still widely available as a treatment for any type of illness: Elizabeth T.'s first attempt to let blood was, after all, at a chemist's, where the practice was presumably still being offered.[59] Indeed, Isabella Beeton's famous *Book of Household Management* (1861) contained instructions on the performance of bleeding, to be used at home in 'cases of great emergency, such as the strong kind of apoplexy, and when a surgeon cannot possibly be obtained for some considerable time'.[60] Elizabeth T.'s actions were certainly interpreted as symptoms of mental distress. However, the emphasis in her case record was on the existence of a 'supernatural voice' that commanded her to 'go and be cupped'. It was the fact that Elizabeth had responded to this voice by injuring herself that was seen as proof that she was mad, not her efforts to bleed herself.

That self-cutting has only very recently been emphasized in models of self-harm may have something to do with the way in which bleeding has been viewed as therapeutic throughout much of medical history. Bloodletting (along with other so-called 'heroic' remedies such as purging and vomiting) remained a cornerstone of Western therapeutics for over two thousand years. To modern readers, the practice seems largely inexplicable: perhaps associated with religious self-punishment, or a 'placebo effect'.[61] This presents a skewed vision of pre-modern therapeutics, judging them outside their historical contexts by evaluating past practices in relation to modern assumptions about efficacy. Yet what has often confused twentieth-century researchers is the way in which the emergence of new scientific theories about the body did not necessarily lead to the abandonment of practices like bloodletting. Indeed, bloodletting was almost entirely abandoned by physicians in mid-nineteenth-century Europe without ever really being challenged by scientific medicine. Here, however, I shall look

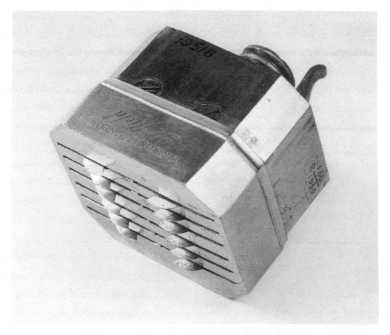

Automatic scarifier by W. H. Hutchison, Sheffield, 19th century.

mainly at bloodletting in the sixteenth and seventeenth centuries, when it retained popularity despite major challenges to the anatomical and physiological theories of the ancients.

Bleeding, bloodletting, phlebotomy and venesection were all terms for the medicinal practice of opening a vein to remove a certain amount of blood. Techniques have varied across history, including the use of medicinal leeches, the opening of a vein with a lancet or fleam and such ingenious eighteenth-century devices as the 'scarificator'. The scarificator or scarifier – an 'artificial leech' – contained a number of small blades on a spring mechanism. The switch wound the spring, which would be primed before the small, brass box was placed against the skin and the spring released, making a number of shallow cuts in the skin. Blood could be collected in a bleeding bowl, and the amount taken was often measured, varying from a few ounces to a pint or more.

Bloodletting can be dated back at least to Hippocratic medicine. Hippocrates – the so-called 'father of medicine' in ancient Greece – has long been associated with humoral medicine.[62] In this model, which retained popularity across the Western world until at least the Renaissance, humours were regarded as regulating the body in health and illness. Illness was caused by an imbalance in these fluids – blood, black bile, yellow bile and phlegm – and could only be cured by correcting the balance. The Hippocratic corpus, however, suggested a variety of ways to do this, with a particular focus on purgatives (inducing diarrhoea or vomiting).[63] It was Galen who promoted bloodletting above and beyond other methods of balancing the humours, as acknowledged by the handful of Renaissance physicians who denounced bloodletting by putting 'Galenists' on trial for the 'Abuses and Disrepute they have brought upon the whole Art of Physick'.[64]

Galen, born in 129 CE, was a Greek citizen from Pergamum, in modern-day Turkey. He studied medicine in the famous school of Alexandria (among other places) and achieved great fame as a doctor in Rome through his flamboyant demonstrations of skill and anatomical knowledge as much as for his theories and texts.[65] Galen justified his use of phlebotomy by claiming a Hippocratic heritage for the procedure; however, it was in Galen's own time that bloodletting became the primary intervention across a variety of ailments.[66] This may have been due in part to Galen's influence as a self-publicist. However, Roman encyclopaedist Celsus (c. 25 BCE– c. 50 CE) had already stated that bloodletting was becoming increasingly prevalent, just before Galen's time: 'It is not new to let blood by cutting a vein, but that there is hardly any disease in which blood is not let, is new.'[67] Through three treatises on venesection, as well as frequent references in other works, Galen became the major authority on bloodletting in the post-classical world. Galen, like some of the Hippocratics, saw bloodletting as a natural process. Evacuation of excess fluid occurred regularly in nature through menstruation and haemorrhage. When weakness left nature unable to perform these necessary actions, it was left to the physician to do so. Galen recommended bleeding for a number of reasons. It might be that the blood contained too much of one of the other three humours (a disease-causing *cacochymia*), or that there was simply an excess of blood itself (a *plethos*), which caused the classic signs of inflammation. Sometimes bleeding was recommended to prevent either of these things occurring, particularly in individuals prone to plethora. Revulsion and derivation, meanwhile, were both methods of diverting blood flow from the site of disease (or haemorrhage) – derivation by directing it to a nearby part of the body, revulsion by sending it to a site far away from the original problem.[68]

In the Renaissance, a bloodletting controversy developed, not because of the place of bleeding in the medical corpus but over the specific methods of bloodletting employed and the rationale behind them – particularly the importance of revulsion and derivation. This fierce debate became strongly linked to a revival of interest in ancient medicine in the late fifteenth and early sixteenth century, with the publication of Latin editions of Galen and Hippocrates, and the adoption of classical works into university teaching. Medical practice by this time had deviated from the teachings of antiquity, especially through the contributions of Arabic medicine, such as the *Canon* of Avicenna (Ibn Sīnā), one of the most widely taught volumes. Byzantine encyclopaedists removed any sense of controversy from Galen's

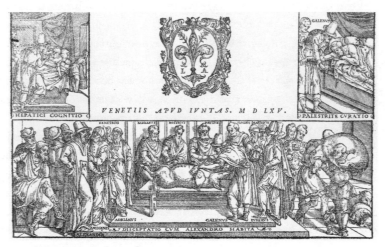

An etching showing Galen publicly vivisecting a pig, from an Italian edition of Galen's *Opera omnia latine in septem classes digesta* (1565).

work on venesection, making his views appear uncontested when they enjoyed a resurgence in the Western world.[69] Yet Galen was challenged on a number of counts during the Renaissance: first by Dutch anatomist Andreas Vesalius (1514–1564), whose famous dissections of human cadavers in Padua questioned Galenic anatomy, which was based on the dissection of animals. As writer Bernard de Mandeville put it two centuries later, Galen's anatomy was proven wrong 'in no less than 106 places'![70] Mandeville's claim, made in a text discussing the 'art of physick', was intended to remind his readers not to rely on Galen, indicating how long-lasting Galenic medicine was. While the publication of Vesalius' work in Padua has been seen as a major advance in medical knowledge, it did nothing to reduce the popularity of bleeding as a remedy.

Vesalius, despite his new anatomical knowledge, did not question the principles on which bloodletting was based, and essentially remained a Galenist in practice. So too did William Harvey, although his discovery of the circulation of the blood might have been expected to prove the biggest challenge to bloodletting. After all, in the ancient world, it was considered that blood moved only one way: both veins and arteries carried blood away from the organs, where it was generated. Cutting a vein further from the heart than the lesion to be treated would, it was thought, increase the amount of blood flowing through that area, carrying any congested material with it. Harvey (1578–1657) was the son of a wealthy merchant, and educated at Cambridge and then Padua. He continued to practise anatomy on his return to England, and carried out a large number of dissections, mostly of animals. His key text, *De motu cordis et sanguinis* (On the Motion of the Heart and Blood), was based on this work. Harvey extrapolated from the movements of the heart in dying animals to explain the circulation of the blood around the rest of the body. His ideas were widely accepted within several decades. While they did not overturn bloodletting as a practice, the site of venesection became less important. 'It's all one in which Arm the Vein be open'd,' London physician Thomas Willis claimed in the mid-1600s, 'though it's now commonly done on the side affected [by pleurisy].'[71]

For Harvey, if the same blood circulated around the body, this meant that any blockage in the system would have particularly damaging effects. Rapid removal of congestion thus became the major reason for bloodletting, in order to ensure that the circulation continued uninterrupted. Indeed, rather than overturning ancient theories, Harvey actually used classical ideas to prove his discoveries – and his own experiments to indicate why bleeding might be successful. The nature of the blood itself was 'disposed from slight causes, such as cold, alarm, horror, and the like, to collect in its source, to concentrate like parts to a whole' and thus cause a dangerous plethora.[72] For Harvey, the response of the blood to external influences was the very reason why the pulse from the heart was needed to drive it through the arteries. His experiments on directional flow showed how the blood could congest in particular vessels when 'access to them is open but the egress from them is closed' – and, if ancient writers were to be believed, this was 'the cause of all tumefaction' (swelling).[73] Bloodletting thus remained popular, among those who supported Galenic theory as well as those who opposed it. Even some physicians who argued against the existence of the four humours regarded the discovery of the circulation as proving the importance of bloodletting, to allow the blood to flow

> equally from the whole Body to its wide Orifice, upon the free Emission of which not only the Plethorick Disposition is taken away, but the greater Vessels being every where emptied by this means, the Blood stagnating in any place is restor'd again to Motion.[74]

Bloodletting remained a popular and widely used therapy well into the nineteenth century and particularly in rural areas, even beyond. In the early 1800s, some asylum doctors thought that mental illness might be relieved by sudden blood loss. William Ellis spoke in 1838 of a sailor apparently relieved of insanity by the 'sudden good effects of a very large and copious bleeding' after cutting his throat, while James Cowles Prichard claimed that the American physician Dr Rush had reported several similar cases of sudden cure.[75] In 1846, the painter Benjamin Haydon shot himself and then cut his throat, believing the bleeding would relieve his 'diseased brain'.[76] While few alienists still claimed benefits for bloodletting in insanity by 1860, the method of treatment remained strong in the public mind, and widely available. Throughout the nineteenth century, patients at Bethlem Hospital continued to claim that bleeding constituted self-treatment, whether to bring on menstruation or, like Elizabeth T., to relieve pressure in the head.[77] As late as 1900, 56-year-old Alexander M. declared 'that he had bled himself with a razor, because medical men were not now allowed to bleed & this relieved his head'.[78] Given the proximity of these explanations to recent medical models of disease, it hardly seems surprising that patients like Alexander refused to accept the word of their doctors that their acts were irrational or, indeed, that they were mad at all. In all three examples outlined above, self-injury was accepted as part of a religious, spiritual or medical framework, sometimes for a considerable time. In the cases of early Christian castration and flagellation in the Middle Ages, these practices were later judged heretical primarily because they threatened an established social and political order, and not for spiritual reasons. In both eras, the hierarchical structure was dominated by the Church and religious teachings. By the 1600s, secular models of human functioning were growing in prominence, particularly within science and medicine. Yet we nonetheless find a model of therapeutic injury, in the practice of medicinal bloodletting. This not only remained in use despite shifts in anatomical understanding, it even *gained* in popularity, due to the new notion that the circulation of the blood was central to health and disease.

All three practices outlined above have at least one significant difference from modern psychiatric models of self-inflicted injury. Self-castration in antiquity was part of a widespread practice that had both commercial and spiritual elements. Contemporaries did not distinguish whether castration was performed by an individual or carried out by someone else – even, frequently, whether it was done by force or choice. The act of castration was of far less importance than the role the eunuch played within society; indeed, social roles in general were emphasized above and beyond the

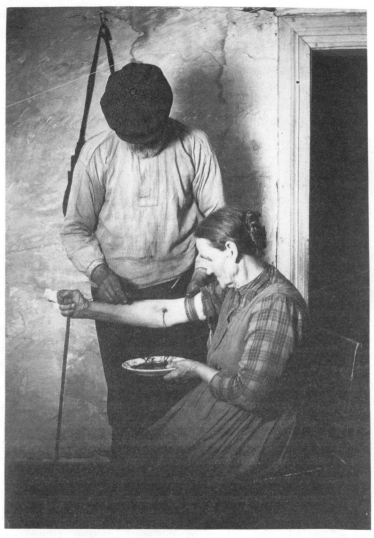

A bloodletting scene in rural Norway, photographed by Nils Keyland for the Nordic Museum Archive, 1922. Keyland was an ethnologist and cultural historian who documented the old Finnish culture in his native Värmland in the early 20th century.

individual. Neither was castration necessarily associated with madness or frenzy, unlike the modern connection between self-castration and psychotic states.[79] Instead, it had a variety of social and political meanings across the later Roman Empire and in early Christianity. The processions of flagellants in the Middle Ages also offer quite a different model from today's definitions. Private and, later, group flagellation only rose to prominence in the medieval era. The celebratory manner in which self-wounding became adopted in religious worship in the Middle Ages was very different from later understandings of flagellation as a perverse and pathological practice. Although it may be hard for us today to understand how flagellant communities functioned, the group element of the ritual was certainly important to lay participants. The very *public* nature of this practice differed completely from modern assumptions about self-harm.

Therapeutic bloodletting, meanwhile, was a key part of Western medical practice for almost two thousand years. Bleeding was viewed as a regular, natural process that aided bodily functioning. If it did not occur naturally, medical intervention was required. Although self-performed bloodletting was not usually recommended, domestic texts in the nineteenth century explained how to carry out the procedure, in case a surgeon could not be found. This way of thinking about bleeding remained associated with self-harm by patients in the late eighteenth and early nineteenth centuries, even where doctors had abandoned it. The Victorian psychiatric model of self-mutilation, then, was very different from modern ones, as we shall see in the next chapter.

TWO

MORBID IMPULSE AND MORAL INSANITY
The Emergence of Self-mutilation in Late Nineteenth-century Psychiatry

In January 1845, the *Cornwall Royal Gazette* reported the 'distressing' self-mutilation of 'a very handsome and accomplished young woman'. Nineteen-year-old Jesse McKenzie had for many months 'devoted herself to the reading of scriptures', becoming 'extremely melancholy'. She remained at home, however, until, in front of her mother and aunt, she plucked out one of her eyes and threw it on the ground, telling her relatives, 'if thy right eye offend thee, pluck it out.' It was this that led to Jesse's detention in Hanwell Asylum, described as a 'confirmed maniac'.[1] Jesse's case lies somewhere between the instances of self-injury outlined in the previous chapter and the understanding of self-mutilation within a psychiatric context that emerged in later decades. It was not a given conclusion in 1845 that an act of self-inflicted violence would result in asylum admission, or even be considered explicit evidence of mental illness. As the asylum system expanded in the middle decades of the nineteenth century, the association between psychiatry and self-injury became increasingly prevalent. The modern understanding of self-harm as a specific category of abnormal individual behaviour emerged in this period. As we shall see, however, it was shaped quite differently from later models. In this chapter, I briefly explain the context in which self-mutilation was categorized: the expanding asylum system and the emerging psychiatric profession. I describe how 'self-mutilation' emerged from the interest clinicians had in classifying and defining 'insane' behaviour. But why was a particular model of self-harm adopted at this time? And what led psychiatrists to draw parallels between different forms of self-injury – ranging from hair-plucking to limb amputation – to create an overarching category?

These connections cannot be explained simply by the existence of a psychiatric system, and we must look beyond psychiatry into law, medicine, psychology and scientific practice to answer these questions. One important context for the creation of a specific category of self-mutilation is the widespread publicity given to a tendency in legal cases to attribute suicidal acts to mental illness. This began in the eighteenth century, but became increasingly associated with psychiatry as the nineteenth century progressed. In later years, it was often assumed that Victorian writers made no distinction between suicidal and non-suicidal self-injury. However, this was not the case. Psychiatrists in the late nineteenth century frequently argued that self-mutilation was *not* carried out for suicidal motives, although they differed in the ways they applied alternative meaning to these acts. Was self-mutilation, they wondered, a 'morbid instinct', showing evidence of a 'perversion of the will' in a particular individual? Or did it have a wider meaning, which might shed light on the psychology of human motivation more generally? In Jesse McKenzie's case, the religious motives for her act failed to explain the sudden and seemingly impulsive behaviour, suggesting that it might have been the result of a nerve impulse that she was unable to control, or that she was not even consciously aware of. Some psychiatrists, however, considered that, however illogical, the motives of their patients were as valid as the physiological process by which a self-injurious act might have occurred. The tension between these two models – of 'uncontrollable impulse' and conscious or unconscious motive – continues to impact understandings of self-harm today. Both were rooted in Victorian science and culture, and we can better understand these two concepts by exploring them in the era in which they emerged. Two of the late Victorian and Edwardian explanations for self-harm directly founded on these conflicting ideas will be explored in more detail in the next two chapters. Here, however, I concentrate on the formation of the category of 'self-mutilation' and its impact within and outside asylum psychiatry.

Domestic bureaucracy: a brief history of the asylum system

The asylum system expanded rapidly in nineteenth-century Britain and western Europe. While so-called private madhouses (and some charitable hospitals) had existed before this period, the passing of the Lunacy Act and County Asylums Act of 1845 meant that every county in England and Wales was legally required to build a public pauper lunatic asylum. These rapidly expanded in number and size through the second half of the nineteenth century, with the total number of 'certified lunatics' in England and Wales rising from 11,272 in 1844 to over 80,000 by 1900.[2] Alongside this emerged the profession of the medically trained asylum psychiatrist – or 'alienist', as such doctors were called at the time. In the eighteenth and early nineteenth centuries, asylum superintendents had often been lay practitioners, whose institutions were based either on a religious-philanthropic framework (such as the Quaker York Retreat) or run at a financial profit.[3] Medically trained practitioners like John Conolly (1794–1866) and James Cowles Prichard (1786–1848) worked hard to raise the profile of their field. By the 1850s, most institutions across the West employed qualified physicians to oversee their operations. In Britain, these doctors set up a professional body in 1841 – the Association of Medical Officers of Asylums and Hospitals for the Insane (from 1865 known as the Medico-Psychological Association) – and, in 1853, they started their own journal, the *Journal of Mental Science*.[4] By the end of the nineteenth century, the Association had almost six hundred members, and this rapid expansion has been seen as evidence of the determination alienists had to become specialists in 'psychological medicine', defining their field by publishing their theories and practice. Psychiatry became viewed as a medical specialty.[5]

Despite this, much of nineteenth-century psychiatric therapy continued to be based on the concept of 'moral treatment' that was introduced around 1800 by the Tuke family in York and Philippe Pinel in Paris. Moral treatment emphasized the importance of recuperation in a domestic setting, with kindness and consideration shown to patients and the use of recreation and employment. At the Quaker York Retreat, religious sentiment was also a key element of treatment. In his 1892 essay 'Reform in the Treatment of the Insane', the alienist Daniel Hack Tuke (grandson of the Retreat's founder, William Tuke) claimed that moral treatment was based on the idea that the insane were not absolutely deprived of reason, and thus could be motivated by 'hope, feeling and honour'.[6] While some historians have claimed moral treatment was a means of 'social control' (an effort by doctors and other authority figures to impose a framework of values onto patients), others have viewed it as the forerunner of psychological therapies.[7] Indeed, while physicians in the last few decades of the nineteenth century came to view moral treatment as synonymous with the 'homishness' of the asylum environment, which emphasized bourgeois ideals of domestic family life, others described it as 'the influence of mind upon mind', and therefore 'intellectual and emotional treatment'.[8] In this way, therapies introduced by lay practitioners were 'medicalized' (given a new explanation couched in medical terms) and incorporated into biological and psychological explanations of insanity by a generation of medically trained alienists.

There are two ways in which the medical model of asylum practice in this period provides an important context to the story of self-harm: first, the legacy of moral treatment, in particular the 'non-restraint' system; second, the well-documented efforts of asylum professionals to classify (and thus define) their field. The English non-restraint movement is often absent from popular histories of the asylum, but it was a major force in psychiatric development of this period.[9] In 1838, Robert Gardiner Hill at the Lincoln Asylum claimed to have dispensed with mechanical restraint entirely and, the following year, his system achieved widespread publicity when it was adopted by the well-known asylum reformer John Conolly at Hanwell.[10] It is easy, in retrospect, to view the declining use of restraint as evidence of an increasingly humanitarian approach to mental illness; however, the situation wasn't quite so simple. Debate raged in medical journals – and sometimes the general press – as to the benefits or otherwise of the non-restraint system. Those who advocated it claimed it to be the *only*

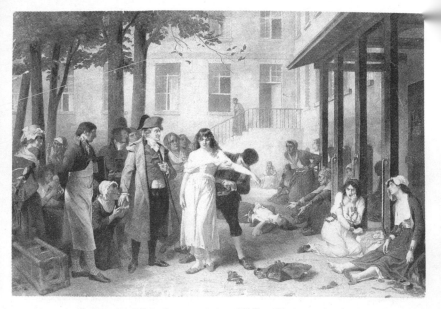

Etching showing the famous painting of Philippe Pinel removing the chains from patients at the Salpêtrière Hospital, Paris. This heavily romanticized depiction has been much criticized by historians. The approach was actually implemented by Jean-Baptiste Pussin, who became Pinel's assistant after the doctor witnessed his work at the Bicêtre Hospital. Gravure by Goupil after a painting by Tony Robert-Fleury, 1876.

humane method of treatment, and tended to contrast their approach with references to past brutality. Other doctors, however, were more circumspect. They claimed that dispensing with restraints might actually cause harm to vulnerable patients, requiring high levels of manual handling and the use of alternative methods of control, including the padded cell and sedatives. In fact, the term 'chemical restraint', to describe over-reliance on medication, emerged in this period.[11]

But why should restraint be required at all in an asylum, where patients were already confined by locked doors? The risk of suicidal and self-injurious behaviour was one of the main arguments used against non-restraint in the mid- and late nineteenth century. The widespread adoption of the practice by 1850 was therefore followed by greater attention to suicidal behaviour in asylums. Efforts to categorize patients as suicidal had practical and professional consequences. Classification was a major impetus across late Victorian scientific fields, in particular within the natural and biological sciences.[12] Within psychiatry, it created a language used by the new medical experts that set them apart from their lay predecessors, while also carving out a specialism distinct from other fields of medicine. The influence of physiological and neurological approaches to mental illness (especially concepts of mind based on brain biology) also encouraged this development of an increasingly technical language. Yet, unlike the natural and biological sciences, psychiatric categorization was rooted not in anatomy but in descriptive terms, applicable to symptoms rather than overarching categories. Contemporary practitioners were not unaware of this peculiarity, and largely regarded it as indicative of the youthful state of psychiatry as a science. They considered that with increasing research, such as microscopic investigation of brain samples, would come greater knowledge.[13] In the interim, however, the classification of symptoms served a distinctly practical purpose. This was also one of the reasons for distinguishing suicidal and other forms of self-injurious behaviour from each other.

Suicidal or self-mutilating? The creation of a category

In October 1900, Harriett T. was admitted to the Bethlem Royal Hospital from Holloway Prison, where she had been held on remand since her 'attempted suicide' a week previously. A fifty-year-old single woman, Harriett was described as of

> fair height, well made & well nourished ... [with] fairish hair which has lately been shaved on the top of her head, as she attempted suicide a short time ago by cutting her scalp.[14]

The 'delusions of persecution' Harriett exhibited in prison saw her very quickly transferred to Bethlem. However, the 'suicidal' act that led to her arrest – a scalp wound well away from any major blood vessels – was not something usually considered suicidal by alienists. Nonetheless, doctors at Bethlem attributed her wound to suicidal thoughts, just as the police, hospital and prison authorities had done. Cases like this emphasize the close relation of self-mutilation to the study of suicide. In another patient, a similar wound might have been interpreted as 'self-mutilation', leading to the important question: how does an act become defined as one or the other?

From January 1844, admission papers to the Bethlem Royal Hospital enquired whether a patient was 'disposed to suicide, or otherwise to self-injury', suggesting separate, albeit related, symptoms of mental disorder.[15] Self-injury, while ostensibly distinct from suicide, referred to a wide variety of acts, including refusal of food and attempted suicide, as indicated by the diversity of answers in the hospital papers. Many patients were listed merely as 'suicidal', often with no further detail appearing elsewhere. Other entries, however, gave information on suicide attempts or, alternatively, what might appear to a modern reader to be non-suicidal forms of self-injury. For example, in 1853, it is stated that 23-year-old Henry M. 'picks himself' and 'has now several sore places on his head, face and legs from picking and scratching himself', while Sophia W. has 'a disposition to injure herself by knocking her head against the wall and biting herself'.[16] It was often admitted that the distinction from suicide was 'perhaps a some-what artificial distinction', although nonetheless 'there is a distinction.'[17] The acts described as self-mutilation varied from disabling to relatively minor injuries. By the 1890s – the decade in which the first British med-ical definition of 'self-mutilation' was published – the term incorporated flesh-picking, biting, hair-plucking, punching or knocking against objects, cutting or otherwise removing part of the body, swallowing or inserting foreign bodies such as needles, and eating rubbish.[18]

It doesn't seem that the term 'self-mutilation' was much used before it was introduced in a medical context. In 1755, when Samuel Johnson first published his famous *A Dictionary of the English Language*, he indicated that the word 'self' was 'much used in composition'.[19] Johnson did not include 'self-mutilation' or 'self-injury' in his list of compositions; nor did John Ash in his *New and Complete Dictionary of the English Language* of 1775 (among 114 compounds of self-). Nineteenth-century dictionaries, medical or otherwise (except Tuke's *Dictionary of Psychological Medicine*), also did not include 'self-mutilation', despite a seemingly ever-increasing number of derivatives of 'self' from the mere eight in Bailey's *Etymological Dictionary* (1730). By the publication of what became the *Oxford English Dictionary* (*OED*), these 'self-' compounds ran to several densely printed pages. It was only in the *Supplement* to the *OED* (1933) that 'self-mutilation' was first included, as an 'obvious compound' of 'self'.[20] From the decision to exclude 'self-mutilation' from the first edition but include it in the 1933 supplement, we might assume an increasing use of the term within the public domain. Indeed, use of the term did slowly increase across a variety of publications, and we even see a small jump in use of the term between 1932 and 1934, around the publication of the *OED Supplement*.

This increased use was not necessarily as a psychiatric term, however. The *OED*'s contributors were almost all volunteers, from a variety of backgrounds.[21] While several of the books chosen by the editors as important sources did fall within the field of psychiatry (including Maudsley's *Physiology and Pathology of Mind*, first published 1867, and Tuke and Bucknill's *Manual of Psychological Medicine*, first published 1858), the lack of clarity within psychiatric definitions is indicated by quotations chosen from these medical works. The term 'self-destruction' was illustrated in the *OED* by one of many quotations from Clifford Allbutt's *System of Medicine* (1899), by the alienist Henry Rayner on 'Melancholia and Hypochondriasis': 'Very commonly attempts at self-destruction or self-injury are made.'[22] Five pages earlier, in the full article, Rayner made a similar point, but with different wording: 'Perversion of self-feeling may culminate in self-loathing or hatred . . . resulting in neglect of health, or even in self-mutilation and self-destruction.' That neither quote was suggested as illustrative of either 'self-injury' or 'self-mutilation' indicated both the lack of agreement over terminology within psychiatry, as well as the ongoing perception in some circles that self-injurious behaviour was akin to suicide, and did not need separate definition. However, in his article, Rayner did distinguish between suicide (intentional self-destruction) and 'self-homicide' (death following self-mutilation *without* suicidal intent), emphasizing the importance of exploring the patient's motive to differentiate between the two.

Although Rayner did not suggest *why* this distinction was important, the legal and ethical context of suicide suggests one answer. The 'suicidal' act of Harriett T. – like those of many others – had initially been framed legally, and she had been arrested. Suicide had long been a crime in many Western countries, with harsh penalties enacted in England from the Middle Ages onwards. These included burial at a crossroads or on a highway, with the body pierced through with a wooden stake; the property of a confirmed suicide was also forfeited to the crown. Many of these laws, however, were only rigorously enforced in the sixteenth and seventeenth centuries.[23] During the late seventeenth and eighteenth centuries, coroners' juries increasingly returned a verdict of non compos mentis in suicide trials. This was rooted in the belief that the law was unjustly punitive to the surviving family of a suicide, potentially leaving them in poverty, as well as shifting ethical ideas concerning the justifiability of suicide. Suicide largely became seen as a secular, rather than a religious, issue. By the nineteenth century, the widespread belief that suicide was evidence of an 'unsound mind' (supported by the verdicts of juries, rather than the other way around) meant that the topic was regularly debated by asylum practitioners.

Mid-nineteenth-century alienists frequently played on public anxiety about suicide to promote their institutions as protective.[24] Conversely, however, the Commissioners in Lunacy (state-appointed asylum inspectors) and the popular press perceived any suicide *in* an institution as tantamount to neglect. Creating a distinction between self-mutilation and suicidal behaviour could provide a buffer against these accusations. In the Ipswich Asylum Annual Report for 1871, the superintendent discussed a case in which a patient died several weeks after having torn out his eye, stating, 'the only remark I should wish to make upon this case is that I never considered it one of suicide, but simply one of self-mutilation.'[25] Self-mutilation,

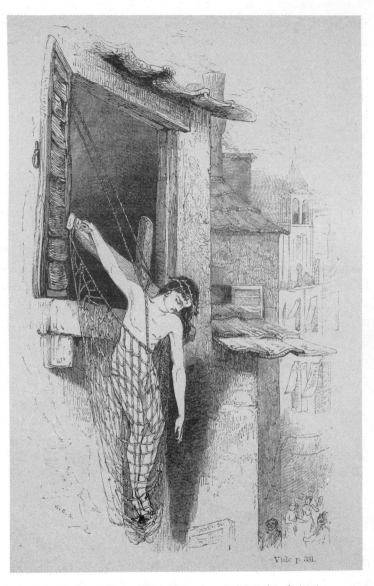

Vide p. 381.

Frontispiece to Forbes Winslow's *Anatomy of Suicide* (1840), showing
the self-crucifixion attempt of Matthew Lovat in Venice. Lovat physically
recovered from the ordeal but remained of 'melancholy caste'.

then, although related to suicide, *could* be presented quite differently, mo. akin to accidental injury than an intentional act. In the same report from Ipswich, a list of 'accidents' included 'one patient [who] bit off the first joint of her little finger whilst in a state of epileptic delirium'. In the 1880s, the prevention of 'self-mutilation' was emphasized in justifying the return of some forms of mechanical restraint, like so-called 'strong dresses' and 'padded gloves', to asylums. As George Savage, superintendent of Bethlem, put it: 'I am satisfied that many persons who were thus treated were saved from death.'[26] The ways in which suicidal behaviour and self-mutilation were defined and distinguished from each other within the asylum system provide an important context to the emergence of the category of self-mutilation.

Though it is important to note that the pathology of self-mutilation emerged as a topic of interest around the same time as attempted suicide was first criminalized, it was not just the legal context that saw self-mutilation and suicide defined as separate acts.[27] The distinction between suicide and self-mutilation was not something simply waiting to be discovered, but something that needed to be *created*. Indeed, Harriett T.'s story indicates that a broader approach to the subject is required. Harriett's *own* evidence played an important part in the decision to categorize her as suicidal rather than self-mutilating. She told doctors she had been:

> Hypnotized & subjected to X rays by some unknown person; this person told her she was a wicked woman, & must kill herself, hence she made her suicidal attempt, she was alone at the time but distinctly heard this person's voice.[28]

Attention to motive required input from both alienist and patient, suggesting a two-way process of negotiation that offers an interesting perspective on the process of categorization within the Victorian asylum. Thomas Brushfield, the Superintendent of Brookwood Asylum, emphasized the need to divide the category of 'danger to self' into two kinds: with and without a suicidal motive. Certain acts, for example castration,

...ggested to alienists that the motive for self-injury was *not* a suicidal one. Nonetheless, Brushfield changed his mind about one patient who declared his attempt at castration *had* been suicidal in intent. Similarly, the alienist reclassified a female patient who had been admitted as 'suicidal', asserting that 'her motive for doing this [cutting off her hand] was a non-suicidal one' resulting from the 'primary suggestion' of reading a scriptural quotation, which prompted 'auditory hallucinations' commanding the commission of the act. The doctor related these hallucinations to the patient's life experiences, also viewed as the potential cause of her illness: long-term grief over the loss of a child.[29] In practice, then, alienists applied a variety of different criteria – legal, medical, physiological, cultural and environmental – in determining the motives of their patients.

An interest in motive was also apparent in the main Victorian medical definition of self-mutilation in Britain: a five-page article by alienist James Adam (1834–1908) for Tuke's *Dictionary of Psychological Medicine* (1892). A medical graduate, Adam chose to specialize in psychiatry after an early career as an army medical officer, serving in the Indian Mutiny of 1857. He subsequently traced a path through several large English and Scottish pauper asylums before purchasing West Malling Place, a small private asylum in Kent, in 1883. The alienist remained here, treating a small circle of upper-class patients, until his death in 1908, upon which his obituary remarked that his publications on self-mutilation showed an interest in the 'scientific side of his life's work'.[30] Given that Adam published little else, it is entirely possible that the obituarist struggled to find much else to say about him. However, it is interesting that Adam chose self-mutilation as a speciality, for, unlike many colleagues, his writings on the topic were not incorporated into teaching lectures or textbooks, but intended to stand alone.

Adam began his definition of self-mutilation by legitimizing the topic as an important area for scientific inquiry through retrospective diagnosis. He gave an account of cases dating back to 'the earliest ages' to indicate the universal nature of the pathology described. These early acts were then compared and contrasted with those observed by the Victorian alienist.

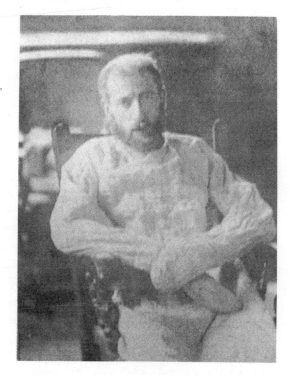

This photograph from the Bethlem Royal Hospital casebook shows Robert H. He was made to wear padded gloves in 1884, to stop him rubbing away the hair from the top of his head. Robert was described as 'vacant', although he had periods of lucidity, during which he played cards and talked rationally.

Adam claimed that the best way to throw 'additional light . . . upon the obscurity which surrounds the whole subject' was through 'an endeavour to trace some of the motives which have prompted to the commission of the acts at various periods of history, and under various religious conditions.'[31] He sought to better understand normal psychology through comparison of motives, as well as the relation of the individual to society under particular circumstances. Indeed, self-mutilation did not necessarily indicate insanity for Adam, although the 'borderland' between madness and sound mind was a shady area, reflected in his typically imprecise claim that:

All the states of mind leading to self-mutilation, self-torture, &c., hitherto considered, are compatible with reputed sanity, although they are to insanity near akin, and generally indicate more or less mental derangement.[32]

Despite its vagueness, this proximity between self-mutilation and sanity was widely agreed on by Victorian alienists, reinforcing the argument that attitudes to self-mutilation are not necessarily fixed or obvious. For late nineteenth-century writers, self-mutilation could be carried out by sane individuals through religious conviction – although, like the 'borderland', conviction was difficult to define. Adam claimed that self-mutilation through religious delusion indicated outright insanity, but nowhere did he suggest how conviction and delusion might be differentiated. Other sane motives for self-mutilation included as a demonstration of endurance and strength of will, as attempted suicide and in order to manipulate others.[33] In insanity, these explanations could continue to play a part, as might the effect of hallucinations or delusions (illustrated by the example of a patient who plucked out her eyes to prevent disturbing hallucinations). However, Adam concentrated particularly on one further explanation for insane self-mutilation, the 'sexual self-mutilation' that will be discussed in detail in the next chapter.

But how did Adam reach his conclusions? Were they formed by 'object-ive' description of his patients, or were other factors involved in the way he framed self-mutilation and highlighted particular behaviours? It would be misleading to view historical concepts of self-mutilation solely through published material. After all, the alienists who theorized on the topic were all in asylum practice, and their ideas were formed and shaped by the context in which they worked. While small private asylums like Adam's offer little material for contextualization, much more can be gleaned from the records of the medium-sized Bethlem Royal Hospital, whose superintendents in the last few decades of the century all contributed to writings on self-mutilation. From a simple statistical standpoint, it is useful to explore through these records whether alienists who wrote about self-mutilation were merely reporting the behaviours that occurred most frequently in their institutions. Between 1840 and 1900, a total of 69 papers using the term 'self-mutilation' were published in three major British medical journals (the *Journal of Mental Science*, *The Lancet* and the *British Medical Journal*). These papers referred to 89 instances of self-mutilation, with just over a quarter of these (24) being castration or genital injury. As shown by the grey bars in the chart below, this made castration the dominant form of self-inflicted injury published in medical journals of the mid- and late nineteenth century. In addition, a number of articles described amputation and enucleation (plucking out an eye). A few, predominantly in the *Journal of Mental Science*, referenced 'minor mutilations' (as Adam called them): skin-picking and hair-plucking.

The black bars in the chart show the prevalence of behaviours recorded in the Bethlem case records. Between 1880 and 1900, a total of 592 patients at Bethlem (11 per cent of the total patient population) carried out some form of self-inflicted injury.[34] While nearly half of the published papers relate to castration, amputation and enucleation, less than 10 per cent of the Bethlem cases detail similar acts. Far more prevalent in this twenty-year

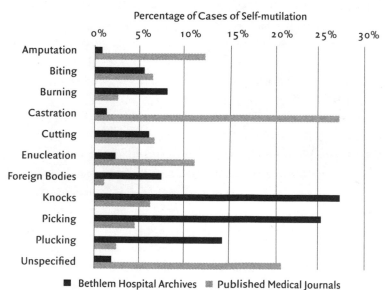

Types of self-mutilation in medical journals compared to Bethlem Royal Hospital cases.

period are the large number of individuals picking their skin, pulling out their hair or knocking themselves against walls, floor or furniture.

Publications on self-inflicted injury did not simply describe what was observed within asylums. These texts concentrated on dramatic acts: writers and journal editors assumed that extremes would be of most interest to readers. This practice can easily be taken today as evidence that these behaviours *were* more prevalent. It could also, as we shall see in the following chapter, mislead contemporaries into perceiving certain acts (castration) as occurring far more frequently than practice suggested. An understanding of self-inflicted injury was therefore not constructed through definitions of a linguistic term *or* through statistical occurrence of behaviours, but instead was a complex interplay of factors within an institution. These included the practical maintenance of order and prevention of harm within the asylum, as well as interaction between doctors and patients in determining the focus of inquiry: the 'motive' of the patient informed the decision as to whether an act was classified as suicidal or self-injurious. Yet this motive could also shed light on a wider understanding of human behaviour, and the topic was seen to provide evidence of the existence of 'natural instincts' in man by indicating how these might be perverted by insanity. Thus, the motive behind self-mutilation was not explored solely in order to differentiate such acts from suicide, but could be regarded as an end in itself.

The hysterical lioness: self-mutilation and morbid instincts

On 18 May 1884, a 'fine lioness' in the Dublin Zoological Gardens was discovered to have eaten six inches of her tail during the night. Just over a week later, she removed most of the rest of her tail and, later in the summer, part of her right hind paw. Her food was changed, she was given drugs to ease constipation, and bitter substances were put onto her tail and paw to try and stop the gnawing. None of these seemed to have any effect, and eventually the wound on her foot was so large that it was decided to put the animal down.[35] The surgeon P. Abraham, who presented the case to the Irish Academy of Medicine, was so intrigued by the lack of explanation for the lioness's behaviour that he corresponded with zookeepers across Europe, gathering together similar cases. He discovered that such habits were 'not uncommon' among other animals in confinement despite being, as one listener claimed during the discussion following, 'so foreign to animal instinct'. Interestingly, while this could have led to the conclusion that the unnatural environment of captivity *caused* the development of morbid behaviour, explanations given tended to ascribe human disorders to these animals. Abraham concluded that such behaviours – which he also recorded in a variety of other large cats and carnivorous animals, and occasionally in monkeys – were caused by 'mental derangement'. He further noted that 'the carnivora which have "taken on" in this way have been nearly always females', and usually young or at the menopause. This suggested to him that 'we may look upon this perversion of taste . . . as one of the manifestations in the lower animals of that Protean affection which we call "hysteria".'[36]

An assumption that self-mutilation contravened the laws of animal and human nature was widespread in this era, and a number of writers who explored self-injury came from a background in the natural sciences. For many people, this idea of self-injury as a morbid or perverse instinct led to the foregone conclusion that anyone exhibiting such behaviour must be insane. Hysteria, however, was regarded as a nervous disorder – on the borderland between sanity and outright madness, making it difficult to classify. Self-mutilation was variously portrayed as indicating an absence of the sensation of pain, a lack of volition or will to resist impulsive behaviour or a diminished interest in self-preservation. The first explanation was most popular in Germany. Wilhelm Griesinger (1817–1868), a German neurologist and psychiatrist, developed a model of self-mutilation as an 'anomaly of sensibility', part of his overall rejection of traditional psychological and metaphysical classifications of mental disorder. Instead, he divided irregularities into 'anomalies of sensibility' and 'disorder[s] of the motor power'. Self-mutilation, for Griesinger, became marked by 'decreased sensibility, by anaesthesia or analgesia'. He cited a patient who, in part from wantonness, and in part to compel the attendant to send for the physician, had deliberately smashed the first phalanx of his thumb with a brick. This man told me he had not suffered the least pain.[37]

For Griesinger, elevating the status of the physiological response meant that the direct motive for self-mutilation could be discarded: the lack of pain was the cause, not the patient's desired result. Ten years later, forensic psychiatrist Richard von Krafft-Ebing also claimed that the 'loss of the pain-sense is of great significance in insanity,' seeing it as a direct cause of self-inflicted injury.[38] For these physicians, the absence of pain became a *directly* stimulating factor in self-mutilation.

Griesinger's classification of insanity was not adopted outright in British psychiatry. However, the view that self-injury was based on the influence of an 'insane impulse' often appeared in British texts in the 1860s and '70s. 'Impulse' tended to refer to a loosely defined stimulus to the nervous system that might cause someone to respond without consciously considering their actions. Insane impulses were regarded as contravening natural laws, like the self-mutilation of the Dublin lioness. The alienist and botanist William Carmichael McIntosh used natural history as a model for exploring the 'morbid impulse'.[39] He sought a universal explanation for so-called 'perverted impulses' (including self-mutilation) in damage to the faculties of volition (the will) and emotion. McIntosh's model used the physiological principles of Thomas Laycock (who had taught him at Edinburgh and remained a friend) in an evolutionary hierarchy of classification, influenced by writers like Darwin and the psychologist Herbert Spencer.[40] His concept of 'morbid impulse' reflected the idea that human behaviour was regulated by the dual processes of impulse and inhibition. Both terms were used as scientific descriptions of nervous action: however, they also had socio-evolutionary connotations. Impulsive behaviour was especially attributed to animals and 'savages', while 'self-control' was regarded by many as a marker of civilization.

When McIntosh divided morbid instincts into four types in relation to the natural instinct they were assumed to contravene, these reflected those emphasized by middle-class Victorian men as indicating civilized (that is, Western) status. Some of these were physiological – first 'alimentary' and then 'sexual' – but they were followed by less explicitly biological functions: the domestic, personal and social. Self-mutilation came under the category of the personal. While stressing that wider factors than physiology played a part in the recognition and development of 'perversions' – for 'their occurrence is found to be regulated by the degree of civilisation, mode of life . . . and the prevailing tendencies of the age, which indelibly stamps them with its characteristic features' – McIntosh nonetheless related every morbid impulse to a corresponding natural process, indicating that both should be regarded in absolute terms.[41]

The emergence of definitions of self-mutilation fitted into an ethos in which volition, self-control and brain biology were emphasized within scientific and popular language. Self-mutilation could be characterized as a 'morbid instinct' (representative of 'delirium' or extreme intellectual disorder) or as an example of 'uncontrollable impulse'. These descriptions appealed due to their scientific respectability, as portrayed in McIntosh's work through a correlation between morbid impulse and reflex functioning and the use of comparative examples from the animal world. Similarly, Bethlem's Theo Hyslop claimed that loss of control in asylum patients provided direct evidence of the existence of the will in the normal self, illustrating this with two examples of self-injurious behaviour:

A patient was brought to Bethlem bound hand and foot, at his own request, in order to prevent self-mutilation, which proved an ungovernable impulse to him. Another patient begged and implored that mechanical restraint might be employed to prevent him injuring himself.[42]

This comparison to 'normal' behaviour frequently had a cultural dimension, and descriptions of non-Western, culturally sanctioned mutilations were often compared to insane acts of self-injury in Western countries to imply the universal nature of such behaviour. In 1897, the American

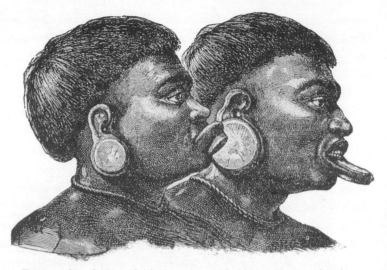

This image from Gould and Pyle's *Anomalies and Curiosities of Medicine* (1897) was intended to illustrate 'the ludicrous custom of piercing the ears for the wearing of ornaments, typical of savagery and found in all indigenous African tribes, [which] is universally prevalent among our own people'. The tribe pictured, the Botocudo or Aimoré people, was actually South American.

ophthalmologists George Gould and Walter Pyle, for example, included a section on self-mutilation in their *Anomalies and Curiosities of Medicine*, drawing on anthropology to describe a wide variety of 'peculiar custom[s] among savages', including facial piercings, scarification or castration for religious or ceremonial purposes.[43] This comparative technique was also adopted by British alienists, such as James Adam, and McIntosh's framework came from a similar model.

However, analogy to the natural world did *not* as a matter of course lead to the obvious conclusion that self-mutilation in man was pathological. Indeed, McIntosh asserted that self-mutilation could be a natural process in certain animals. Referring to the 'wonderful power of self-mutilation' in crustaceans (his own special study), he indicated that mutilations in nature often served a purpose: 'Under ordinary circumstances . . . such self-mutilations in the crustacea are intended for the safety of the animal, whereas in man, for the most part, they are essentially morbid.'[44] In other words, self-mutilation in man was unnatural (and therefore pathological) *because* it appeared to serve no purpose. He referred similarly to suicide, claiming that:

> Man in a state of nature seldom or never commits suicide, because his instincts and impulses are natural, even though they may be exaggerated, whereas in civilization nothing is more common.[45]

Statements like this indicate the complexity of Victorian notions of self-mutilation: it was not necessarily an obvious conclusion that self-mutilation in man was 'morbid', either through description of acts *or* by analogy to the natural world: other factors influenced McIntosh's decision to draw a distinction between human and animal life, attributing a *use* to self-mutilation within nature, while regarding it as indicative of disease in mankind.

Although McIntosh did not elaborate on the morbid nature of self-mutilation in man – listing self-injurious acts without any attempt at explanation – some later medical writers related self-injury directly to the *effects* of civilization: a response to an unnatural environment, which, it was supposed, resulted in a failure of natural selection. This idea characterized what is known as 'degenerationist' literature in Britain following the publication of William Greg's 'On the Failure of "Natural Selection" in the Case of Man'. While some writers portrayed self-mutilation as representative of a primitive state, others used the topic to comment on the increasing fear of national decline across Europe in the final decades of the nineteenth century, as expressed in fields such as criminology, sociology and aesthetics. This ethos shifted self-mutilation from a topic connected with a progressive notion of purposeful evolution within nature (as it was, for the most part, in McIntosh's paper), to one instead associated with pessimistic theories of decline. This sociocultural evolutionary perspective helps to explain how, for nineteenth-century alienists writing on self-mutilation, hair-plucking and skin-picking could be categorized alongside the more physically destructive behaviours of castration, amputation and enucleation.

Just as evolutionary development was thought to progress along a gradual scale, alienists suggested that there was a progression of self-mutilation, from major injuries through to the 'nervous, fidgety, restless habits' that 'less perhaps in magnitude, are common among nervous people who are not insane'.[46] Indeed, the extent of such behaviour at any given time was regarded as a 'valuable criterion' of a patient's nervous condition: an indication that the 'excitable', 'emotional' or 'reserved' (and therefore particularly susceptible) patient had lost all self-control and was in danger of outright insanity. In effect, self-mutilation was thought to make the internal state of insanity externally visible to the physician, in the same way that the physical characteristics and modes of life in so-called 'savage' populations were correlated with their mental and moral make-up by anthropologists.

For nineteenth-century writers, connections between self-mutilation and social behaviour were bound up in an evolutionary approach to culture and biology, which attempted to classify impulses on a straightforward hierarchy. But where did self-mutilation fit? Was a desire to injure oneself evidence of the emergence of a primitive impulse or an intentional protest against or unconscious response to the rapid changes of the industrial age? Elements of both these ideas can be seen in the way 22-year-old Mary S. was diagnosed at Bethlem. Recorded as suffering from 'hysterical mania', Mary was regarded as impulsive with 'but little control over her emotions'. This was shown by her tendency to pull out her hair, as depicted in the photograph opposite. However, the image was also thought to emphasize Mary's preoccupied and isolated state: 'Patient keeps standing up in the position indicated in the photograph, continually picking her head. Remains by herself, doesn't talk.'[47] Alienists remained uncertain how to diagnose or classify self-mutilation. In 1892, James Shaw suggested in his textbook that 'self-injury apart from suicidal tendency' could be prompted by 'excitement, terror, delusions, or unconsciousness' and hence occur in 'acute mania; pubescent insanity; agitated melancholia; puerperal insanity; monomania; epileptic insanity; [and] delirium tremens' – in other words, almost every psychiatric classification![48]

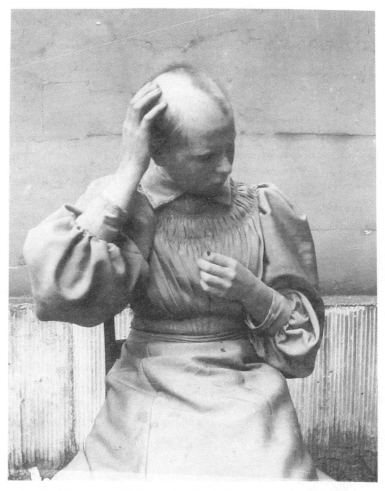

Mary S. photographed at Bethlem in 1895. After pulling out most of her hair, Mary was discharged uncured; however, she visited the hospital a year later, apparently fully recovered physically and mentally.

The confusion between the two models of self-mutilation – impulsive or cognitive; primitive or degenerationist – is highlighted particularly in a highly publicized case of the early 1880s. The mystery surrounding a young Staffordshire farmer brought the topic of self-mutilation firmly to the forefront of the public mind. The case of Isaac Brooks also caused confusion among alienists as to whether self-mutilation was evidence of outright insanity. Following this case, those diagnoses perceived as being on the 'borderlands of insanity', such as moral insanity or hysteria, were increasingly put forward as explanations for individual acts of self-inflicted injury.

The Isaac Brooks enigma: uncontrollable impulse or mental motive?

Isaac Brooks was a stonemason and small farmer from Leek, in Staffordshire. He was unmarried and lived with family, including his mother and his illegitimate son (the child's mother was dead). In 1879, then aged 29, Brooks called the local doctor (Francis Warrington) to attend to a cut wound on the scrotum, from which one of his testicles protruded. When asked to explain the injury, the young man claimed he had been attacked and wounded by three men, whom he later named as local farmers. Two were subsequently arrested and sentenced to ten years' imprisonment for the crime. The whole story, including a second, identical, injury eighteen months later, only appeared in print after Brooks's death in December 1881. On his deathbed, the farmer signed a full confession stating that the men were innocent and, according to initial (mistaken) reports, that his injuries were self-inflicted.[49] The newly formed Press Association ensured the wide distribution of the story and, in early January 1882, it appeared in newspapers around Britain, from London to Liverpool, Glasgow to Leeds and Sheffield to Birmingham. From an initial focus on the miscarriage of justice, most reports quickly moved on to speculate about the character and habits of Isaac Brooks himself, and how these related to what was widely agreed to be an act of self-mutilation. As a commentary in *The Lancet* stated: 'There cannot be the slightest doubt in the mind of any one . . . that the case was throughout one of self-mutilation from insanity'.[50]

This categorical statement – repeated verbatim in many newspapers – indicates that the idea of 'self-mutilation from insanity' was well-established by 1882. Indeed, alienists quickly diagnosed Brooks, even though he had never been in an asylum or shown any unsoundness of mind during his life. The combination of self-mutilation and false accusation appeared to be 'a definite plan of lying and mischief-making [which] seems to be the symptom of moral insanity'.[51] One anonymous alienist supported this with examples from his own asylum experience, of patients who had injured themselves apparently to accuse others. He went on to describe other instances of self-inflicted injury, implying a similar background of moral insanity and manipulation in all such cases.

Moral insanity was a diagnosis introduced by the alienist and anthropologist James Cowles Prichard in 1833, and incorporated into his 1835 *Treatise on Insanity*. It described a defect in moral or emotional capacity in an individual who otherwise showed no sign of intellectual impairment. While modern readers often assume the term is evidence of the strict social sanctions of the Victorian era, 'moral' was never intended to equate directly to social correctness but was a far looser term, implying emotional upheaval and often extreme behaviour, which seemed at odds with the patient's personality or intelligence.[52] Take, for example, a case submitted by Daniel Hack Tuke to the *Journal of Mental Science* of 1885. This described a patient, W.B., born in Wales but living in Canada. W.B. was described as a 'pleasant, agreeable sort of fellow' who 'has a mind equal, if not superior, to that of the average of his class in life'; nonetheless, he had spent much of his life either in prison or an asylum.[53] From an early age he tortured animals and other children, with a favourite pastime being to cut the throats of horses. When in an institution, he continued to torture and sometimes seriously injure those around him: on one occasion he attempted to castrate a helpless fellow patient with a table knife; on another he was found to have caught a kitten and tortured it until 'the floor was besmeared with blood.' Yet, despite his unrepentant cruelty, W.B. did not seem irrational:

> If so situated that he could not indulge his evil propensities, he was a quiet and useful man, but he could not be trusted. He had a fair education, and enjoyed reading newspapers, letters, etc., sent to him.[54]

W.B. confused doctors, as had Isaac Brooks, poetically described by Dr Warrington as 'an enigma in life and a puzzle in death'.[55] Despite outwardly possessing the qualities expected of a civilized man – 'useful', educated and 'anxious to be well dressed' – both men nonetheless engaged in behaviour regarded as impulsive and uncivilized.[56]

Prichard regarded moral insanity as having a metaphysical or religious dimension. In later years, this was often repackaged by alienists in secular terms. Religious or not, late nineteenth-century scientists and philosophers shared great concern for the future of humanity, equating morality with physical and mental evolution. For these writers, Isaac Brooks and W.B. represented a threat framed in biological and evolutionary terms, placing ideals of social order within a natural scientific framework to become a 'great fundamental law alike of Nature and Christian morals'.[57] Thus, 'breaches of the conventional as well as the moral laws of society may be but symptoms of disorder or disease of the higher nervous system.'[58] George Savage illustrated this statement with examples of the 'malingering and mischief-making' he connected with hysteria and hypochondriasis. In particular, 'it is not at all uncommon to meet with hysterical young women who put themselves to great personal torture without any apparent object.' Miss M, for example, a 'bright, pretty and accomplished' girl, had been sending threatening anonymous letters to relatives,

> saying many things which were not true ... Beside all this, some time before, she had had a peculiar skin affection, which was proved to have been produced by herself by burning with hair-curlers.

Miss M's self-mutilation was explained via the diagnosis of moral insanity, which nonetheless saw her described as deceitful. Cases like this were taken as evidence of the 'self-culture' of civilization, an increasing tendency for individuals to focus on their own desires at the expense of those around them.[59]

The Isaac Brooks case drew together evolutionary interpretations of self-mutilation with the diagnosis of moral insanity. Brooks's state of mind was judged solely on his actions – in this instance an attempt at self-castration and a false accusation against others. Indeed, given that the farmer had already died, there was no other way his state of mind *could* be judged. The physical and mental models for explaining his acts sat awkwardly side by side in both medical and popular accounts. One author in the *Journal of Mental Science* considered that Brooks's 'madness' must have begun with a physical change, resulting perhaps from puberty, which might cause 'a loss of control of the lower nervous centres, so that sexual excess, or abuse of some kind, has been indulged in'. Subsequently,

> This constant and exhausting strain increases nervous weakness, and the patients lose more and more their self-control; they become weak, and, like weak people generally, suspicious.[60]

This description ensured that a physical explanation of insanity could be advanced, while nonetheless maintaining the responsibility of the patient, who, it is suggested, would not have been affected had he not 'indulged'. Thus, the location of Brooks's wound became seen as 'evidence' of his motivation: a complicated mixture of nervous weakness and mental guilt.

This analogy between physical and mental cause was even more apparent in lay reports, as shown in the manner in which Brooks's death itself was reported. Brooks's doctor reported the cause of death as blood loss from a second injury. However, newspaper accounts avoided mentioning any direct cause of death whatsoever, instead making an explicit connection between Brooks's death and the trial. *The Guardian* claimed that 'from the time of the trial Brooks went "downhill". He seemed oppressed by some mental trouble.'[61] Some local newspapers took this description even further. The *Sheffield and Rotherham Independent*, one of the most eager followers of the story, claimed that:

> [M]ental trouble . . . fast fed itself upon his physical system, and caused him to resemble an animated skeleton. So marked indeed was the change, that so long ago as last September, the Rev. Richd. Smith,

Vicar of Rushton, seeing him wandering aimlessly amongst the graves in the picturesque churchyard was so struck by his appearance that he asked him if his sufferings arose from a belief that he had sworn away the liberty of innocent men. Brooks denied that this was the case ... There were those, however, who openly attributed his wasting away to remorse, and that they were right will soon be seen.[62]

Here, Brooks's confession was regarded as proof that his death was indeed a direct result of inner turmoil (guilt), which in turn caused physical wasting. Thus, for many people, Brooks's alleged guilt was strongly connected to physical, nervous weakness, albeit associated with a moral cause.

As well as the tendency to suggest a combined psychological and biological account of motivation, which confusingly referred to both impulse and idea, medical and popular accounts also situated this within a wider, social context. Reporters emphasized the effects Brooks's self-mutilation had had on the surrounding community, as well as making regular reference to his son, a potential biological threat if the hereditary nature of mental illness was to be believed. Indeed, in a period which saw the growing popularity of moralizing journalistic crusades, such as W. T. Stead's 'Maiden Tribute of Modern Babylon' (published in the *Pall Mall Gazette* in 1885), reporters increasingly tended to provide explicit social comment in their texts.[63] Here, it was not just Brooks the individual who was viewed as problematic; instead, he was held up as symptomatic of the age, his act representative of a wider selfishness. Retrospective analysis of Brooks's character emphasized his 'solitary' nature. As the *Journal of Mental Science* put it:

The man was single, and lived a very subjective life; he was just the type of man in whom all the evils of civilization seem to accumulate, great sensibility, with loss of power of control, an emotional but ill-ruled machine. A solitary man, thinking himself misunderstood and neglected, building castles in the air, finding the times out of joint, and from this idea conceiving that he has enemies and persecutors.[64]

Here we can see both the impulsive and mental elements attributed to self-inflicted injury at this time. By relating Brooks's self-mutilation to his rejection of the surrounding community, his act was portrayed as the ultimate act of selfish preoccupation. If, as many writers at this time held, individual development reached its peak in social feeling, then those, like Brooks, who were thought to have failed to develop such characteristics might pose a national threat.

In this chapter, I have explained how the category of self-mutilation was defined and constituted in the late Victorian period, through a combination of biological, psychological and social concerns. Despite the breadth of views we have seen, self-injury was largely (and newly) associated with psychiatry in this period, and the ideas and attitudes that emerged were couched in much more explicitly medical terms than most of those sketched out in the previous chapter. First, self-mutilation was categorized as a symptom of mental disorder, primarily through a conscious effort to distinguish it from suicidal behaviour. There were both practical and legal reasons for doing this. Unlike suicide (and, newly in the Victorian era, attempted suicide), self-mutilation was not a crime. Occurrences of self-mutilation in the asylum were also slightly less likely to be seen as a sign of poor care than those of suicide, and alienists adopted the term as a means of protection against bad publicity for their institutions.

However, self-inflicted injury could still result in death and, if a major injury occurred to a patient within an asylum, there was little practical need to decide whether the motive of the individual was to commit suicide or not. Thus, the interest in motive in self-mutilation was also part of a wider interest within late nineteenth-century psychiatry in attempting to understand normal psychology through the acts of the insane. There were three main explanations for self-mutilation in this period. First, a purely physiological model explained self-injury in terms of the absence of the sensation of pain. While this explanation attracted some interest in Germany, it was never popular in Britain, where explanations tended to be made on a much broader socio-environmental model. Biological understandings of human functioning were still important, however, and self-mutilation might be viewed as the effect of 'nervous impulse'. Acts of self-injury in those certified insane were judged to prove the existence of 'the will' in healthy individuals. This nervous model also fitted into the natural sciences, where 'morbid instincts' were viewed as a perversion of natural order, as exemplified by analogy to animal behaviour. The explanations for animal self-mutilation, however, were often made in terms of human models of nervous disorder. This set self-mutilation within a broader, socio-evolutionary understanding of human and animal functioning.

It was widely agreed among alienists that self-mutilation *was* evidence of perversion, primarily through diagnoses such as hysteria and moral insanity. However, there was little agreement as to what this implied for human behaviour more generally. Did instances of self-injury in the animal kingdom suggest that such acts were evidence of a reversion to a primitive state? This, it seemed to some, was supported by the 'mutilations' Darwin and others described in 'savages' where 'hardly any part of the body, which can be unnaturally modified, has escaped.'[65] Others, however, depicted self-injury as indicative of the 'self-culture' produced by the 'artificial relationships of society', the main explanation in the case of Isaac Brooks, which implied that self-mutilation was symbolic of selfish degeneration.[66] The difficulty of reconciling these views emerges still more clearly in the two models of self-mutilation laid out in the following two chapters: the view of 'sexual self-mutilation' in men as an impulsive act alongside the 'motiveless malingering' associated with hysteria.

THREE

SEXUAL SELF-MUTILATION
Masturbation, Masculinity and Self-control in Late Victorian Britain

I n the wake of the Isaac Brooks reports detailed in the previous chapter, one medical writer categorically claimed that this episode was 'no isolated one', for 'there are many well-authenticated cases of youths and men of all ages who have sometimes successfully, at others unsuccessfully, performed this painful operation upon themselves.'[1] Although no evidence was given to back the statement up, comments like this were often taken at face value. Nearly twenty years later, when American doctors George Gould and Walter Pyle published *Anomalies and Curiosities of Medicine*, the authors used fifty years of articles on self-inflicted injury to claim that:

> Self-mutilation in man is almost invariably the result of meditation over the generative function, and the great majority of cases of this nature are avulsions or amputations of some parts of the genitalia.[2]

Self-castration, in the last decades of the nineteenth century, became the paradigm for self-mutilation – in a similar way that self-cutting did in the later twentieth century (see Chapter Six). Sometimes the terms 'self-castration' and 'self-mutilation' were even used interchangeably. In the index catalogue to the U.S. Surgeon-General's medical library (1910), the entry for 'self-mutilation' pointed readers to associated listings for 'sexual instinct (perversion of)' and 'Skoptsy' (a Russian religious cult that practised ritual castration), suggesting a particular link between the three terms.[3] The articles listed nonetheless included a large number focusing on other types of self-inflicted injury, including amputation and enucleation. As we have seen, castration was not particularly common in asylums or hospitals, compared to other forms of self-injury. So why was there such keen interest in male genital self-injury at this time? And in what ways was self-castration explained and understood?

Today, it might seem obvious to connect castration with gender dysphoria or anxiety over sexual identity: perhaps we might consider it an attempt to alter one's biological sex. However, as I have shown, we cannot assume that maleness has always been thought directly related to the biological sex organs, or even to be affected by their absence. Indeed, late Victorian writers had quite a different way of viewing self-castration than the modern category of gender dysphoria; it was usually depicted as an egotistical – and therefore characteristically male – act. In this chapter I explore this very different model of masculinity and sexuality through the Victorian category of 'sexual self-mutilation'. I begin with a brief background on the shifting definition of castration, emphasizing the diversity of ways in which castration has been viewed in relation to sex and gender. Then I describe the 'sexual self-mutilation' outlined by the psychiatrist James Adam in 1892, focusing on one particular patient who was key to Adam's description of self-castration. I then set this in the context of the era: the potential threat that 'male lust' was thought to pose to Western civilization and the associated view that self-mutilation formed part of a catalogue of male 'perversions'. These sexual perversions were increasingly debated by authors such as the famous German-Austrian forensic psychiatrist Richard von Krafft-Ebing (1840–1902), whose Psychopathia Sexualis introduced the terms 'sadism' and 'masochism' into our vocabulary. By viewing a (heterosexual) interest in sex as the basis for individual growth and social cohesion, psychiatrists depicted castration as a social threat, which could only be countered by a model of masculinity that emphasized self-control and sexual restraint.

'A frequent cause of insanity in young men': definitions of castration and sexual mutilation

Some earlier approaches to castration have already been outlined in Chapter One: as an effort to preserve the life-giving male 'pneuma' and as part of a 'genderless ideal' of early Christianity. But what does the term castration actually mean? The *Oxford English Dictionary* gives the primary definition as 'the removing of the testicles'. This explanation seems so obvious that it is easy to assume that this is what castration has always meant. Yet, in nineteenth-century texts, the term was also applied to operations carried out on women: ovariotomy – the removal of one or both ovaries – and the briefly popular, controversial medical practice of clitoridectomy – the removal of the clitoris.[4] It could also be used to mean ablation of the testicles *or* amputation of the penis, and there was rarely clear differentiation between these two acts. While this might seem surprising today, following a century of endocrinological research into 'sex hormones', there was no obvious reason to distinguish between injuries that impaired sexual function in the late nineteenth century. The sex organs were generally believed to influence the body through the central nervous system, not by means of chemical secretion. If this was so, then damage to any part of the genitals could affect this process, thus significantly altering the individual who had been castrated.[5]

Another element of Victorian medical writing on castration that may seem surprising to modern readers is that there was often little interest in whether or not the operation was successful in preventing sexual function, suggesting that this was not the fundamental importance of castration to contemporaries. Today, we tend to assume that castration causes impotence and a related loss of secondary sex characteristics (although even this is challenged by routine procedures like vasectomy).[6] As has been shown, however, at various times castration has also been considered to *enhance* masculinity (by ensuring that a man would not waste the 'vital force' essential to his male status) and to have no specific effect whatsoever on a man's fundamental being.[7] In the nineteenth century, genital procedures like circumcision were also being increasingly advised on health (rather than religious) grounds for male infants, particularly in the United States, where it had become a routine procedure by the turn of the twentieth century.[8] Castration, then, does not necessarily imply impotence and loss, and we should be wary of interpreting historical material to support the modern assumption that it does. Certainly, this interpretation is by no means obvious in the definition of 'sexual self-mutilation' put forward by James Adam in 1892.

Adam's interest in writing up and classifying self-mutilation was seemingly inspired by the high-profile Brooks case, which indicated the 'importance of the subject in its general as well as its medico-legal aspect'.[9] The alienist's first article included an account of two cases of self-injury – enucleation in a female patient and castration in a male. Ten years later, he had collected another study of the latter, and this led him to present them as part of a general model:

> The following are cases of sexual self-mutilation; similar ones are given in Krafft-Ebing's 'Psychopathia Sexualis,' by Moll, and by some of the French authors, more particularly in their systematic works on mental diseases.[10]

Although Adam did not draw any specific conclusions about the meaning of the cases he outlined, this introductory statement, setting them in the context of continental research, is revealing. Unlike enucleation, amputation or injuries caused by burning – which he presented as straightforward individual case studies – Adam considered sexual mutilation to be part of a broader field of scientific research. Looking in more detail at these two cases indicates the varied ways in which castration could be understood: not least in the fact that one related to the removal of the testicles and the other the penis.

Adam's first case was an eighteen-year-old farmer – the 'tall and hand-some' W.B. – who was admitted to the Southern Counties Asylum in Dumfries six days after he had 'completely and cleanly removed the whole of the penis' with a sharp penknife.[11] Interestingly, this act had not been the decisive factor in W.B.'s certification, for he was only stated as having been insane for four days (two days after his self-mutilation). Indeed, Dr Taylor Monteath, who attended to W.B.'s wounds, declared the young man 'quite rational at that time', although noting that he 'seemed much dejected in spirit, and expressed his regret several times to both his mother and myself for what he had done'.[12] Dr Monteath considered that the youth's admission that he had masturbated was explanation enough for his self-mutilation. To modern eyes, this might appear to be an irrationally excessive response to a harmless pastime; however, masturbation was certainly not considered this way in the late Victorian period.

In the eighteenth century, so-called self-abuse became conceptualized as a disease. John Marten's *Onania; or, The Heinous Sin of Self-pollution* (1712) was influential in suggesting that 'solitary sex' had become a social problem by causing physical wasting, lethargy, impotence and even death in large numbers of young men.[13] Although masturbation had previously been regarded as a physical and moral concern, it had not been singled out as *the* sexual vice but was one of a number of ways, including excessive sexual intercourse, in which essential fluids (and thus energy) might be lost.

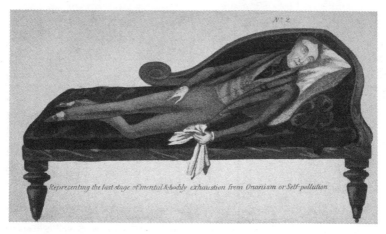

Representing the last stage of mental & bodily exhaustion from Onanism or Self-pollution

Illustration from *The Secret Companion* by Robert Brodie (1845), a medical text warning about the potential dangers of masturbation. Here we are shown the 'last stage of mental & bodily exhaustion from Onanism or Self-pollution'.

An increased focus on the pathology of masturbation in this period was part of a new philosophical understanding of the relationship between the individual and society, which encouraged greater attention to self-imposed restraint. Masturbation, in this context, became viewed as evidence of an individual who had *lost* self-control and was thus also unable to contribute to society.[14] Concern over the damaging effects of masturbation, like belief in bloodletting, faded in the twentieth century without any direct medical recantation of the theory.[15] By the second half of the nineteenth century, alienists specifically related masturbation to mental illness, although there was some debate as to whether it was a cause or a symptom.[16] In 1861, Robert Ritchie (superintendent of Bethnal House Asylum, London) published 'An Inquiry into a Frequent Cause of Insanity in Young Men'.[17] The 'frequent cause' was masturbation and Ritchie posited a link between self-abuse and self-inflicted injury, drawing attention to it three times in his short article. He considered that self-mutilation indicated 'an unsound reasoning power, the visiting on the supposed offending organs the faults of the ill-regulated mind'.[18] This statement suggested a shift from viewing the pathology of masturbation as a physical problem to a mental one: part of a new under-standing of body and mind as regulated by nervous impulse, which could be controlled by mental volition. Yet medical remedies for masturbation none-theless ranged from cauterization to uncomfortable restraining devices – all focusing on the 'offending organs' rather than mental regulation, and still in use in some asylums into the twentieth century. At the enormous Middlesex County Asylum at Colney Hatch (later Friern Hospital), blistering the penis was a weekly ritual in the early twentieth century, and castration was even suggested as a long-term preventive.[19]

The ongoing concern over the dangers of masturbation, and the advocacy of radical cures for a practice that many still believed could result in death, sets the concerns of many asylum patients of this period – like Adam's young farmer – in a very different context from our modern assumptions. It was quite plausible for young Frederick B. (admitted to Bethlem in 1886) to interpret masturbation as suicidal; it was recorded that he says 'he has tried to kill himself by masturbation.'[20] The physicians did not

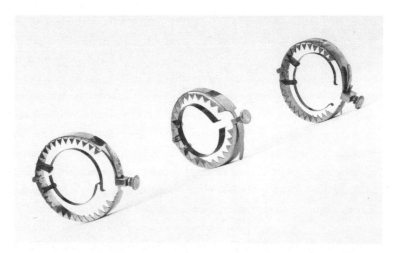

Anti-masturbation devices. These were designed to prevent the wearer from stimulating himself, and are of a design that was often used in psychiatric institutions; c. 1880-1920.

interpret their patient's behaviour in the same way, for he was not listed as suicidal. Instead, it was claimed that Frederick's 'general mental condition seems to be that of brooding over the state of his sexual organs with hypochondriasis'. Such a comment is suggestive of the shifting position of most alienists on masturbation. Through the later nineteenth century, many doctors moved from viewing self-abuse as a physical to a mental cause of insanity. Thus, physicians came to associate masturbation with sexual hypochondriasis, and the sex organs accordingly shifted from being the physical site of disease (for which castration was a potential cure) to a psychological fixation of the patient (with castration similarly indicative of the patient's obsessive state of mind). Thus James Adam laid the blame for W.B.'s actions on external suggestion rather than the physical effects of masturbation, for 'he had been reading some quack publications on nervous debility, and also Salvation Army publications, which roused within him strong convictions of his wickedness.'[21]

The other case that was influential for Adam's model bore few similarities to the eighteen-year-old farmer: in class and background, in age or in the context of his injury. Nonetheless, the site of the wound meant that the alienist absorbed both into his general model. Captain Henry P. H. was confined in West Malling Place asylum in April 1871, over a decade before Adam arrived there. He was 65 years old, and had first been diagnosed with mania thirty years previously, when he was sent to Brook House in Clapton. Around the same time, the Captain was retired from the Bengal Army on half pay. In between asylum admissions, he lived with his unmarried sister, Ellen, in Yateley, Hampshire, until her death in 1862. Four years after Ellen's death, the Captain 'removed the testes & part of the scrotum . . . having the impression he must become a Eunuch to preach to a tribe in the North of India'. Henry's explanations were interpreted in his case notes as religious and sexual delusions:

> Although a Eunuch in this country he would not be thought so in India for they would say 'he might have connection with their Wifes [sic] & Daughters to amuse them.' Such scandal as this would be ignominious to a Missionary. This appears one objection to his returning to India and he thinks now he might meet with a Lady who would live with him without being desirous of cohabitation – 'A kind of Spiritual Wife.' There he thinks he could live happily.[22]

When Adam classified Henry as a case of 'sexual self-mutilation', he implied that the Captain's sexual instincts inspired the 'fit of religious enthusiasm and excitement' which prompted the act itself. In mutilating himself, Henry had prevented proper reproductive function, and his desire for a 'Spiritual Wife' was regarded as a related delusion. The term may well refer to the 1868 book *Spiritual Wives* by the historian and traveller William Hepworth Dixon. Dixon compared 'celibate love' to polygamy, suggesting that *both* were equally misguided and damaging to civilization.[23] Indeed, for much of the nineteenth century, celibacy was regarded as more problematic by many Protestants than sex for purposes other than procreation.[24]

Yet an understanding of motive was complicated by Henry's connections with India. In the *Dictionary*, Adam began by noting that the Captain 'had been many years resident in the East, and had come to acquire many Eastern languages and ways', suggesting that exposure to foreign culture had influenced his act.[25] Indeed, Henry's own acknowledgement of the culturally specific meaning of eunuchism, as indicated in the above quote, is revealing. It was a popular assumption in the West that eunuchs were primarily guardians in harems: their castration meant that they would not be able to impregnate the inhabitants. Yet, as the Captain notes, many eunuchs were still able to 'have connection': removal of the testicles did not generally prevent erection, merely procreation. The complicated cultural relationship between sex and gender was further emphasized in this period by anthropological investigations of 'Eastern' cultures. In the same year that Henry was admitted to West Malling Place, the British Governor-General enforced the Criminal Tribes Act in northern India. This effectively criminalized people purely due to membership of a particular group. Among those included were the *hijda*, often translated as the 'third gender': a tribe of 'natural eunuchs' who dressed in women's clothing.[26] Their activity blurred the distinction between the physical creation of a eunuch through castration and his social persona through the adoption of a female role: as the author of a report to the Anthropological Institute noted, the *hijda* were not necessarily castrated or congenitally abnormal.

Adam certainly emphasized the role of 'Eastern' religions and culture in the origins of an impulse towards self-mutilation in mankind.[27] Thus, he used the Captain's case to suggest the dangerous nature of primitive cultures to those exposed to them: the Christian missionary might be affected by the very group he wished to convert. Yet this association with Eastern influences was striking in its absence from the notes on Henry's behaviour in the privileged West Malling Place environment, where he was 'overbearing in his conversation and conduct' and believed he was the proprietor. Case notes indicated the relative freedom a wealthy, elderly gentleman in an elite rural asylum might have. He was permitted to walk off the premises unattended, and slept alone in a single room. Although the doctors suggested that the Captain's health would be affected by his taking daily walks, even in cold weather, it was remarked that 'he is so perverse you cannot get him to remain indoors or take anything except what he feels

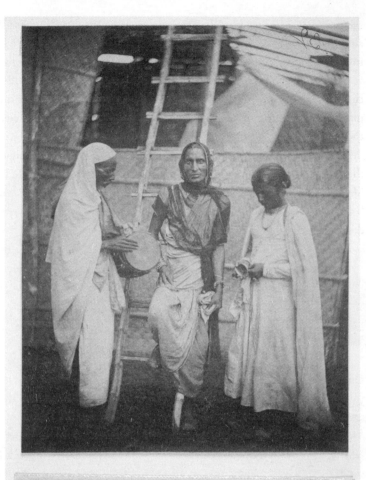

Gurmah, Khunsa or Hijra, reputed hermaphrodite, Eastern Bengal.

A reputed hermaphrodite and companions, taken by an unknown photographer in the early 1860s in eastern Bengal. This image is associated with the British government's increasing interest in the 19th century in gathering information on the races, customs, costumes and occupations of its colonial interests.

inclined.'[28] Rather than implying the Eastern ways Henry had supposedly acquired, or even his status as a certified lunatic, Captain Henry P. H. instead appeared as certain of his domain as any wealthy imperial officer.

Self-castration alone was not considered evidence of insanity in either the case of W.B. or Henry P. H. However, it *could* be deemed to constitute madness in some circumstances. In 1877, a young boot-riveter admitted to the Newcastle-upon-Tyne Borough Lunatic Asylum was diagnosed with 'Monomania with Self-Mutilation and a Suicidal Tendency', implying that these two symptoms were prominent.[29] Indeed, the onset of W.H.S.'s illness dated from his self-mutilation (the removal of a testicle) just one day before. Yet, like W. B., W.H.S. was quiet – even 'rational' – and happily described the infliction of his injury:

> He answered questions rationally, and stated that he had mutilated himself with a table knife, and that, in consequence of it being blunt, he had made four or five cuts before effecting his purpose. He stated that he considered it proper to remove the organ, and asked reporter if he was going to remove the other testicle.[30]

Unlike W.B., W.H.S. did not regret his actions, and thus his impulse towards self-mutilation was viewed as the basis of his illness, a 'distinct and especial' monomaniacal delusion.

Although self-castration was the paradigm for self-mutilation in this period, there is no evidence to suggest that it was common practice. It was rarely recorded in asylum annual reports and not much more often in patient casebooks. From 1880 to 1900, just five patients at the Bethlem Royal Hospital attempted castration, and only three acts resulted in (minor) injury. Although 'sexual self-mutilation' was primarily associated in published works with men, just as many female patients as male ones mutilated their genitals while at Bethlem. Psychiatric explanations for self-mutilation need to be viewed in this context, rather than taken at face value. In the cases of W.B. and Henry P. H., certain religious, sexual and social concerns highlighted by alienists *did* make an appearance: in particular, religious 'enthusiasm' and Henry's connection with 'the East', the location (as James Adam saw it) of the origin of the human impulse towards self-mutilation. Yet Henry's life and behaviour in the asylum complicated this story, as did his continued insistence that his actions were justified. Although in Henry's case this was thought evidence of an ongoing delusional state, W.H.S. by contrast recovered his health without appearing overly concerned by his injuries or showing any particular regret. It is just as easy to find examples in asylum records in which the expectations of alienists were *not* confirmed as those in which they were. We cannot, then, find an explanation as to why self-castration was emphasized within psychiatric practice. Instead, we must look at broader medical and social concerns about sex and masculinity to understand how and why alienists defined sexual self-mutilation.

Impulse, sexuality and desire: from masturbation to inversion

Victorian attitudes to sex and sexuality have a recognized place in modern cultural stereotypes: to be 'Victorian' is usually synonymous with being prudish or sexually repressed. This repression is usually perceived to have eased around the beginning of the twentieth century, when the emergence of scientific sexual research accompanied a progressive advance to modern 'enlightened' notions of sex and sexuality. Yet these assumptions can be questioned on many levels: indeed, the widespread discussion of sex in the second half of the nineteenth century shows that many Victorians were *very* interested in sex.[31] Projecting modern ideas of sexuality back onto the nineteenth century is problematic, for the very concept of *possessing* sexuality cannot be considered a natural given from which our analysis departs; instead, 'sexuality' is created and shaped by cultural ideas and attitudes.[32] Victorian writers paid close attention to categorizing and containing what they regarded as sexual deviance – most notably creating newly medical views of 'the homosexual' (in Victorian terms, the 'invert' or 'Urning'). In 1885, the infamous Labouchere Amendment to the Criminal Law Amendment Act newly criminalized acts of 'gross indecency' between two men, whether 'in public or private'.[33] Previously, only sodomy had been a crime – and, moreover, one that was notoriously difficult to prove, as in the Boulton and Park trial of 1871. This case made public the existence of a group of cross-dressing 'Mary-Annes' (as Ernest 'Stella' Boulton and Frederick 'Fanny' Park and their associates called themselves) in London's West End. However, doctors could not determine any medical evidence of anal intercourse and the trial collapsed.[34] The Labouchere Amendment received much attention in subsequent years through several prominent scandals, including the discovery of a male brothel in Cleveland Street in 1889 and the Oscar Wilde trials of 1895. Yet a lot of attention was also paid to so-called 'normal' sexuality in this period, revealing the existence of numerous concerns about male sexual desire – and, indeed, male health in general – in the late nineteenth and early twentieth centuries.[35] Fear over venereal disease, concerns about the effects of masturbation and the need for sex education, and political agitation by both men and women around the sexual 'double standard' show that 'normality' could be a fraught and contentious topic.

Social and political concerns around self-injury thus need to be viewed in relation to notions of sex and gender in this period. Pulling out hair, for example, was usually associated with insanity in women. At Bethlem, far more women engaged in hair-plucking than men (73 per cent of these patients were female). As with many other insane behaviours – undressing in public, the destruction of property or eating 'ravenously' – these injuries were interpreted by male doctors as a rejection of social propriety, and much more worthy of note in female patients. Long hair in women is 'universally admired', claimed the evolutionary anthropologist Winwood Reade, connecting hair directly to femininity.[36] Hair not only symbolized ideals of beauty but also other elements of 'proper' behaviour in the Victorian era. In the Sherlock Holmes adventure 'The Copper Beeches', the detective is consulted by Violet Hunter, a governess who has been offered a surprisingly lucrative position on the condition that she cut off her hair. Miss Hunter is horrified by the suggestion: her prospective employer's words sound almost obscene. 'I could hardly believe my ears ... I could not dream of sacrificing [my hair] in this off-hand fashion,' she declares.[37] Eventually, the governess decides she cannot afford such principles, and does as she is asked. Although on the surface this tale might appear to be a mildly misogynistic comment on the vanity of women, more was implied. Holmes repeatedly tells Watson that 'no sister of his should ever have accepted such a situation,' and the absence of any family to advise and protect Miss Hunter emphasizes the governess's vulnerability.[38] In cutting her hair in return for payment, it is suggested, Violet Hunter has prostituted herself. Indeed, cutting the hair short might even be classified as self-mutilation. In 1893, thirty-year-old Edith B. was admitted to Bethlem after having, under an impulse, 'cut off all her hair, cut her hand, and her foot'.[39] By grouping these three acts together, apparently compelled by the same drive, it was implied that hair-cutting was similar to wounding any other part of the body.

The rejection of feminine beauty through hair-plucking made such women seem politically dangerous, like the 'manly women' and 'glorified spinsters' described in lurid terms by the press: women who cut their hair short and had other goals in life than marriage.[40] Perhaps some Victorian female patients explicitly intended this reaction. At Bethlem, 25-year-old Alice G., for example, was 'very boyish and untidy', with short hair.[41] The rejection of prescribed gender roles also made these women seem sexually dubious: in many cases, hair-cutting or -plucking was explicitly linked to female sexuality. The young Annie B. 'cut her hair short and shortened her dress',[42] an act of childish rebellion that was also sexually provocative. Beginning to wear long dresses was a sign of womanhood for the bourgeois Victorian girl, yet short dresses were also associated with the lower classes – Annie expressed a desire to look like a servant. The idea of domestic service might hold a tantalizing prospect of independence (whatever the reality) for young middle-class women, some of whom apparently welcomed asylum admission as an escape from overbearing parents. Ada S. described her home life as 'very quiet and irksome' because 'her parents allow her to have very little company.' Bethlem Hospital, however, offered Ada the opportunity to socialize, and 'she greatly enjoys the music and the tennis she gets here.'[43]

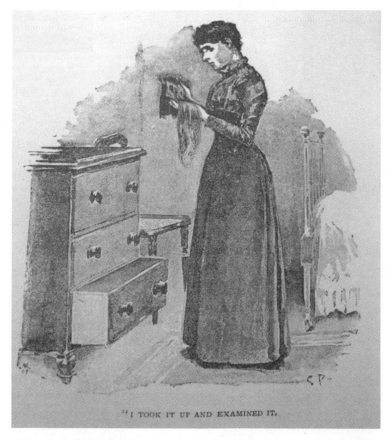

"I TOOK IT UP AND EXAMINED IT."

Illustration by Sydney Paget for 'The Copper Beeches', showing the moment the newly shorn Violet Hunter discovers a strange coil of hair – matching her own – in one of the drawers in her room.

Since lust was viewed as a male attribute, women who seemed to exhibit sexual desire – including prostitutes – were seen as 'unsexed', in the words of physician and sex writer William Acton.[44] Yet many late Victorian women identified with the prostitute victims of the Ripper murders.[45] From September 1888, a large number of patients admitted to Bethlem held delusions about the Whitechapel murders, which were widely and luridly reported. Yet there was a clear gender divide. Male patients feared that they were suspected of being the murderer ('Jack the Ripper', as the press named him), while women openly identified with the victims. In some cases this supported a link between self-mutilation and 'deviant' sexuality. Annie G., a 25-year-old teacher, was admitted to Bethlem in early 1889. Her delusions centred on the idea 'that she was to be cut-up – unsexed – like the Whitechapel victims'. Annie heard 'gentlemen's voices', particularly those 'of a person "lost" to her': hinted to be a former lover. Her doctors connected Annie G. and the murdered prostitutes by making assumptions about her past behaviour: 'with ideas of this nature there is a considerable admixture of the sexual element.' Later, when the 'erotic and troublesome' schoolteacher attempted to injure her genitals, this was simply regarded as further evidence of her sexual deviance, with Annie's 'erotic' ideas thought to have predisposed her towards self-mutilation.[46]

The large number of excellent feminist histories of the late nineteenth century can lead to the impression, by omission, that prescribed gender roles were only problematic for Victorian women.[47] Yet the connection between the 'unsexed' prostitute and self-mutilation reminds us that 'sexual self-mutilation' was generally viewed as a peculiarly *male* behaviour. Social histories have considered the last decades of the nineteenth century to be a time of great change – even crisis – for earlier models of masculinity, through changes in the workplace (the rise of desk and service jobs for the middle classes and the decline of manual labour) and the home (the presumption that fathers should take greater interest in their children and domestic life). Male–female marital relations became of prominent importance in this period. In psychiatry, marriage was described as productive of altruistic emotions: the bedrock of a secular society.[48] Alienists upheld the importance of marriage for maintaining mental health, and it was even suggested as a remedy for 'nervous' disorders like hysteria and hypochondriasis. When the 25-year-old teacher Alice Rose M. was admitted to Bethlem as a voluntary boarder in 1895, she had been subject to nervous symptoms for four years. Previously, Alice had consulted the eminent neurologist Victor Horsley, but refused to follow his advice of 'rest & marriage'.[49]

Relationships with the opposite sex and, in particular, the care of children were thought to be emotionally beneficial for unstable people, though not all, as George Savage put it:

The sexual function is the function which develops altruism, so without children the parents become egotistical, and egotism and insanity are not far apart.[50]

This connection of procreative marriage with healthy social relations relied on pre-existing religious models of society, as well as the suggestion of evolutionary biologists, like Darwin, that man had evolved as a 'social' animal, with sexual selection an important part of this.[51] Continental sex research fitted neatly within this commitment to altruism, emotion and social feeling as vital for civilization. Richard von Krafft-Ebing, for example, claimed sexual life was central to human existence, in his magnum opus *Psychopathia Sexualis* (1886):

Sexual life is no doubt the one mighty factor in the individual and social relations of man that discloses his powers of activity, of acquiring property, of establishing a home, and of awakening altruistic sentiments towards a person of the opposite sex, and towards his own issue as well as towards the whole human race.[52]

Many people today regard sex as an important element of a romantic relationship. However, it seems unlikely that most would assume a person was *required* to be sexually active in order to develop altruistic feeling. Yet this is just what many late Victorians claimed, a suggestion that only makes sense within the anthropological and evolutionary context of nineteenth-century thought, by which civilization was regarded as progressing from smaller to larger units. In this model, intimate personal relationships were a stepping stone towards the family, which in turn was claimed to enable an individual to appreciate a wider human sphere, from village or tribe to humanity as a whole. But what, according to Victorian doctors, would happen if this 'healthy' sexual drive were absent or altered? And how was this illustrated or explained by the concept of sexual self-mutilation?

The basis for social advancement: sexology and self-mutilation

The assumption that heterosexual relationships were vital for the progress of civilization can be prominently seen in the new field of sexual pathology that emerged at this time, particularly in Continental Europe. This would later become known as the science of sexology, a term popularized by the British writer Havelock Ellis (1859–1939), whose *Studies in the Psychology of Sex* reached seven volumes. Although Ellis was not well known in Britain in the 1890s (the first of the 'studies' was not published until 1897), there was certainly awareness among alienists of other work on sexual pathology. Thus, when James Adam referred readers on self-mutilation to examples by Krafft-Ebing and Albert Moll (1862–1939), he addressed a field that many of his contemporaries could be expected to have encountered, even if they were not actively writing in it themselves. Krafft-Ebing is today most famous for his compilation *Psychopathia Sexualis*. Through an ever-increasing collection of case studies (from 51 in the first volume to over three hundred in the twelfth edition), the German psychiatrist catalogued a variety of 'perversions' of the sexual drive. While particularly concerned with what he termed 'antipathic sexual instinct' (homosexuality), Krafft-Ebing also wrote about sexual anaesthesia and hyperaesthesia (absence of or excessive sexual desire) and fetishism (spelled 'fetichism' at the time), as well as introducing the terms 'sadism' and 'masochism'. The book was first published in German in 1886, but there were eleven revised editions over the next fifteen years, in which the content expanded enormously.[53] Before 1900, *Psychopathia Sexualis* was also translated into Russian, Italian, English, Hungarian and French.[54] Albert Moll, meanwhile, was a physician from Berlin who published *Die Konträre Sexualempfindung* (The Contrary Sexual Feeling) in 1891. This focused largely on homosexuality, differentiating (as did Krafft-Ebing) between 'innate' and 'acquired' homosexuality. In 1897, Moll's *Untersuchungen über die Libido sexualis*

(Investigations Concerning the Libido Sexualis) challenged the idea t
conception was the purpose of the sexual act: instead, he noted that it w.
merely a coincidental by-product of *some* sexual acts, for even heterosexual
vaginal intercourse did not always – or even often – result in pregnancy.[55]

Moll's works were not available in English, and *Psychopathia Sexualis* was
not translated until the seventh edition; however, this did not mean they
were inaccessible to British psychiatrists. As educated, upper-middle-class
professionals, many alienists would have been fluent in French and
German. Indeed, *Psychopathia Sexualis* was reviewed in the *Journal of
Mental Science* eighteen months before the English translation was issued.[56]
This review expressed concern at the supposedly indecent nature of Krafft-
Ebing's work. However, this did not prevent James Adam suggesting his
cases as further reading on sexual self-mutilation. How, though, did Krafft-
Ebing and his associates understand or classify self-mutilation? Today, we
might expect to find a connection with sadomasochism: indeed, certain
psychoanalysts later invoked this concept to explain self-mutilation, as
explored in Chapter Five.[57]

Sadism and masochism were introduced in the fifth German edition
of *Psychopathia Sexualis* to refer, respectively, to sexual desire associated
with violence or the infliction of pain, and that connected with submission
to another person (to the extent of humiliation or abuse). Krafft-Ebing
regarded both perversions as mostly seen in men and claimed that female
cases (particularly of masochism, which he considered 'natural' in women)
were rare. Sadism could be understood as an exaggeration of masculine
dominance, while masochism was its female counterpart – a 'pathological
growth of specific feminine mental elements' which, in men, was frequently
connected with homosexuality.[58] This final link explains why references to
masochism do *not* appear in texts on sexual self-mutilation prior to 1913,
despite being available as a possible explanation for self-inflicted injury.[59]
For late nineteenth-century psychiatrists, *homosexuality* was the primary
perversion of sexual instinct. From the second German edition onwards,
Psychopathia Sexualis contained 'especial reference to the antipathic sexual
instinct' and, by the twelfth edition, Krafft-Ebing came to conclude that

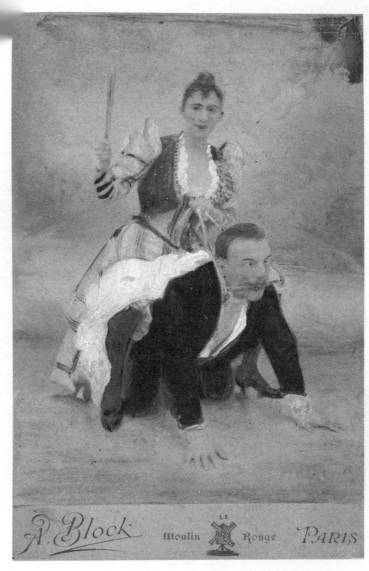

Erotic postcard from a collection owned by Richard von Krafft-Ebing, the German-Austrian forensic psychiatrist, as part of his systematic study of sexual deviation. Note that the passive partner in this scenario is male: he is being ridden and possibly caned by a dominant female. For Krafft-Ebing, this was a subversion of the natural order.

'masochism is, properly speaking, only a rudimentary form of antipathic sexual instinct.'[60]

It is thus not surprising that, as a sexual perversion, castration was most often discussed in relation to cases of homosexuality (usually known in England as 'sexual inversion'). After all, the entry in Tuke's *Dictionary* for 'sexual perversion', which also referred to sexology, dealt almost exclusively with homosexuality.[61] This brief, morally superior survey supported Havelock Ellis's later complaint that the problem with English psychiatrists was not necessarily that they considered homosexuality to be pathological, but that they refused to discuss the topic at all.[62] Certainly, although alienists sanctimoniously claimed to have little experience in the area, homosexual feelings were expressed by a number of patients in Bethlem during the 1880s and 1890s (whether as a contributing factor to their troubles or as a symptom of illness). In the majority of cases, however, the experiences and desires described by these patients were ascribed little significance, and often dismissed as delusions. Only in one instance did a patient receive a diagnosis of 'Sexual Perversion'; however, there were other occasions on which patients presented autobiographical confessions to their doctors. Masturbation continued to be of far more concern in asylums than so-called 'unnatural' sexual behaviour, for patients as well as superintendents. Thus, when the artist Henry H. claimed he should be castrated for his 'sexual perversion', it was masturbation that he meant.[63] A similar concern with masturbation appeared in the accounts of sexual behaviour sent to Krafft-Ebing, in which some patients claimed that indulgence in homosexual or masochistic practices was important to protect them from the far greater danger of masturbation. For most Victorians, a sexual encounter with another person was physically and morally superior to 'solitary sex', and it is entirely possible that their doctors, associating sex with altruism, agreed.

The young Catholic novice Theodore B., admitted in June 1893, received the only diagnosis of 'Sexual Perversion' at Bethlem.[64] On his recent return from a monastery, the young man told his father that 'a man had fallen in love with him' and further insisted that he was, in fact, a woman. His father reported that Theodore said that he had always had the feeling that he was a woman & had a woman's instincts, became excited, talked incessantly about having an amputation which w[oul]d enable him to dress & act as a woman.

This idea associated the cultural trappings of femininity with physical form (which we have already encountered in Western understandings of the *hijda*). This fitted closely within the trope of gender inversion and cross-dressing commonly associated with homosexuality in this period.[65] Theodore

prays that his external genitals may be removed & that if they are not removed he will either remove them himself or commit suicide. He says that he is pregnant & that they (external genitals) disgust him.

Like many of Krafft-Ebing's patients, Theodore insistently asserted the 'higher' nature of his feelings, telling Dr Craig that 'men love him as they do women' and stressing that no 'unnatural offences of any kind' had taken place. Craig appeared sceptical about this; nonetheless, the physician focused mainly on the patient's belief that he was a woman, rather than his sexual practices. When Theodore ceased to declare himself female, and explained the claim that he was pregnant by 'a sensitive feeling in the right side', the young man was deemed to be recovering. Although removed by his father after just four days in Bethlem, Theodore was discharged as 'relieved' – a rapid turnaround for a patient admitted under an Urgency Order.

Castration was not always seen as evidence of homosexual desires, however. It was also associated with the absence of sexual feeling, a perversion regarded as equally dangerous. One of Krafft-Ebing's earliest published cases detailed attempted self-mutilation. E., a thirty-year-old journeyman painter, was diagnosed with 'sexual anaesthesia'. Krafft-Ebing was called as a medical witness after E. was arrested

while trying to cut off the scrotum of a boy he had caught in the woods. He gave as a motive for this act that he wished to cut into it in order that the world should not multiply. Often in his youth, with like purpose, he had cut into his own genitals.[66]

Voicing the Malthusian belief that population growth would inevitably outstrip natural resources, E. acted on fears that were widespread, for he 'declared that it would be better to castrate all children than to allow others to come into the world that could only be fated to endure poverty and misery'.[67] On Krafft-Ebing's testimony, E. was judged insane and sent to an asylum rather than prison. This judgement meant that E.'s concerns about his own childhood poverty were dismissed as irrational. Instead, Krafft-Ebing's emphasis lay in an association between E.'s violent acts (to himself and others), his lack of desire for 'normal' sexual intercourse, and his personality. Given the writer's strong belief in the altruistic potential of sexual activity, it is hardly surprising that he found E. 'selfish and weak-minded' and a lover of solitude. Conclusively, Krafft-Ebing declared that 'social feelings are absolutely foreign to him.' E. certainly did possess physical feeling: Krafft-Ebing noted that his attempts at 'self-emasculation' had not been carried out because of pain. Absence of sexual feeling was not a physical phenomenon and people with sexual anaesthesia were not impotent; however 'the corresponding emotions of sexual life are absolutely wanting.'[68]

Krafft-Ebing's judgement was contrary to that voiced by E. For E., his act of violence *was* socially motivated, aiming to benefit humanity in its entirety. Rather than being pathological, his attempts at self-castration were efforts at cure, an idea also put forward in non-criminal cases.[69] In one of these, castration was carried out. A seventeen-year-old student told Krafft-Ebing that his neurasthenia (nervous exhaustion) was caused by masturbation. When hypnosis failed to help, the student said he wished to be castrated. Although the psychiatrist advised against the procedure, the patient had his testicles removed by a willing surgeon. When his symptoms continued, he visited Krafft-Ebing again, this time considering amputation of the penis. Apparently, the psychiatrist persuaded the boy against such a course, although whether this advice was ultimately taken is, of course, impossible to know.[70] What these cases *do* indicate, however, is that castration was considered – and sometimes even performed – for a variety of perceived sexual problems throughout the nineteenth century, and possibly beyond.

'Indifferent to his environment': the Skoptsy and the psychology of castration

For physicians, castration was increasingly portrayed as a dangerous and pathological act which could alter the entire character of an individual:

> The man bereft of his virility is morose and spiteful, egotistic, jealous, contrary, listless, has but little self-respect or sense of honor, and is cowardly. Analogies are seen in the Skopzens, who, after their castration, change for the worse.[71]

Generalizations of this kind related castration to a broader psychological change than that of gender inversion, claiming that anthropological investigation of the Skoptsy (Skopzens) proved this connection. This Russian religious group emerged in the late eighteenth century as one of a number of sects that broke away from the Russian Orthodox Church.[72] The Skoptsy were persecuted particularly severely following the discovery of their practice of ritual castration in 1772. The sect later became one of the most oft-cited instances of castration in Western medical literature, providing much of the material for later investigation of the physiological consequences of 'Eunuchism'.[73] Although castration was not literally self-performed, the Skoptsy's acts were usually considered within the remit of self-mutilation.[74] Thus, an article in the *Medical Press* of 1888 compared self-mutilation in Western asylums with 'religious fanaticism in Russia', even though the British cases described were of enucleation rather than castration.[75]

It was not until the late nineteenth century that the Skoptsy came to attention in western Europe, following a series of open trials. Reports showed the close relation made by Western commentators between castration and

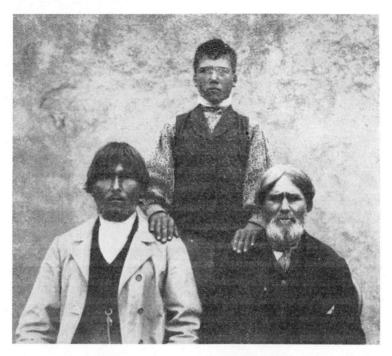

Photograph of three male Skoptsy in the early 1900s. The beards of the men seated indicate that they were castrated after puberty. Western photographs often depicted several generations of Skoptsy, drawing attention to the physical differences caused by the age at castration.

character. The trial of a wealthy gentleman named Plotitzine was reported in a number of local newspapers. Headlines made use of the rhetoric of the 'self-mutilator' as a type of person: three papers titled the story 'Russian Self-mutilators and their Treasure'.[76] This stereotype emphasized the idea that the sect were insular and money-loving. These views of the Skoptsy were based on anti-Semitic rhetoric and suggested that, having renounced human ties, the sect devoted themselves instead to the pursuit of gain. This was not by any means a foregone conclusion: after all, Krafft-Ebing had regarded the sexual instinct as a *requirement* for the drive to acquire wealth![77] It did, however, fit into Western discourses that associated the sexual instinct with altruism and love for humanity, and the reverse with a selfish way of life. In general, the Skoptsy came to be associated – socially, financially and psychologically, as well as sexually – with selfishness.

It was specifically the physical act of castration that was thought to have changed the character of the Skoptsy. This was a common assumption about eunuchism in Victorian evolutionary psychology. Darwin thought that eunuchs were inferior to other males,[78] while psychologist Henry Maudsley declared, with characteristic forthrightness, that:

> The physical degeneration of a sexual impotency is surely reflected in a corresponding moral degradation ... The perfect moral man must be of perfect physical development. Eunuchs are said to be the vilest creatures of the human race, cowards, deceitful, envious and vicious.[79]

Western descriptions of the Skoptsy invariably vilified them for their secrecy and love of gain, without wondering whether this was true or, even if it was, whether these traits had been caused by their life of exile, rather than the process of castration. The Russian writer Evgeny Pelikan

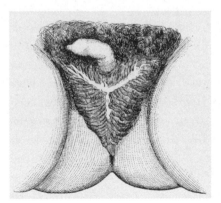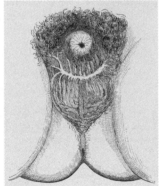

Both images here show castration of male Skoptsy: the 'minor seal' involved the removal of the testicles and scrotum, while the major, or 'royal', seal included amputation of the penis. These etchings from Evgeny Pelikan were reproduced by Gould and Pyle, who assumed the 'royal' seal showed female genitalia, indicating their belief that castration meant removal of the testes and not the penis.

was particularly influential for these portrayals of the Skoptsy in the West. Pelikan (1824–1884) was a professor of forensic medicine in St Petersburg, and his use of case studies emerged from this medico-legal context. Many Skoptsy claimed at trial that they had been castrated 'accidentally', and so Pelikan's writings focused on medical evidence to contradict this, as well as other ways of physically identifying Skoptsy, whether castrated before or after puberty.[80] The two forms of castration practised were detailed in his work. The 'minor seal' involved removal of the testicles and scrotum, while the major, or 'royal', seal included amputation of the penis. Female Skoptsy also underwent a physical indoctrination: the breasts were scarred, and sometimes removed, as was the labia and, occasionally, the clitoris.[81] Interest in the physical appearance of the Skoptsy was a major feature of attention in western Europe. At the Anthropological Society, Barnard Davis showed an anatomical preparation 'which exhibits the radical excision of the sexual organs of a male Scoptsi' in conjunction with 'photographs . . . of rich individual Scoptsis at Bucharest'.[82] These pictures were thought to show the ways in which castration altered character. Thus, Davis noted the 'peculiar mildness and want of force in their countenances'.

This emphasis on physical and behavioural change through mutilation tended to concentrate on the male Skoptsy. Although trial records revealed that many women were mutilated as well as men, and the two sexes were generally treated similarly in Russian legal proceedings, it was the castration of the male Skoptsy that formed the sole topic of discussion in the West.[83] This was very similar to the way in which accounts of sexual self-mutilation were treated in asylums. There were just as many instances of female genital self-injury as male in Bethlem during the last two decades of the nineteenth century, yet the only published article that referenced sexual mutilation in women declared it was unusual.[84] Similarly, it was masculine assumption that led psychiatrists to conclude that 'modesty and custom naturally constitute, in women, insurmountable obstacles to the expression of perverse sexual instinct.'[85] However, in line with such assumptions, the concept of sexual self-mutilation spoke to Western doctors about the role of sexuality in the formation of masculinity and associated concerns with the regulation of male sexual desire. Victorian men were more closely associated with their sex drive than women, and thus the social consequences of the *loss* of sexual function were deemed far greater in men than in women.[86] Indeed, the element of Pelikan's text that particularly resonated with Western commentators was his suggestion that the loss of sexual ability in the Skoptsy might be a source of social danger, for the regulation of sexual desire also controlled other elements of male behaviour:

> Once he becomes sexually active, the normal man starts to find the opposite sex attractive: the first instinctive call of love also inspires him with the urge to noble action and great deeds and with devotion to the fatherland. The young man castrated before puberty knows none of this: he remains indifferent to his environment, lacking the smallest germ of noble aspiration, sense of duty, or civic obligation.[87]

Thus, in western Europe, it was not the religious rituals of the Skoptsy that commentators reflected on, but instead the threat they appeared to pose to society. Interestingly, the Skoptsy ritual was never a solitary one: like the medieval flagellants, the group rite of castration drew the community together.[88] Yet James Adam declared that 'fanatics' were dangerous in having 'withdrawn from the society of man', while fellow alienist Charles Mercier claimed that an 'orphan celibate' could not experience the 'social emotions' of ethical and patriotic duty.[89] This description indicates once again why the character of the Skoptsy was frequently associated with the physical act of castration. Even when 'eunuchism' became reclassified as an 'endocrine disease' in the twentieth century, the associated psychological profile continued to emphasize traits like withdrawal and egotism: a 'tendency to introversion with infantilistic traits and abnormalities of behaviour of "limelight" nature due to over-compensation of inferiority complex'.[90] Although this psychoanalytic language would have been foreign to nineteenth-century psychiatrists, the underlying message was very similar: eunuchs failed to develop the altruism associated with the growth of normal sexual function during puberty. From this perspective, the castrated man could not fail to be selfish, turning castration itself into an egotistical act.

In this chapter I have drawn together examples of self-castration and other forms of ritual mutilation. However, it should certainly not be assumed that castration was widespread in late nineteenth-century Europe. Instead, I have sought to account for the much higher level of *discussion* about castration – particularly self-performed – relative to the rate at which it was actually carried out. In the first place, I explored the importance of case studies, within and outside the asylum, in creating a concept of 'sexual self-mutilation'. The existence of cases of genital self-injury does not, however, indicate why castration was emphasized over other forms of self-mutilation, or why it acquired associations with a selfish, passive and introverted character. Neither can this be explained by the assumption that castration is 'necessarily' about loss of masculinity. Indeed, the Victorian concern over masturbation challenges this notion, for castration – even where self-performed – could certainly be regarded as preferable to the slow death or decline into insanity often attributed to masturbation. Some physicians do appear to have suggested – and even carried out – this radical cure, along with the lesser surgery of circumcision. Within psychiatry, however, there was a greater emphasis on the psychological and sociological origin of mental illness – particularly among those alienists most interested in self-mutilation. This perspective meant that physical therapies – such as castration and other forms of sexual surgery – no longer seemed appropriate. Sexuality began to be considered a mental state, and thus more deeply embedded in the individual character than could be altered by surgical intervention. From this, it fell that self-castration was pathological in and of itself.

Yet, in order to understand how the character of the eunuch could arouse such censure, the broader context of socio-evolutionary approaches to civilization needs to be taken into account. Like other male 'disorders' – including hypochondriasis, masturbation and homosexuality – castration in the late nineteenth century was claimed to alter the character of the individual, encouraging a selfish self-obsession. These concerns were strongly rooted in contemporary ideals of masculinity, of which self-control was an essential element. In the later nineteenth century, the acquisition of this control was connected with sexual health. As the man developed sexually so, it was assumed, did he develop socially, so that the 'natural' selfishness of the male sex would blossom into altruism. Self-castration, in this context, was presented as the ultimate act of selfish preoccupation: a refusal to perform a useful social function. Anthropological and sexological examples appeared to support this contention, offering evidence that castration altered behaviour, leaving the eunuch passive, inert, disinterested in society and focused on personal gain: an individualist view that failed to take into account the social context of the castrated man. Castration was also assumed to be *about* sex, unlike some of the classical examples in Chapter One. When a mass trial of Skoptsy was carried out at Kharkov in 1910, physicians described it as 'mass sexual psychosis'.[91]

Many of the Skoptsy could not understand why they were shunned by broader society. Nikifor Petrovich Latyshev (1863–*c*. 1939), a self-appointed chronicler of the sect, speculated in his later life on the cause of hostility towards the Skoptsy:

> Judging by my life, my proper life, I'm a great guy! My exemplary decent behaviour admits me everywhere. What qualities are missing for me to be accepted as human. Better be a drunk, a hooligan, roué, drifter, loafer or malingerer – but not castrated! Nothing is more shameful among humankind. I've felt this on my own hide for 75 years.[92]

That castration has not always been believed to make a man less than human – or even less masculine – indicates that the topic of sexual self-mutilation in late nineteenth-century England was related to concerns in a large number of other fields: psychiatric, psychological, anthropological and sexological. Although this model of self-mutilation may seem bizarre today, 'sexual self-mutilation' certainly has a legacy. Consider, for example, the ongoing characterization of self-harm as a feminine trait (and of men who injure themselves as effeminate), which will be explored at greater length in the next chapter. Gender identity disorder was recently amended to gender dysphoria in the *DSM-5*; however, definitions through much of the twentieth century assumed 'sexual perversion' was associated with any desire to physically change the sex assigned at birth.[93] Our sex need not necessarily be related to our sexuality, although this is often taken as a given today. The description of sexual self-mutilation in the late nineteenth century was part of a growing interest in defining the physical and psychological character of an individual by his or her sexual preferences, a process that remains widespread in the Western world today.

FOUR

MOTIVELESS MALINGERERS
Multiple Personality, Attention-seeking and Hysteria around 1900

In the summer of 1875, Mrs Helen Miller, a thirty-year-old 'intelligent German Jewess', was transferred from Sing Sing prison to the New York State Asylum for Insane Criminals after she, in her own words, 'began to "cut up"'. Mrs Miller had been sentenced to five years in prison for grand larceny, just a few months after she was last discharged from the asylum. According to the physician's report, the patient's actions were due to her being 'anxious to be transferred to the Asylum'; however, once admitted, she continued to injure herself over the next few years, usually by cutting her arms with pieces of glass. Helen Miller's behaviour was considered unusual, not least due to her chosen method of self-injury. As her physician, Walter Channing, noted, self-cutting was rarely described in articles in British or American journals; instead burning, scalding, hair-plucking and castration were 'the favorite methods'. So what was the explanation for Helen's strange behaviour? The patient's age, her sex, her frequent episodes of unexplained medical symptoms (including choking and painful menstruation) and a past indicative of kleptomania all suggested a diagnosis of hysteria. Helen's acts were not suicidal, her doctor declared; instead, they were acts of 'simulation' – intended, it was thought, to attract attention.[1]

An oft-cited modern cliché of self-harm is the assumption that the practice is manipulative of others. In particular, this view has been associated with a diagnosis of borderline personality disorder, one symptom of which is self-inflicted injury. Those labelled with this diagnosis may find it hard to access treatment, with their behaviour stigmatized as inherently selfish, encapsulated in the negative concept of 'attention-seeking'. While some claim that this view has altered in recent years, others refute this suggestion.[2] But how did the idea that inflicting damage on one's own body is manipulative of others first occur? It is not a foregone conclusion that injuring oneself will have an effect on anyone else. Although some of the nineteenth-century literature on self-mutilation, outlined in Chapter Two, did assume that these behaviours had selfish motives, much did not; this was still less the case in the prehistory of self-harm. The connection between self-inflicted injury and manipulative behaviour was constructed within late nineteenth-century psychiatry, entangled in a variety of other social and political concerns. At the turn of the twentieth century it gained many associations that have remained a part of later models of self-harm; most of these were transferred from the diagnosis of hysteria.

In this chapter I begin by outlining the ways in which self-mutilation first became associated with hysteria. What did hysteria mean to Victorian and Edwardian doctors and their patients? I go on to show how the notion of hysterical self-injury emerged from attention to the 'fasting girls' of the mid-Victorian period, when abstinence, lesions – such as religious stigmata – and associated mental states were increasingly explained in physiological and behavioural, rather than spiritual, terms. There was no obvious connection between these cases and the disparate accounts of self-injury related in this chapter, other than that made by the medical profession at the time: the paradigm of hysteria. In particular, I look at the 'needle girls' of the late nineteenth century, and the way their actions were framed as 'motiveless malingering'. This phrase indicates the wider context around self-injury, which developed further in the early twentieth century, particularly in relation to so-called *dermatitis artefacta*. While the concept of 'needle girls' was primarily based on assumptions about gendered attributes, 'hysterical malingering' had broader economic and political associations, related to the supposed spread of malingering. This concept – of feigned or self-inflicted illness in order to avoid work or duty – had long been a military concern, but was increasingly applied to civilian populations around the turn of the twentieth century, usually men. Female 'self-mutilators' were differentiated from their male counterparts through the assumption that their acts were 'motiveless' or 'unconscious'. Their behaviour was judged as proof that women were 'naturally' manipulative, indicating that approaches to self-injury are of broad social, economic and political relevance.

Self-mutilation and hysteria: from bodily to mental symptoms

The concept of hysteria has a lengthy history, which can be dated back to some of the oldest surviving documents in medical history, from around 1900 BCE.[3] Yet the notion of hysteria as a constant disease entity is problematic, for, throughout the centuries, models of illness and the symptoms presented by patients have altered significantly. Indeed, the very *term* hysteria may be questionable. The use of the word in ancient texts was often added in nineteenth-century translations, reflecting the keen interest in both hysteria and retrospective diagnosis in this period.[4] In ancient Greek medicine, there *was* no clearly defined concept of hysteria, although later writers assumed that the Greek term had long been applied to a disorder thought to reside within the female reproductive anatomy (the so-called 'wandering womb'). By the seventeenth century, however, doctors regarded hysteria as a distinct disease entity, and began to explore a neurological framework for it, seeing it as the female counterpart to male hypochondriasis. Hysteria, like hypochondriasis, became a 'neurosis': a disease of the nerves, rather than the womb (hypochondriasis was similarly named after the region of the body in which it was supposed to originate – the digestive regions, or hypochondrium).[5] This did not mean that hysteria was thought to be psychological, and its symptoms psychosomatic: for a long while, neuroses were considered physiological disorders, caused by lesions in the nervous system. By the nineteenth century, this 'nervous' model was well established, and hysteria was regarded by many as a distinct and unchanging disease. Nonetheless, the medical concept of hysteria remained extremely broad: general practitioners, alienists, neurologists and surgeons were all involved in the treatment of hysterical patients, whose symptoms might vary from mild malaise or weakness to complaints of paralysis or cutaneous anaesthesia and the grand fits made famous by Jean-Martin Charcot at the Salpêtrière Hospital in late nineteenth-century Paris. In practice, hysteria was often used as a way of explaining any phenomenon that did not fit neatly within an organic model of disease, and competing models of the disorder were often used in combination, so that late nineteenth-century practitioners might suggest a mixture of neurological, behavioural and psychological interpretations of their patients' symptoms.

In Helen Miller's case, it was almost immediately decided that her efforts at self-mutilation were a hysterical symptom. Indeed, as with many cases of hysteria in the late nineteenth century, her doctors reported the details that confirmed this diagnosis, while ignoring those that didn't. Marriage, for example, was often suggested as a *cure* for hysteria but Helen's husband was never mentioned. Instead, Dr Channing wrote to

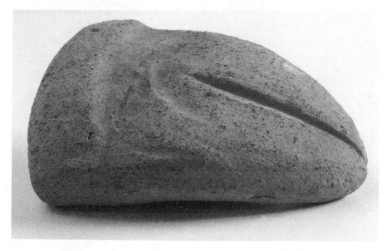

Roman votive offering in the shape of a vulva. These clay-baked body parts were offered to the gods to request a cure for a disease or other ailment afflicting that part of the body.

Helen's previous physicians for evidence of her mental state. An unnamed New York doctor provided a detailed account of his own encounters with the patient, from the first time he had treated Mrs Miller seven years previously. She had sought his assistance for painful menstruation as well as to help 'break her of the opium habit'. Surprisingly, Helen's addiction to opium was also barely mentioned – perhaps because her physicians concluded that, despite this, she had not led 'a fast life'. Opium was widely available at this time, and addiction was less commonly associated with hysteria than another trait, on which Helen's background history focused: a compulsion to steal.

Kleptomania, the morbid propensity towards theft (often of useless items), was first named and described by the French physician Charles Marc in 1840.[6] Although the existence of monomania (a disorder focused around one specific symptom) was questioned by the late nineteenth century, the existence of a morbid desire to steal was nonetheless regarded as a disease of modern life. In J. Baker's entry in the *Dictionary of Psychological Medicine*, the alienist associated kleptomania with normal psychology: 'A desire to acquire is natural to everyone. This feeling in persons of well-regulated minds and honest conceptions is kept under the control of the will.'[7] Theft, however, was either a sign of dishonesty or a neurotic condition (the inability to resist the urge to steal). Some suggested that environmental factors also applied. The tendency of department stores to display clothes on open shelves exacerbated 'a not unnatural tendency to steal articles of clothing . . . Perhaps the openness of many of the Stores is a temptation too great to be resisted.'[8] Helen Miller was arrested a number of times for stealing from various doctors, and 'her last trial was for stealing a stuffed canary and a microscope lens.' As she stole items of little or no purpose or value, neurosis was considered a more likely explanation than dishonesty in her case. Despite viewing her guilt in the last crime as unproven, her doctor nonetheless confirmed that 'I believe her to be a kleptomaniac, if one ever existed, and probably her rooms are filled with things taken from doctor's offices.'[9] It was also claimed that these 'thieving propensities' were shown during Helen's time in hospital. She would pick

Cartoon from *Punch* (1861) spoofing the idea of medical diagnosis of kleptomania. Note that the thief is male, lampooning the application of the kleptomania diagnosis to theft by middle-class women.

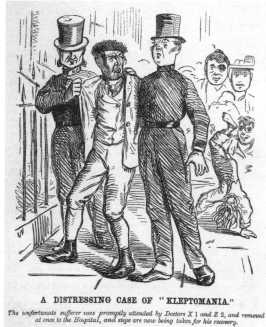

A DISTRESSING CASE OF "KLEPTOMANIA."

The unfortunate sufferer was promptly attended by Doctors X 1 and Z 2, and removed at once to the Hospital, and steps are now being taken for his recovery.

up any useless item she saw and insist, if challenged, that the object belonged to her.

Other symptoms associated with hysteria were the physical symptoms of other illnesses: hysteria was a 'protean disease' that could mimic almost any other condition.[10] It was only a failure to find a bodily cause for an ailment (or the presence of a pre-existing 'nervous' condition) that meant a diagnosis of hysteria was assumed. Victorian hysteria has thus been compared to modern 'psychosomatic' conditions, such as chronic fatigue syndrome or irritable bowel syndrome.[11] However, to make these comparisons runs the risk of missing the things that were distinctly Victorian about the associations between hysteria and self-inflicted injury. In Helen's case, this was shown in the way her symptoms were considered, at one and the same time, as marks of genuine physical illness *and* efforts to manipulate others. For the past two years, it was recorded, she has been very hysterical, having frequent attacks of choking, globus hystericus, and imagined at one time that she had a spool in her throat, and could only swallow through the hole in the middle.

Although these symptoms might have seemed outside the patient's control, manipulation was nonetheless hinted at by Helen's treatment. When she refused food for several days on account of her symptoms, 'no attention was paid to her, and she recovered.'[12]

Receiving the attention of others was widely considered to be the main aim of the hysterical patient. Helen visited countless doctors, and reportedly 'took a special pride in having the attention of the physicians directed towards her'. In the asylum, this affected her behaviour, so that, when she felt herself 'an object of surgical interest', Helen worked hard on the wards, was 'tranquil and rational', intelligent and cheerful. Despite this shift in her behaviour, the doctors don't seem to have made any particular effort to determine *why* Mrs Miller might desire medical attention – or, indeed, any attention whatever. Her past life and case history were considered of far less relevance than her 'hysterical' propensities, and self-mutilation was seen as the strongest evidence of her state:

> In the present case the hysterical element was always present. The wounds were made as lacerated as possible, the garments were covered unnecessarily with blood, and a time of day chosen when help was sure to be at hand. Everything was done to produce as much effect as possible. Though the muscles were sometimes hacked to the bone, an artery sufficiently large to require ligation was never injured.[13]

Although Helen Miller was not known to have had any specific anatomical knowledge, the assumption was made that she somehow knew how to avoid harming herself significantly, a conclusion that highlighted the 'manipulative' nature of her wounds. While hysteria was still conceptualized as a disease at this time, it was simultaneously viewed as a type of character or personality with manipulative and deceitful tendencies. Helen Miller's actions were interpreted through this framework, leading to a direct association between self-harm and deceit. Similar connections were made in other cases of self-harm linked to hysteria, particularly in the so-called motiveless malingering of needle girls.

Needle girls: the foreign body and the motiveless malingerer

In December 1850, Dr Budd reported the supposedly typical case of a hysterical young woman in *The Lancet*. Budd's patient was 36 years old – a little older than the standard hysteric – but nonetheless unmarried. Adverse life experiences – the death of her father alongside 'certain ill treatment which she met with' (probably a euphemism for sexual or other abuse) – had, a few years earlier, caused an outbreak of insanity. However, the patient had recovered, and had been looked after for five years by some 'kind-hearted ladies'. This was viewed as a sign of her hysterical tendencies (rather than the genuine kindness of others), for 'hysterical patients are extremely fond of attracting attention and sympathy.'[14] When admitted to King's College Hospital, Budd's patient was suffering from severe stomach pains and fits of vomiting. However, Dr Budd quickly found the cause, when he examined the outside of the stomach and felt 'hard and resisting bodies' below and 'little white scars . . . scattered about' on the surface of the skin. Over the next ten days, about fifty needles were removed from the patient's abdomen. She claimed (after 'much persuasion, and even threatening') that she had thrust all the needles into her skin during the 'fit of insanity' five years before. Budd refused to credit this story, as the needles appeared to have been thrust in at different times. The entire case was published under the title 'The Mania of Thrusting Needles into the Flesh'. This cast the topic as a 'monomania', in the same field as kleptomania. Could such acts, the article enquired, be committed 'under the mere influence of hysteria', or must outright insanity play a role? Over the next four decades, doctors and surgeons increasingly came to favour the former explanation and, in 1897, two American doctors coined a name for this phenomenon: 'needle girls'.

These doctors, Gould and Pyle, retrospectively applied the name 'needle girls' to a collection of cases published over the preceding fifty years. This name was presumably coined by the authors to play on widespread interest in the aforementioned 'fasting girls' (on whom they also included a section). The notion of hysterical self-injury thus appears to have emerged from attention to the fasting girls of the mid-Victorian period, including the well-publicized Welsh Fasting Girl, Sarah Jacob. In cases of purportedly mystical abstinence, lesions (such as religious stigmata) and euphoric mental states, symptoms were increasingly explained in physiological and behavioural, rather than spiritual, terms in this era. These often contradictory explanations stemmed from a prior understanding that such cases must (and therefore could) be explained as 'natural'.

Needle girls, Gould and Pyle stated, carried out a 'peculiar type of self-mutilation . . . sometimes seen in hysteric persons' of 'piercing their flesh with numerous needles or pins'.[15] The descriptions cited focused on the work of the surgical detective, rather than the patient, and any motives underlying self-inflicted injury were subsumed under the broad banner of hysteria, in itself regarded as sufficient explanation. In 1862, for example, Ernest Hart, surgeon to the West London Hospital, reported a case under the telling title 'Hysteria: Wilful Self-infliction of Injury'. Hart described a 'young girl of good appearance and superior education' who entered the hospital with an abscess of the forefinger. The surgeon removed several pieces of needle and, although 'no suspicion was then excited as to her peculiar habit . . . there is little doubt that the needles were wilfully introduced and broken into the flesh'. The end of the finger was eventually amputated; however, the patient continued to return regularly to the hospital, presenting damage to the stump. As evidence of her fickle, manipulative nature, Hart complained that: 'At the same time she managed to have several of her teeth extracted, and was taking medicine as a physician's out-patient.' Although his patient 'energetically' denied producing the symptoms herself, Hart was convinced of it, and solved the problem by *sealing* the bandages.[16]

In Hart's analysis, as in other 'needle girl' reports, the patient was clearly presented as controlling her situation. Even when she could be regarded as the passive recipient of damage inflicted by another – as in the surgical extraction of her teeth – Hart described her as the active subject, 'managing' the situation, until she was eventually outwitted by the surgeon's ingenious technical ability and forced to submit to medical cure. Other surgeons described patients as 'highly neurotic, sly, and deceitful',[17] and some concluded that any such case was evidence of 'hysterical deception',[18] making self-inflicted injury synonymous with deceit. This approach stemmed from the Victorian concept of the hysterical temperament, defined by such negative character traits.[19] Ultimately, it was the ingenious nature of the protective surgical treatment – or the skill in removing foreign bodies – that was of more interest than the patient herself.

It is noticeable, however, that such 'hysterical' patients did not always – or even often – come into contact with alienists or asylums. Indeed, while self-inflicted injury was sometimes considered a sign of unstable mental condition, even this might be re-evaluated over time. Between 1898 and 1909, Beatrice A. was admitted to the Royal London Hospital on four occasions, having inserted hairpins into her bladder. On her first admission, then aged 24, it was noted that the patient 'has had foreign bodies removed thrice before'.[20] Initially a waitress and later a milliner by trade, Beatrice appears to have been fairly well educated: her letters, it was claimed, are 'very skilfully done'.[21] In 1898, however, the motive for the patient's injury was regarded as obvious. Beatrice was as 'mad as a hatter (Sister Mary says so)'![22] This 'diagnosis' was presumably made on the basis that she openly admitted intentionally inserting a curling pin and doubled-up hairpin into her bladder. Nonetheless, Beatrice was discharged cured, without being referred to a hospital physician (as was the usual case with hysteria) *or* an asylum, and, when she was readmitted in 1906, absolutely no reference was made to her mental state. Again, the hairpin was extracted and she was discharged: the rapid solution of a surgical puzzle. The same emphasis on human biology rather than psychology can be seen in museum specimens from the same period, collected to show the way a foreign body has been transformed by its journey through the human body, rather than the reasons for its insertion.

In 1909, Beatrice's case was described more extensively. Hinting in moralistic tones at deceit, since no symptoms of insanity were observed, it was noted that 'this patient writes letters describing her case & purposely to be seen by a medical man. Once admitted & the hair pin is removed she will make full confession & solemn promises not to do it again.' Since it had already been stated that Beatrice returned repeatedly, this note suggested the patient to be deceitful. Yet the description did not end here, for Beatrice was candid now that she was being asked about her behaviour. She informed the surgeons:

> That she formerly suffered from an impulse to throw herself out
> [of] windows & once did it. Many years ago however she gave this
> up for the now harmless amusement of putting hairpins into her
> bladder. She was quite willing to discuss her mental state, says she
> has no other peculiarities and that the introduction of the hairpin
> has no relation to sexual feelings.[23]

Her unusual explanation appears to have perturbed Beatrice A.'s surgeons, located, as it was, somewhere between the rational and the irrational.

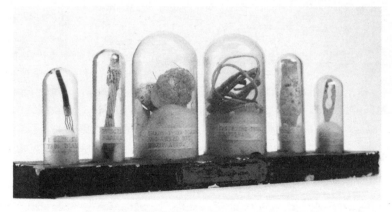

Foreign bodies removed from the bladder, kept in the UCL Pathology Collections. Most pathology collections contain such items, of interest to medical science not for what they are but the journey they have taken through the human body.

Inserting hairpins did indeed seem less dangerous than falling from a height, but why might she need to do *either*? The next time Beatrice appeared in the receiving room (about a month later), she was told she would not be admitted, and an offer was made, seemingly punitively, to remove the pin immediately, but without anaesthetic. The patient refused and was sent away, lost to the medical record.

It is impossible to draw any conclusions as to the life experiences or state of mind that might have lain behind Beatrice A.'s admittedly peculiar 'harmless amusement'. What we *can* state, however, is that this record serves as a rare occurrence of surgical interest in the reasons behind self-inflicted injury. By the 1930s, the influence of psychoanalysis had led surgeons to suggest that exploring foreign bodies offered 'a wide field for the study of human nature'.[24] In 1909, however, the association of Beatrice's mental state with complaints about her failure to keep her word suggests that interest in her psychology was bound up in notions that the behaviour of the female (hysterical) patient was rooted in a 'peculiar perversion of mind', for 'we know that hysterical women cheat in all manner of ways'.[25] These concerns coloured much of the debate around hysterical mutilation, and were further complicated by the difficulty of drawing a line between hysteria and feigned illness. Even in psychological texts, the assumption was that 'hysterical individuals not uncommonly inflict injuries upon themselves, probably from a desire to obtain the sympathy of others.'[26]

The hysterical self-mutilator, then, tended to be described as a 'motiveless malingerer'. Malingering was increasingly a topic of medical and social interest at this time. The last few decades of the nineteenth century saw a rapidly increasing concern with the concept of malingering, as well as use of the term itself. In three key medical journals (*Journal of Mental Science, British Medical Journal* and *The Lancet*), the number of articles containing the term soared from less than thirty in 1851 to nearly three hundred in the first decade of the twentieth century. Similar increase in use occurred in textbooks and newspapers. Malingering had initially been described as a military phenomenon. However, it was the application of the concept to civilian populations that accounted for a large proportion of the increased use. This concern over civilian malingering has been explained by the rise of health insurance systems across Europe: the introduction of accident insurance in Germany in 1871 and the Employers' Liability Act of 1880 and subsequent Workmen's Compensation Acts in the United Kingdom.[27] These worker insurance schemes represented a broad shift in understandings of responsibility, from a model of obligation (in which responsibility for accident and compensation lay with the employer, unless employee negligence could be proved) to one of collective responsibility. In the latter model, insurers measured the statistical probability of an accident occurring against its severity to determine both the cost of insurance and any payout. The method seemed to be free of judgement or blame. However, the expense of such a system, and the means of assessing the worker's right to a claim, made the issue of malingering class-oriented from the outset. The malingerer was invariably the worker, not the employer, and he (and not his employer) would be the person accused of attempting to cheat the system.

While later writers, such as the outspoken Sir John Collie (1860–1935), made much of the financial impact of malingering, the topic continued to be framed morally in medical circles, particularly in relation to hysteria. In 1870, inspired by the death of the Welsh Fasting Girl the previous year, the *British Medical Journal* (*BMJ*) published a series of articles by practitioners on the topic of feigned disease and malingering. Interestingly, these articles pre-dated the economic legislation outlined above.[28] The majority of writers in the 1870s regarded 'motiveless malingering' (as the *BMJ* termed it) as an entirely new topic of medical inquiry. The very terminology used here indicates an important element of the debate. Motiveless malingerers were to be distinguished from those in whom the reason for self-inflicted injury was thought obvious: evasion of duty, or financial gain. By analogy, however, the assumption was made that the hysterical patient *must* have an underlying motive. The term 'motiveless malingering' was adopted for distinction's sake, while

by no means intending to imply that the will ever really acts without motive, but merely that in these cases the motive cannot be quoted

This First World War cartoon by John Hassall appeared in a British pamphlet. It illustrates a mocking suggestion that 'the only persons who are making a respectable income in London now are the bone-breakers', who help young men to avoid military service. The pamphlet was a pastiche, but the joke could not work without widespread awareness of a concept of malingering in this period.

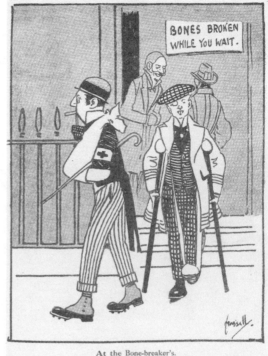

At the Bone-breaker's.

beforehand as explaining the act, but has to be sought after the fact has been established by other means.[29]

Uncovering this motive, however, was a more complicated task than physical treatment of the wounds:

> Motiveless malingerers ... are almost invariably of the class of those known as 'hysterical'. In other words, they are of the female sex, arrived at the age of puberty and unmarried. Hysterical in any more definite sense they seldom are; on the contrary, those guilty of these tricks have often been previously considered by their friends to be of remarkably calm and well-balanced temperament.[30]

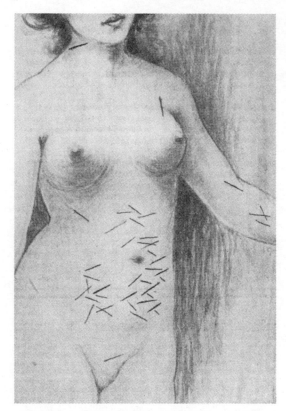

This illustration was reproduced in an article by Alexander Nicoll, to indicate the locations from which he removed needles from his female patient. Illustrations such as this emphasised a focus on the body of the patient rather than the mental state.

The absence of nervous symptoms or a disposition to deceit caused problems for the physician in detecting this type of malingering. Unlike the male malingerer, who might give himself away with his suspicious manner or guilty expression, the only way of uncovering the hysterical malingerer was often in the wounds themselves: hence images focused on the objects removed, rather than the patient. However, the context of malingering led many surgeons to ignore the issue of causation entirely. Even the writer of the article on 'motiveless malingerers' did not, it seems, expect to find the answer as to why patients 'assume their maladies without any ostensible object in sight, and often to the destruction, apparently, of their social happiness'.

In retrospect, we might well find the absence of much interest in *why* patients presented with swallowed or otherwise inserted foreign bodies surprising, particularly given the keen attention to the relation of mind and body within purported religious phenomena. Yet, although attention to fasting girls and stigmata appears to have encouraged speculation about needle girls, the latter cases were generally presented in a purely surgical context. For the surgeon, dealing with the immediate bodily problem was the concern, after which a patient could be discharged as cured. The separation between medical and surgical cases in the Royal London Hospital exacerbated this divide; it was relatively rare for patients to pass from surgeon to physician and vice versa. For many surgeons, claims that their patients were hysterical seem to have been used simply to explain any difficulty in curing the immediate problem. Nonetheless, there are some hints at a wider puzzle in some of the cases discussed. The example of Beatrice A., at the turn of the twentieth century, indicates a growing belief that the question 'why?' could not necessarily be answered by the patient. For certain physicians and alienists, if not necessarily surgeons, the concept of the unconscious became an increasingly popular explanation of this problem. This is most apparent in the treatment of so-called *dermatitis artefacta*: skin lesions produced artificially by the patient.

The psyche on the skin: from motiveless to unconscious malingering

Of the papers on 'motiveless malingering' published in the *BMJ* in 1870, three dealt with 'feigned or hysterical diseases of the skin'.[31] Similar examples appeared in dermatology textbooks and, at the end of the century, this form of self-injury was the only one to receive a dedicated entry in Clifford Allbutt's *System of Medicine*.[32] Some physicians claimed that such cases 'were nearly always of the nature of mechanical or chemical irritation of the skin', although others thought lesions might appear spontaneously due to mental distress: the effect of a peculiarly delicate state of both skin and imagination in neurotics.[33] In the 1930s, after four decades of studying the topic, London dermatologist Henry MacCormac suggested that 'autophytic dermatitis' (commonly called *dermatitis artefacta* or *dermatitis factitia*) was 'by no means a modern phenomenon', although 'the strain and increasing effort which characterize present conditions have very clearly increased its incidence.'[34] This connection between self-injury and the stresses of modern life arose repeatedly through the twentieth century: during MacCormac's early career, modernity was also viewed as the cause of specific nervous diseases, like neurasthenia.[35] MacCormac divided his patients into four groups, primarily by what he saw as their motive for self-injury: hysterical, malingering, mischief (predominantly attributed to children) and 'phantom dermatoses' (a patient's belief that a complaint was more extensive than the doctor perceived it to be). He spent far longer exploring the first class than the other three, of which, he claimed, investigation was relatively easy. 'Hysterics' were a far more complicated issue:

Recognition and disclosure of the true state of affairs, far from bringing the matter to an end, in most cases only raises new and perplexing problems . . . for these eruptive processes are not skin diseases as ordinarily understood, except in the malingering class, but rather a reflection upon the skin of a disordered condition of the mind.[36]

While interest in the physical nature of self-inflicted wounds certainly continued, two important (and interconnected) ideas associated with self-inflicted injury emerged in Britain in this era. First was the suggestion that self-mutilation might be performed 'unconsciously', so that the patient himself was not actually aware that he had done it. These notions were firmly rooted in new psychological explanations for behaviour that attributed an important role to mental stimuli and contexts of which the patient was unaware. Today, this is most frequently attributed to Freudian psychoanalysis; however, it was through the psychotherapeutic approach of Pierre Janet (1859–1947) that unconscious states were connected to self-inflicted injury by French and British practitioners. Malingering, it was increasingly assumed, was conscious simulation of illness, while self-mutilation in hysteria was its counterpart in the 'unconscious'. These concerns later became bound up in discussion of war neuroses during the First World War, although much of the interest in the unconscious certainly pre-dated wartime psychiatry and psychology. There was also a second, closely related, implication of Janet's model of psychasthenia (obsessional behaviour) in hysterical self-injury: the idea of double personality.

Janet was a pupil of the neurologist Jean-Martin Charcot (1825–1893), who had famously experimented on hysterical patients at the Salpêtrière Hospital in Paris. He classified a number of 'stages' of hysteria, many of which he produced artificially through hypnosis: according to Charcot, only hysterics could be hypnotized. Charcot himself does not appear to have had any particular interest in self-injury, and the topic was absent from his clinical lectures. Like the British surgeons referred to earlier, the French neurologist instead emphasized the simulation and 'desire to deceive' in hysterical cases, and it is probable that he saw self-mutilation as evidence of this trait.[37] Janet certainly regarded himself as departing from the thoughts of his teacher who, he felt, had laid far too much emphasis on the role of anaesthesia in hysteria. Anaesthesia, Janet declared, was not causational but only held diagnostic relevance, a shift in view that was important for regarding self-inflicted injury as holding greater meaning than merely a response to a lack of physical sensation, as other neurologists had thought (described in Chapter Two).[38] One of Janet's aims through his career was to bring together the natural sciences with philosophy, psychology and spiritualism.[39] Self-mutilation seemed to sit on this boundary, somewhere between natural and pathological process and psychological motivation. In 'On the Pathogenesis of Some Impulsions', Janet recorded his observations of patients who exhibited 'certain useless, bizarre and even dangerous acts' (including self-mutilation) which they found extremely difficult to resist. Rather than a physical basis for self-injurious acts, Janet's explanations focused on mental phenomena – what's more, those that were outside the individual's conscious control.[40]

In his early works, Janet described two cases of self-inflicted injury as 'tics'. In 1898, for example, he reported the case of a ten-year-old girl who was dominated by an *idée fixe*, under which she tore at her skin, despite showing every sign of intelligence and possessing a normal degree of cutaneous sensation.[41] Five years later, he connected such tics with psychasthenia, through the case of a young girl who pulled out her hair to such an extent that she was required to wear a wig.[42] The attribution of psychasthenia suggested that it was a pre-existing state of nervous malaise that prevented patients from resisting their impulses to self-injury. By 1906, self-mutilation achieved greater prominence in Janet's framework. The above examples are simply two among hundreds of case studies of psychasthenic symptoms. In 1906, however, he described at length a young 'girl' of twenty, Ne., who

> cannot stop herself from burning her hands and feet; her pleasure, when she is alone, consists in taking a kettle of boiling water, and pouring it, drop by drop, on the skin of her extremities.

The gratification of impulse produced pleasure for the patient, even when it also caused pain, rejecting a simplistic physical model of self-inflicted injury. This Janet made explicit by directly refuting the explanation he thought likely to be made by his contemporaries:

> We have here, you will say, an insane person who has a mystical delirium and who is anaesthetic. By no means; she is a young girl, intelligent and instructed, who is not at all delirious, at least when she is being examined, and who has preserved all her sensibilities.[43]

Ne., then, could not be regarded as insane – or even necessarily hysterical – and the physical symptoms of hysteria (including cutaneous anaesthesia) were not the explanation of her injuries.

Janet regarded the physical pain felt by his patient as a secondary result of her injuries: the gratification of impulse was the main reason for Ne.'s self-mutilation. But from whence did the impulse spring? The French doctor associated various forms of obsession – with food, walking, alcohol and self-mutilation – with mental depression. This, he claimed, produced a feeling of incompleteness for the patient, which could only be broken by exciting acts. He illustrated this with several lengthy accounts from Ne.'s letters, seemingly impressed with her insight. Ne. declared that her state of depression made mental effort difficult for her, and thus she could only obtain pleasure from the impact of physical change on her body. This she described as 'awakening' her and giving her a sensation of control and independence. Finally, she wrote:

> Why do you speak of my desire for mortification? It is my parents who believe that, but it is absurd. It would be a mortification if it brought only suffering, but I enjoy this suffering; it gives me back my mind; it prevents my thoughts from stopping; what would not one do to attain such happiness?[44]

For Ne., self-mutilation was both a physical *and* a mental therapy for her unpleasant state. Janet himself laid greater emphasis on the mental aspect of her symptoms. Since he regarded her self-infliction of wounds as pathological, and her underlying illness as mental, this supported the contention that *any* physical intervention into her condition must constitute improper treatment.

Indeed, artefact injury *did* result in serious surgical intervention. In 1908, Georges Dieulafoy, professor of pathology at the Hôtel-Dieu de Paris, gave a lengthy report of an unusual case. Dieulafoy's patient was 'un garçon' of thirty who suffered from a gangrenous affection of the skin for two and a half years. He had consulted numerous doctors and surgeons before ending up at the Hôtel-Dieu. On one occasion, the patient even agreed to have most of his arm amputated, and had contemplated further operations. Despite this drastic intervention, Dieulafoy came to the conclusion that the man's injuries were self-inflicted. In order to prove this diagnosis, he had portions of the skin tested for the presence of corrosive substances and, when these tests proved positive, arranged a confrontation with the patient, in the presence of his employer. The patient's confession was secured when Dieulafoy assured him that he would not be held responsible for his actions, which were the result of a morbid mental state. However, if he persisted in the deception now that it had been uncovered he would *become* a dishonest man! This call to honour – whereby patients were considered deceitful only once an 'unconscious' process was revealed – appears to have been common in this period. Even in those diagnosed as mentally ill, doctors expected patients to give – and keep – their word that they would not injure themselves.[45] Apparently shocked, Dieulafoy's patient readily agreed, stating that he had been compelled to create the wounds just as a 'morphinomaniac' was compelled to inject morphine:

> I was, he said, dominated by a fixed idea, of which I could not rid myself. I allowed my arm to be amputated, and I well believe that one day would come when, in order to continue the deception, I would have allowed the amputation of my leg.[46]

Unlike Janet's cases, Dieulafoy claimed his patient was easily cured: all that was needed was for the doctor to reveal the true nature of the wounds, and the patient recovered. Thus, the case was reported in the press as 'A Medical Puzzle Solved'.[47]

Other doctors, however, were beginning to doubt that cure was so easy. Some, like Janet, suggested that lengthy psychotherapy was required to reveal the unconscious roots of the patient's need to injure him or herself. By the 1920s, the London physician Frederick Parkes Weber (1863–1962) began to refer such patients for psychotherapeutic treatment. This allowed the general practitioner to absolve himself of responsibility for his patient, who instead became 'a psychological problem'.[48] Although there were few places in early twentieth-century Britain where such treatment was offered, this did not prevent some doctors looking for other sources of emotional support for their patients: sympathetic family members and nurses were both thought well placed to discuss a patient's 'troubles'.[49] What's more, physicians began to show increased interest in the *outcome* of hospital treatment. In 1925, Henry MacCormac found himself embarrassed by a student's innocent question as to what ultimately happened to patients presenting with self-inflicted lesions. Accordingly, he set about a follow-up study. The dermatologist wrote to all patients he had treated for artificial dermatitis during the years 1913–25. MacCormac's patients were all unmarried women, the majority between the ages of seventeen and 26, and half had shown symptoms of hysteria 'such as anaesthesia of the palate and patchy anaesthesia and numbness of the skin'.[50] Of course, the extraction of 'genuine hysterical eruptions' (which MacCormac claimed had been his criterion for this study) from other cases was frequently determined along lines of gender and age; a male patient was more likely to be viewed as either a malingerer or having a 'true' dermatitis. The division of malingering into hysterical and unconscious on the one hand, and conscious fraud on the other, was very often made on gender lines.[51]

MacCormac received replies from just half his patients, and one had been readmitted since her first visit. Many, MacCormac claimed, misremembered or had even entirely forgotten their hospital experiences. One young kitchen maid, who had married since her admission aged seventeen, asked:

> if you would inform me if being a married woman as I now am will it affect my leg or will I ever have any trouble with it later on in life?
> . . . I should also like to know if it will have any effect on my future children.

Deciding that the patient's query was genuine, MacCormac suggested that this could be explained by double personality or 'the habit of burying the memory of unpleasant events in the subconscious mind'. Another patient insisted that she had *never* been in the Middlesex Hospital, although her 'name is an uncommon one'! The mysterious mental aspect of these cases, MacCormac concluded, meant that, although all the patients from whom he had received news 'appear to have recovered, or at least discontinued damaging the skin . . . it is hardly likely that they will eventually become normal individuals'. If the patient's issues were unconscious, this meant they could re-emerge at any point.[52]

The reference to double personality (also called 'double consciousness' or 'multiple personality') is an interesting one. The attention to this phenomenon in France is fairly well documented. Pierre Janet had begun experimenting on the splitting of consciousness in 1885, when he encountered Léonie B., a 45-year-old woman who transformed into another personality, which she called Léontine. Under hypnosis, a third personality emerged.[53] Another famous case was Reverend Ansel Bourne, an American born-again preacher who disappeared, only to be found two months later running a shop in Pennsylvania under the name John Brown. When hypnotized, Brown's memories returned. In 1890, psychologist William James published material from his interview with Bourne in his classic textbook, *Principles of Psychology*.[54] Bound up in the wider interest in hypnosis and the unconscious in this era, Janet regarded multiple personality as a form of dissociation. The topic was already loosely associated with self-mutilation by the turn of the century. Bethlem Royal Hospital's Theo Hyslop (1863–1933) used one such case to illustrate a paper on 'double consciousness' in 1899. Hyslop was an Associate of the Society for Psychical Research (an organization that aimed to scientifically explore purported spiritual phenomena) and had met Janet in the early 1890s, later corresponding with him.[55] In 'Double Consciousness', Hyslop related Janet's work on the 'anaesthetic hysterical types' of multiple personality, citing particularly his well-known work with Léonie. Hyslop sought to expand the field of research on consciousness through a discussion of cases he felt might 'help to bridge the apparently impassable gap between double consciousness and more ordinary experiences'. These included one instance of self-injurious behaviour.[56]

The 25-year-old teacher Alice Rose M. was admitted to Bethlem as a voluntary boarder in March 1895. Alice remained in the hospital for only sixteen days before 'her friends took her away as they thought that the other people in the gallery would be bad for her,' yet there are more case notes recorded about her than for many patients who remained a year or more, indicating a high level of interest in her case.[57] Alice, 'an intellectual and highly cultivated lady' of 'restless, nervous disposition', had begun sleepwalking in 1891: 'She used to make a great deal of noise at night, banging at the door, hitting her head on the floor & such like.'[58] Two years later, mesmerism by a friend eased her condition, stopping Alice from 'bang[ing] herself about so much', but in the summer of that year (1893) 'she again started sleeplessness & sleepwalking only she threw herself about more'. Knocking the head or body was incorporated into contemporary understanding of self-mutilation. In Alice's case, changes in her condition seem to have been measured by those around her through the extent of this behaviour. Eventually, Alice developed three separate personalities:

> Her second person she calls 'Nocturna' & herself she calls 'Morison' ... a little later on she seems to have acquired a '3rd state' who used to do all manner of mischief ... Perhaps one of the most important things to be grasped is that Nocturna knows what Morison is doing but Morison does not know what Nocturna is doing and neither of them know what the 3rd state is doing. This has been picked out of 2 hours conversation [with Alice and her friend Miss Kennedy] so that necessarily there are many details wanting.[59]

Despite the absence of detail, and the short duration of Alice's stay at Bethlem, Hyslop nonetheless concluded in his publication that the case was:

> In favour of the hypothesis that dual consciousness is only complete somnambulism. The successive awakening of the senses constitutes a gradation from ordinary sleep to complete somnambulism, which gives to the person studied the appearance of leading a dual life.

From this, he indicated that insanity might be comparable to 'some dream states', with acts like self-mutilation thus committed 'unconsciously'.[60] This notion suggested that there might be a motive behind the self-inflicted injury that was beneath the level of consciousness, even if this were as confused or irrational as in a dream.

Another explanation was that the patient's 'second self' (or underlying consciousness) was, in fact, *more* rational than the primary self, protecting it during insanity or other nervous disorder. Alice, as Hyslop remarked, 'never really hurt herself'. Frederic W. H. Myers, a poet and founder of the Society for Psychical Research, thought there might be 'a supervision – a *subliminal* supervision – exercised over the hysteric's limbs. Part of her personality is still alive to the danger, and modifies her movements, unknown to her supraliminal self.'[61] When the patient's conscious self was insane, the 'second self' might protect against self-mutilation, a 'remarkable feature' in the case of Anna Winsor, sent to the American Society for Psychical Research. The patient's right arm 'became, as it were, the primary possession of the secondary personality' with 'beneficent control' over Anna's attempts to tear out her hair.[62] Myers's conclusions about human personality in this case resulted from the prior assumption that the act of tearing the hair was a perversion of the natural instinct of self-preservation: a similar perspective to that of the naturalists discussed earlier. However, the role of a secondary level of consciousness here was a new element.

The above examples indicate that there was already a background in psychology and psychiatry when dermatologists began connecting *dermatitis artefacta* with multiple personality in the early 1900s. George Pernet (1861–1939), who received his MD in Paris, claimed in 1909 to have been interested in 'the psychological aspect of dermatitis factitia' for 'a good many years'. Invited to speak at a meeting of the American Dermatological Association, Pernet indicated the difficulty of untangling an underlying motive in such cases. His solution was to look to contemporary research on hysteria and unconscious acts, citing, in particular, Janet on multiple personality and the related concept of dissociation taken up by William James and Morton Prince, among others. The attribution of multiple personality in such cases accounted for the failure of many physicians to secure confessions from their patients, and the hostility of patients and their families to a diagnosis of self-injury. A hysterical patient, it was suggested, might not be aware that her wounds

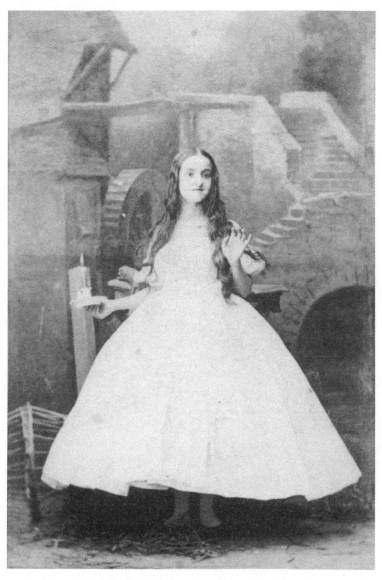

The opera singer Adelina Patti in the title role of Amina, the sleepwalker, in Bellini's *La sonnambula*. Interest in somnambulism was associated with other research into multiple personality, hysteria and the unconscious.

were self-inflicted and 'should be looked upon as mentally rather than physically ill. They mutilated themselves because they could not help it.'[63] Rather than being 'motiveless', these cases were now deemed to be *unconscious*: it was assumed that a motive existed, but was hidden from doctor *and* patient.

When Pernet presented several cases of *dermatitis artefacta* to the Dermatological Section of the Royal Society of Medicine in 1915, debate focused on the 'mysterious mental element in these cases'.[64] One participant suggested a Freudian interpretation: that self-mutilation was evidence of mental repression. From this perspective, self-inflicted skin lesions could be regarded as conversion hysteria: the alteration of an idea into physical stigmata.[65] Another participant, Samuel, recommended treatment with psychoanalysis or hypnosis: if the acts were unconscious, treatment needed to access the patient's unconscious mind. Pernet himself was in broad agreement with this psychological interpretation, although he (like many British practitioners) preferred to use Janet's model rather than, as he put it, 'Freudism'. Frederick Parkes Weber agreed, suggesting that

> of all diseases related to disorders of the psychical system, artificial eruptions in young women most deserve ... study from the psychical point of view, and it would have been a great advantage if the followers of Freud's teaching had concentrated upon this subject much of their psycho-analytic investigations.[66]

However, it remained unusual for cases to be passed between physicians and psychiatrists. Ten years later, the case of a nineteen-year-old girl with linear excoriations on her arms was brought to a similar audience. Unusually, her doctor sent the girl to an alienist, former Bethlem superintendent William H. B. Stoddart. Stoddart, who was treasurer of the Psychoanalytic Society at the time, confirmed that the case was 'one of dual personality, and that the patient was unaware that she produced the lesions herself'. The audience were in widespread agreement that many cases of the kind showed mental stigmata, and . . . raised the question . . . as to whether such cases should not be sent to the mental specialist rather than to the dermatologist.[67]

This psychological view of self-inflicted skin injury was purported to absolve the patient from blame for the condition: if the acts were unconscious, then an individual couldn't be held responsible. However, in practice this was not entirely the case, most often because hysteria remained always in the background. This meant that so-called 'motiveless' self-mutilation was largely seen as a female behaviour. Moreover, the conclusions made on the topic did not solely apply to those diagnosed with hysteria. In 1911, Frederick Parkes Weber published an article on the relation of hysteria to malingering. He claimed hysteria to be a disorder of the 'tertiary sex characters', by which he meant the psychological characteristics thought to be common to men or women. From this, self-mutilation became an embodiment of female psychology, in that it was given an evolutionary explanation:

> In past ages . . . simulation or deception of various kinds must often
> have been serviceable to the weaker female in protecting herself from
> the stronger (and sometimes cruel) male, as well as in enabling her
> sometimes to get her own way . . . therefore, at the present time the
> facility (instinct) for deception is probably greater in the average
> female than in the average male.[68]

Weber's interest in the psychological nature of self-inflicted injury led him to view it as a female behaviour, rooted in the morally dubious context of deception. The belief that women were 'naturally' deceptive was widespread in this period. It was also evident in the attitudes of doctors to rape, for 'though there are evil men there are more evilly-minded hysterical women.'[69] It was regarded as more likely that a woman would attempt to deceive those around her than that her accusation might be justified. The concept of hysterical deception thus relied on preconceptions about the ature, not just of hysteria as an illness, but of women in general. This caused physicians to minimize the possibility that self-injury might have occurred in response to external circumstances. When patients referred to 'family troubles', or even detailed experiences of rape or assault, practitioners divorced any self-inflicted injuries from this external context, instead explaining them through the medical diagnosis of hysteria, and female psychology more generally.

In this chapter I have explored the emergence of 'hysterical self-mutilation' at the end of the nineteenth century and the beginning of the twentieth. There are aspects of this topic that may seem more familiar to us today than other aspects of nineteenth-century self-mutilation. Adopting a present-day perspective can mislead us, however, into seeing hysterical self-mutilation as familiar, and thus failing to acknowledge the many ways in which it was

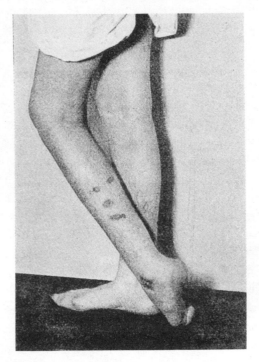

This plate showing the hysterical gait was reproduced in John Collie's *Malingering and Feigned Sickness* (1913) from an earlier medical text on nervous diseases. Collie noted that the marks on the legs were 'scars of self-inflicted burns', associating self-mutilation with both hysteria and malingering.

not. The association of self-injury with hysteria at the turn of the twentie[th] century was increasingly used to provide a psychological framework for phenomena that were previously regarded either in spiritual or physiological terms. In addition, the widespread association of hysteria with manipulation meant that self-inflicted wounds were thought to say something quite specific about an individual, proving their deceitful temperament even where it also showed the fractured state of their inner psyche. Surgical records on 'needle girls', for example, emerged from the conflicted status of hysteria as a diagnosis, somewhere between disease and intentional fraud, creating a connection between self-mutilation and malingering in the later nineteenth century. This link led to the assumption that self-mutilation *must* have a motive, which caused a circular method of reasoning. Physicians found a 'gain' (whether financial or emotional) for their patients because they assumed there must be one. By the early twentieth century, this gain was regarded in explicitly psychological terms. Physicians warned that no 'patient should be bullied out of an artefact dermatitis; the artefact might be cured in that way, but some other psychological disturbance would follow'.[70] The explicit association of self-mutilation with psychological turmoil was new to this era.

We tend to assume today that a psychological approach must be 'progressive', simply because it aligns more neatly with modern understandings of self-harm. However, the new psychological view of self-mutilation in the early twentieth century was perceived in heavily gendered terms, very similar to previous assumptions. In men, as we have seen, self-castration was regarded as evidence of broader national decline and social unrest. In women, as in the cases of hysterical self-mutilation outlined here, self-mutilation was thought to be rooted in individual pathology rather than external factors, explicitly connected to the perceived emotional needs of women. Thus, although the shift in view of hysterical self-mutilation from 'motiveless' to 'unconscious' appeared to absolve the patient from individual blame, she remained culpable by association because of her gender. Hysterical malingering became a comment, by male doctors, about the nature of women as a sex: a reflection of the 'natural' tendency women to deceive and manipulate others. This connection between self-harm and manipulative behaviour remains strong today, and continues to be perceived in gendered terms, for example through the diagnosis of borderline personality disorder, which is much more frequently diagnosed in women. Such ideas gain ready acceptance because we are so unaware of their historical origins that they are accepted as established fact. The historical background to hysteria should lead us to question these concepts in modern psychiatric practice.

FIVE

FOCAL SUICIDE

Hypersexuality, Masochism and the Death Instinct in Psychoanalysis

I n 1942, detective fiction devotees first read about the efforts of the private investigator Toby Dyke and his companion George, hired to find the missing Irma in Elizabeth Ferrars's *Don't Monkey with Murder*.[1] After a confused start, it transpired that Irma was a chimpanzee, brought over from Tobago by the well-known 'psycho-biologist' (as his daughter called him) Dr Paul Virag. As suggested by the title, Irma was found murdered: a crime cunningly committed to cover up the homicide of the elderly Rosa Miall by her ward, Katharine Peach. Although Miss Miall herself never actually appeared in the novel, she was nonetheless at the centre of the plot. The wealthy Miall was an enthusiastic but old-fashioned social improver. She interfered in every aspect of village life in East Leat, and ran a club at which visiting lecturers discussed topics from physiology and economics to alcohol abstinence and eugenics. The latter was her particular concern. The village, Rosa Miall declared, was so isolated that inbreeding had led to mental deficiency, and she had determinedly broken up marriages so that 'there wouldn't be so many mad people in East Leat'.[2]

Some of Miss Miall's concerns, it seems, might have had foundation, in particular the character of the murderous Mrs Peach. Physically beautiful, the thirty-something Katharine Peach was described by Dyke as a 'lovely idiot' who 'turned out to be one of the too abundant mental-deficients of East Leat'.[3] Murder was one proof of her 'bad blood'; however, self-mutilation was another twist. In order to arrange visits from her ɔver (a doctor) to bandage her hand, Mrs Peach had been seen 'poking the point of her scissors into her hand in several places, and laughing.'[4] Katharine Peach was presented as hysterical and mentally deficient, but explicitly *not* mad. Instead, she retained full responsibility for her actions: dangerously manipulative, Mrs Peach was reported to be making herself sick to bring her lover to the house. Her self-mutilation was similarly judged as premeditated.

There is certainly a connection between this fictional depiction of self-harm and the hysterical malingering described in the previous chapter. Indeed, Mrs Peach fitted within Victorian and Edwardian concerns about degenerate heredity and mental deficiency, which in the UK informed the Mental Deficiency Act of 1913. However, the earlier assumption was that defective heredity was externally visible. Beautiful and sexually promiscuous (the plot hung on her foolish marriage and subsequent affairs), Katharine Peach was nonetheless tainted and dangerous. This depiction was very much a product of twentieth-century concerns: female manipulation and sexuality that concealed aggressive tendencies. All of these ideas were bound up in Peach's act of self-inflicted injury, an understanding prominent in psychoanalytic circles in the interwar period. Indeed, psychoanalysis is often where modern researchers assume investigation into self-mutilation began: with Karl A. Menninger's landmark study *Man Against Himself*, published in 1938.[5] Menninger, an American Freudian analyst, regarded self-mutilation as an unconscious mechanism for avoiding suicide, by the concentration of a 'suicidal impulse' on one part of the body as a substitute for the whole. Although Freud himself showed little specific interest in self-injury, later analysts – primarily Louville Emerson, Wilhelm Stekel and Menninger – interpreted self-harm as proving his theories.

In this chapter, I explore two key elements of the psychoanalytic view of self-mutilation that emerged in the United States in this period, both of which are illustrated by the popular presentation of self-injury in *Don't Monkey with Murder*. First, I look at the association between self-harm and female sexuality, and second, the connection made later with the Freudian idea of the 'death instinct'. The connection of self-mutilation to female sexuality was a new one in this era. Although the view of women as manipulative was strongly held in late nineteenth- and early twentieth-century texts on hysterical self-harm, this was not assumed to be related to sexual desire. Indeed, women's sexuality was rarely discussed, even though sex *was* held to be a feature of male self-mutilation, as outlined in Chapter Three. Freud's initial aetiology of hysteria, however, suggested that the disorder resulted from thwarted or repressed sexual desires (usually from childhood). Although Freud and his circle did not apply this model directly to self-mutilation, this connection *was* made in the United States, where interpretations of psychoanalytic theory tended to be less symbolic and more literal than Freud perhaps intended.

Louville Emerson's 'The Case of Miss A' (1913–14) was the first explicit discussion of the psychology of self-harm in a Freudian framework. In this and later works, Emerson developed a more complex internalized understanding of self-inflicted injury than that seen elsewhere, understood first and foremost through his patients' unconscious drives, primarily sexuality. Emerson was not the only psychoanalyst to interpret self-harm in this way. In Germany, Wilhelm Stekel viewed self-injury as an act of both masturbation and masochism. Neither received much wider attention, however, perhaps because Freudian theory was already changing, first with the view of childhood psychosexual trauma as fantasized and then through the introduction of the 'death instinct' in 1920. The death instinct was the starting point for Menninger, whose book and articles on self-mutilation included such diverse cases as a man whose sibling rivalry led him to cut off his luxuriant hair and newspaper accounts of men dying in burglar traps they had themselves built. All of these examples, Menninger claimed, showed mankind's unconscious wish for death. Although Menninger continued to assume there was a sexual element to self-inflicted injury, his understanding of self-mutilation in terms of aggressive rather than sexual drives was more palatable to the general public and, until the publication of Armando Favazza's *Bodies Under Siege* in 1987, *Man Against Himself* remained the major text on the topic.

Although many elements of the psychoanalytic interpretation of self-harm are no longer in vogue – Menninger's contention, for example, that all forms of mutilation were a prototype of self-castration – others have had a more lasting impact. In particular, both Emerson and Menninger promoted the understanding of self-harm as evidence of inner psychological turmoil that is still widely held in the Western world today. Both also viewed the drives that led to self-mutilation in the individual (whether sexual or aggressive) as those that also influenced normal human behaviour. Although presenting self-injury on a sliding scale, from normal to insane acts, was nothing new, psychoanalytic texts promoted this much more adeptly than previous psychiatric models had, by offering a universal explanation of drives and instincts. This idea of conscious and unconscious drives has continued to shape psychological views of self-mutilation in the nearly seventy years since *Man Against Himself* was first published.

Psychosexual trauma and masochism: the case of Miss A

In August 1912, a young female patient at the Boston Psychopathic Hospital had her first session with resident psychoanalyst L. E. Emerson. Honora Downey – Miss A, as she would become known in print – was 23

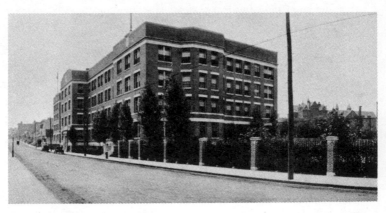

The Boston Psychopathic Hospital, from Lloyd Vernon Briggs's *History of the Psychopathic Hospital, Boston, Massachusetts* (1922).

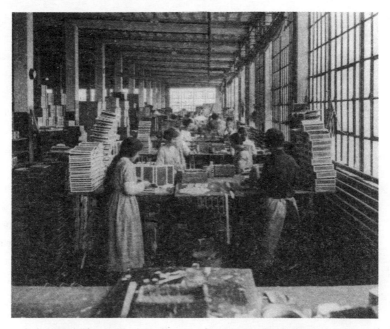

A photograph of women in the work room of an American box factory, c. 1910. Young women worked closely together in these environments, bringing them into a new social setting, outside the home.

years old and from a local working-class family who did not, apparently, know she had been admitted to hospital. Downey had worked in a factory in Boston since being taken out of school at the age of thirteen. By her own account, her life was unhappy. In his notes a few days after the sessions began, Emerson recorded that 'yesterday was the first time she thought life endurable, the first day she was willing to live.'[6] Downey's father terrorized the family throughout her childhood, regularly whipping her brothers – so badly that one contacted the police. Her mother seems to have been largely ineffectual (indeed, she was rarely mentioned in Emerson's notes). Between the ages of eight and fourteen, Downey was sexually abused by an uncle, who 'was accustomed almost daily to masturbate her'.[7] When she was twelve he attempted to rape her. At the age of twenty, one of her brothers offered her money to have sex with him and, at the same age, a cousin tried to assault her. As her analyst bluntly put it, 'her family's sexual morality is suggested by the fact that she said all her brothers but one asked her for "connections" (i.e. coitus).'[8]

The main reason for Downey's admission to hospital was a self-inflicted cut on her left arm. She reported that she had cut herself 28 or 30 times in the last three years, and 'her arm had many other scars, and there was one on her breast.'[9] This, in itself, Emerson did not consider unusual; indeed, his article referred in passing to two other cases he had treated in which self-mutilation occurred. Thus, although 'Miss A' has since been cited as the first case of 'delicate self-cutting' in the clinical literature, Emerson himself felt it had 'no claim to originality'.[10] After all, there were certainly points of comparison with the case of Helen Miller, reported some 25 years earlier (described in the previous chapter). What *was* new, however, was Emerson's method of treatment, alongside a new framework for understanding the aetiology of self-inflicted injury. This framework was embedded in the ideals of psychoanalytic thought, as well as cultural changes in America in the 1910s and '20s.

Louville Eugene Emerson (1873–1939) was born in Maine. His first foray into higher education was to study engineering, but he later became a graduate philosophy student at Harvard, gaining a PhD in experimental psychology in 1909. Less than a decade younger than some of the late Victorian alienists introduced earlier, Emerson was nonetheless more heavily influenced by the cultural changes after the turn of the twentieth century, not least a self-conscious distancing from old-fashioned 'Victorianism' in both Britain and the USA.[11] Another difference between Emerson and his forebears across most of the Western world was his lack of medical background. Most Victorian psychiatrists – and indeed most psychoanalysts, including Freud, Jung, Stekel and Ferenczi – were medically trained, although Freud increasingly came to support lay analysis. This could have put Emerson in a difficult position; however, he was aided by the personal support of Harvard neurologist James Jackson Putnam.[12] It was Putnam who helped Emerson take up clinical practice (which he preferred to teaching dry laboratory psychology), by securing private funds to set him up in a part-time position at the Massachusetts General Hospital in 1911. In 1912, Emerson was also appointed to the staff of the new Boston Psychopathic Hospital.

Psychoanalysis was still a fairly new specialty at this time. In Europe, Freud's work had reached a wider audience only after receiving the support of Eugen Bleuler and Carl Gustav Jung at the Burghölzli: Freud and Jung did not begin their correspondence until 1906.[13] Meanwhile, the Freudian 'circle' began with the founding of the Psychological Wednesday Society by Wilhelm Stekel in 1902 and expanded with the creation of its successor, the Vienna Psychoanalytical Society, in 1908. The journal of the International Psychoanalytical Association, *Zentralblatt für Psychoanalyse*, was established by Stekel and Adler in 1910.[14] None of these early texts contained specific examples of self-mutilation, although some were later reinterpreted in this way. Karl Menninger declared that a 'classical case of neurotic self-mutilation well known to those familiar with psychoanalytic literature involving the nose and teeth is the celebrated Wolf-Man case'.[15]

The Wolf-Man was one of Freud's most well-known case histories, published in 1918 as a case of 'infantile neurosis'. The Wolf-Man – later publicly identified as the Russian aristocrat Sergei Pankejeff – remained famous in later years, partly because one of his childhood dreams was central to Freud's theory of psychosexual development, and partly because the patient himself repudiated Freud's interpretation to the journalist Karin Obholzer.[16] Pankejeff suffered from depression and 'nervous' symptoms; however, to cast him as a case of self-mutilation seems quite a leap, even accepting Menninger's often loose use of the term (the reference appeared following the case of a man with a compulsion for cutting his hair until it was 'repulsively grotesque'). The 'self-mutilation' to which Menninger referred was presumably Pankejeff's contraction of gonorrhoea at the age of eighteen. This infection, Freud stated, caused the patient's health to break down, so that he was entirely dependent on others when he began his psychoanalysis a few years later.[17] Menninger apparently regarded the contraction of venereal disease as self-inflicted, perhaps because Freud saw it as a form of castration. As in Freud's other writings, however, the

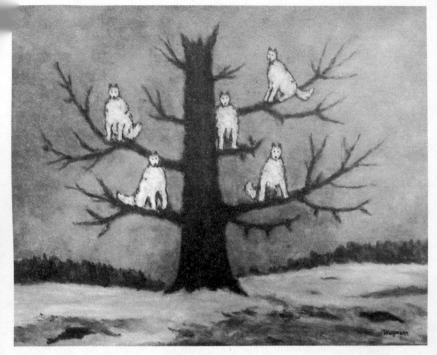

Sergei Pankejeff, *Wolves Sitting in a Tree*, 1964. It was the dream that inspired this painting that gave Pankejeff the nickname 'Wolf-Man', by which Freud referred to him in *History of an Infantile Neurosis*. The childhood dream terrified Pankejeff, who woke screaming after being stared at by these white wolves sitting in a tree outside his bedroom window.

castration remained purely symbolic, even when expanded upon in Ruth Mack Brunswick's later analysis of the same patient.[18] It was only in the texts of American psychoanalysts that examples of physical mutilation were juxtaposed with the functional and symbolic 'mutilations' described by Freud and others.

One could suggest that European psychoanalysts simply did not encounter patients who intentionally injured themselves. Given the cases detailed in the previous three chapters, and the fact that many analysts (such as Jung) began their careers in asylum psychiatry, this seems extremely unlikely, however. Two factors in the United States in this era were particularly important for this connection between actual and symbolic mutilation that does not seem to have occurred widely else-where: first, the influence of Adolf Meyer's doctrine of 'psychobiology', and second, the 'hospital ideal' that emerged in early twentieth-century America. Meyer (1866–1950) was a Swiss-German émigré who arrived in America in 1892. He has been considered the most influential psychiatrist in the U.S., from the time Emerson penned 'The Case of Miss A' until the mid-twentieth century.[19] The doctrine he promoted was founded on ele-ments of late Victorian psychiatry and psychology, in particular that the mind had evolved through adaptation by natural selection. Mental illness was thus characterized as a failure of adaptation. For Meyer, this led to the premise that the physical action of the nervous system and visible, behav-ioural responses were all part of the same system, and could not be treated independently. Meyer was also interested in psychotherapy, and introduced two generations of Americans to Freud. Exploring mental and physical health as part of a single system had important consequences for the health care system in the United States. Asylums began to change their names, adopting a new 'hospital ideal': psychiatric institutions were to be staffed and run like general hospitals, occupying a place somewhere between the old public asylums and the private clinic of the individual nerve specialist.[20] This change made hospitals into scientific centres rather than sites of social welfare. For psychiatrists, psychoanalysis seemed a possible solution to the failures in early twentieth-century asylums, in which increasing numbers of patients were receiving solely custodial care. With its emphasis on sexuality, it also addressed widespread fears of a crisis in sexual morality.[21]

The Boston Psychopathic Hospital was founded in this spirit of thera-peutic optimism, opening its doors in June 1912. Emerson joined the staff the same year. Although psychoanalysis in Europe had largely taken place in private homes and clinics, Emerson regarded the hospital as a useful location for an analyst, as he could treat 'borderland cases' (such as hysteria and psychoneuroses) that were 'medical, surgical, and mental, all at once'. This included psychoanalytic treatment for patients with self-inflicted wounds, for 'surgical attention alone . . . was not adequate to prevent further self-mutilation.'[22] In addition, Emerson held that the hospital could further psychoanalysis as a science, providing research subjects from a variety of different backgrounds and experiences. In reality, his psychoanalytic work was much more focused on the individual than this suggests. However, American clinicians of the 1910s and '20s were far more open than their predecessors about their goals for creating a 'psychiatry of the everyday'.[23] Psychiatric practice had begun to delve into the homes and family lives of patients through new social service departments in hospitals, beginning in 1907.[24] Despite tensions between staff, this was very much a part of the expansion of psychiatry into the everyday, and social workers in return supported the expansion of psychoanalysis. Like social work, psychoanalysis highlighted the significance of life experiences, including incidents from childhood, fantasies and dreams.[25]

As a psychoanalyst, well read in continental theory, it is hardly surprising that Emerson's account of Miss A focused on sexual desire and experiences, including psychosexual trauma, masturbation, sexual guilt and masochism. The first of these was emphasized across most of Emerson's cases. Although Freud, by this time, had come to believe that the psychosexual trauma of childhood was rooted in fantasies rather than actual sexual abuse, Emerson believed the accounts of his patients, and related their experiences alongside the symbolic elements of psychoanalysis. In his analysis of 22-year-old Rachel C. (from 1912 to 1917), the analyst quickly became certain that her hysterical fits and paralyses were a result of sexual trauma, and he uncovered hidden memory after memory of abuse. Of course, Emerson's own certainty in the existence of this cause must have influenced his line of questioning.[26] Honora Downey, however, unlike many of Emerson's other patients, had not forgotten the experiences she recounted to Emerson, and 'no special technique' was required to get her to recall them.[27] Although this meant her case could not be a 'true' Freudian hysteria, Emerson was sure that 'there is no doubt, but that the "indispensable condition," for the later self-mutilation, was the psychosexual trauma of childhood.' This was emphasized in his report of the occasion Downey first cut herself:

One day, about three years ago, as she was cutting bread, her cousin, boarding with her family at the time, attempted a sexual assault. In the scuffle she cut herself with the bread knife ... It happened at the time of this attempted assault the patient was suffering from an intense headache. After cutting herself, however, she noticed that the headache had left.

Emerson presented the headache as secondary to the attempted assault, emphasizing the connection between psychosexual trauma and self-mutilation. When Downey's own written account of her self-cutting omitted the assault entirely (as well as several other sexual details Emerson considered important), the psychoanalyst decided that she had 'suppressed' it. Moreover, his article referred in passing to two other cases he had treated, which, he said, supported his view that self-mutilation was caused by psychosexual trauma during childhood.[28]

However, the notes made during the analysis, as well as the patient's own account, indicate that Downey had a lot more to say about her reasons for cutting, not all of which could be interpreted sexually. She had suffered a 'crazy headache' for three days before the assault, 'and after I had let blood my headache went away, and I thought that the cutting of my wrist, and letting the blood flow had cured it'.[29] The phrase 'let blood' used the therapeutic terminology of bloodletting, and Downey regularly returned to this idea: 'I did think that it would cure my headache, and help to menstruate regularly like other girls did.'[30] Irregular menstruation, in addition to being a sign of pregnancy, was also widely interpreted as a sign of ill-health. Downey told Emerson of the 'common belief' among her female work colleagues that it could lead to consumption (tuberculosis) or insanity. In response, she 'stuck a pen-knife in her Vagina once, to make herself flow'.[31] She was also unhappy with her 'abnormally stout' body, and reported that she 'thought bleeding would reduce fat'.[32] Again, the patient's size had sexual connotations: she disliked the way she looked, but also the fact that she was teased for either being pregnant or loose, for the 'girls in [the] shop used to say fat girls will go it forty diff[erent] ways.'[33]

Although it was Emerson's decision to emphasize sexual trauma as the direct reason for Honora Downey's self-mutilation, there is no reason to doubt that she was the victim of serious abuse. Indeed, her experiences were not unusual. At this time, psychiatrists were just beginning to conceive of the possibility of male sexual assault. Even so, it was rarely clearly separated from the notion of seduction, and both sexes could regard unwanted sexual acts as part of a purportedly natural process.[34] Downey seems to have accepted some of the attentions of male family members as normal. Certainly, the encounter she most resented was at the hands not of her uncle, but of a trusted medical professional, Dr Briggs, who attempted to 'cure her desire to cut herself' by masturbating her.[35] None of this appeared in Emerson's published report – presumably he didn't want to malign a colleague – although Briggs was mentioned numerous times in the notes. Indeed, although Emerson listened to and accepted his patients' stories of sexual abuse, he nonetheless located the drive toward self-mutilation in internal, psychological turmoil, absolving other actors in Downey's story of blame. He even saw self-mutilation as 'symbolic masturbation'. In explaining Miss A's self-cutting, he remarked that 'one could conceive that the sexual craving of the patient was abnormally developed by her early passive masturbation.' By re-casting abuse as 'passive masturbation', Emerson emphasized the role of childhood sexual development (following Freud), but also internalized the experience. Rather than viewing self-harm as a response to unpleasant memories of abuse, we are led to focus on the direct effects of physical manipulation on Honora Downey's sexual development: 'cutting was a sort of symbolical substitute for masturbation.'[36]

There is a connection here with some of the material on male sexuality outlined in Chapter Three, in which self-mutilation was regarded as a form of extreme perversion resulting from masturbation. In 1857, for example, G. M. Jones at the Jersey Hospital had reported a case 'so disgusting' it 'must be said to reduce man below the level of the brute'.[37] Jones's patient was Emile C., a 34-year-old gardener from France, with a severe wound in the scrotum from which one of his testicles protruded – reportedly the only way he could attain sexual excitement due to a long history of onanism. There were many differences between this report – a cautionary tale of the depravity masturbation could lead to – and Emerson's. Jones's emphasis, however, was typical of the mid- and late nineteenth-century contention that self-mutilation in men could be a direct (not symbolic) form of masturbation, an extreme perversion when all others had been exhausted. Indeed, this perception was newly applied to female patients in some instances at the turn of the twentieth century. In 1900, George Monks at the Boston City Hospital reported the removal of hat-pins from the abdomen of a 21-year-old single woman. Although his words were less censorious than Jones's, the context was similar:

> For a long time she had been in the habit of masturbating by massage of the ovaries through the abdominal wall, but, as this finally failed to give her satisfaction, she introduced the hat-pin, as already described.[38]

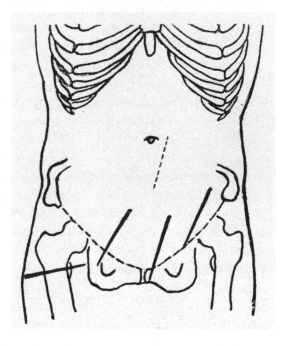

This diagram shows the location of the four needles Monks removed from his patient, reportedly introduced into the abdomen for the purpose of masturbation.

As in the earlier case, it was suggested that excessive masturbation could lead to a failure to achieve orgasm, resulting in sexual perversion in the form of self-injury.

Unlike Honora Downey, Monks's patient was 'mentally stupid'. Although the doctor didn't draw such a conclusion, the fear of sexual activity in so-called 'mental deficients' was a prominent topic at this time.[39] This perceived connection between masturbation and hypersexuality could therefore be seen as socially dangerous. Psychoanalysts tended to question this by regarding masturbation as a normal part of development, connecting early sexual behaviour with other acts including thumb-sucking that were similarly described as 'auto-erotic'.[40] The most outspoken member of Freud's circle on this topic was Wilhelm Stekel (1868–1940). Indeed, one of the major disagreements between Freud and Stekel was about masturbation: Freud believed masturbation could cause harm if carried on at an age after which 'normal' sexual pursuits (that is, heterosexual penetrative intercourse) should have been adopted.[41]

Stekel was one of the key figures in the early psychoanalytic movement, and perhaps the only European analyst who described self-mutilation in his works, in particular *Sadism and Masochism* (1925). Emerson certainly read some of Stekel's texts.[42] Stekel regarded elements of sexual life, particularly masturbation, as symbolic of self-punishment, connecting the 'chronic suicide' of masturbation with asceticism and other forms of self-denial.[43] Stekel claimed that the 'torturing consciousness of guilt' was 'again and again' the source of self-mutilation, 'dictating severe punishment', in which the patient 'combines in one person judge, accused and executioner'.[44] There were certainly elements of this approach in Emerson's outline of Miss A, who, he reported, 'felt disgusted with herself and wished to punish herself, in a way, for her acquiescence as a child in what she instinctively felt were serious misdeeds' (the so-called 'passive masturbation'). The analyst made a similar connection with a scar of the letter 'W' on Downey's leg. This was inflicted after Honora met a man whom she considered marrying; first, however, she told him about her past. 'As was natural,' Emerson reported (indicating his acceptance of some, if not all,

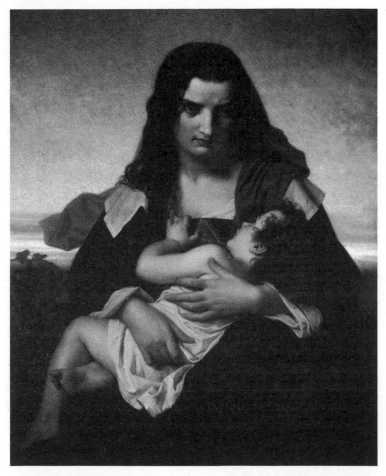

Hugues Merle, *The Scarlet Letter*, 1861. The painting shows Hester Prynne, the female protagonist of the book, with her illegitimate daughter, in a pose reminiscent of depictions of the Madonna and Child. The child's hand partly hides the 'scarlet letter' itself.

of the values of his era), 'he then refused to marry her and called her a whore.' On leaving her lover, Downey drank a glass of her brother's whisky, took his razor and cut the letter 'W' on her leg: 'In this relation Hawthorne's "Scarlet Letter" is interesting', Emerson remarked.[45] The 'scarlet letter' in the book, first published in 1850, was worn throughout by heroine Hester

Prynne. At the end of the text, her lover, Reverend Arthur Dimmesdale, turns out to have a similar symbol burned into his flesh, illustrative of his physical, moral and spiritual breakdown. In the novel, the origins of the wound were debated, although self-injury was given some emphasis: Dimmesdale's 'course of penance' might well have been 'followed out by inflicting a hideous torture on himself'.[46] Of course, this is not to suggest that Hawthorne wrote the character of Dimmesdale as a medical case history. What is interesting here is Emerson's reading of *The Scarlet Letter* as a comparative case of self-mutilation, indicating the underlying guilt and self-inflicted humiliation that he assumed must also be at play in Honora Downey's case, as emphasized in the novel.

Stekel similarly assumed that guilt must form part of 'self-mutilation and self-accusation' in masochism, for

the phenomenon of 'pleasure in pain' leads to the strangest manifestations. Persons inflict wounds upon themselves or accuse themselves unwarrantably of most serious crimes, in order to receive the punishment dictated by the unconscious.[47]

Martin Duberman, who published Emerson's case notes on Downey, similarly assumed her case was 'female masochism'. As we have already seen in Chapter Three, the explanation of self-mutilation as masochism was not an obvious one in late nineteenth- and early twentieth-century Europe, even among those who had read Krafft-Ebing's *Psychopathia Sexualis*. It was, in fact, the psychoanalytic reading of self-mutilation as related sexual experience that first raised the question as to whether self-harm could be considered masochistic. This was not a foregone conclusion. Krafft-Ebing had assumed, as Emerson himself noted, that masochism consisted of 'the desire to experience pain from the sexual object'. However, in self-injury '*object and subject are one*.'[48] Even more confusingly, for Emerson, Krafft-Ebing recorded only two cases of female masochism, one of whom was purportedly insane. The concept of masochism was created, however, in quite a different social and cultural climate from when Louville Emerson was writing. For Krafft-Ebing, accepting a patriarchal structure in which women were subordinated to men (in some cases brutally so), women were by nature masochistic and undertook a passive sexual role. Thus, masochism was 'a pathological growth of specific feminine mental elements', while 'in woman, an inclination to subordination to man . . . is to a certain extent a normal manifestation.'[49] For Emerson and his colleagues, in an era in which new views of women's social and sexual roles were beginning to emerge, masochism *became* a possible explanation for female self-injurious behaviour.

These conclusions about self-mutilation could not have emerged in another era and context. A psychoanalytic reading of self-mutilation newly understood the act – in the case of women at least – as sexual. Cases outside the psychoanalytic realm, such as a neurological report from Chicago in 1911 of a woman who achieved orgasm through the pain of self-inflicted injury, suggest that it was also new contemporary cultural views of young women as sexualized (even aggressively so) that developed this view.[50] This led to a number of different conclusions. The idea that self-inflicted injury was caused by psychosexual trauma sat alongside the somewhat contradictory belief that it was a form of symbolic masturbation and a self-punishment for sexual guilt. Taken together, these motivations suggested a new form of masochism. 'The patient certainly was masochistic,' Emerson bluntly stated in a later paper, 'because she cut herself, many times.'[51] While Krafft-Ebing assumed that women would naturally submit to men, intelligent young women of Honora Downey's generation struggled with the new possibilities open to them. In some ways, these only seemed to make the constraints seem more oppressive. 'I long to do so much, and yet I can do so little,' Downey wrote to Emerson, a view that was no doubt shared by many of her peers. For Downey, the sexual abuse she had suffered was a part of this struggle. Emerson recorded that she 'intends to work, study psychology, write, & do social service. Gives herself 10 yrs to become the equal of Dr Briggs.'[52] While studying psychology was not an attainable goal for a working-class woman in this era, Downey instead trained as a nurse at nearby Waltham Hospital.

Man against himself: self-mutilation and the 'death instinct'

Sexual attitudes also informed some of the early cases described by Karl Menninger, although in *Man Against Himself*, the psychiatrist moved away from this explanation to favour another Freudian drive – the so-called death instinct. In one of his early papers on the topic, however, Menninger described the 'most remarkable case of neurotic self-mutilation' he had ever seen, which he encountered at the Missouri-Kansas Neuropsychiatric Society in January 1930.[53] The 35-year-old mechanic described differed considerably from Miss A, and not just by age and gender. Between the ages of twelve and fourteen, the patient had begun to twitch and jerk his arms. Diagnosed with chorea (a common childhood condition caused by infection), when his symptoms worsened the diagnosis was re-evaluated: Menninger thought it 'probably *Gilles de la Tourette's Disease*'.[54] The mechanic regularly injured himself in these uncontrollable movements: he kicked and slapped himself and had lost three front teeth as a result of

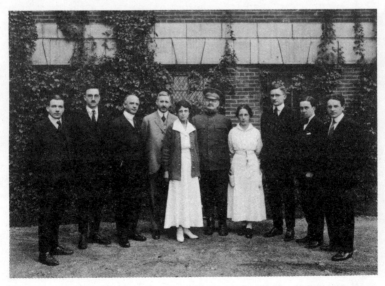

Medical staff at the Boston Psychopathic Hospital in 1918.
Karl Menninger is second from left.

backhand blows with a wrench. His 'hands were covered with the scars of minor injuries. "Whenever I get a knife in my hand", he said, "and naturally I have to do that a lot, I always cut myself; it never fails."'[55]

Initially it seemed that the mechanic's 'jerks, twists, lunges, grimaces, kicks, wriggles, and even barks and whoops' occurred 'in a totally irregular and unpredictable way'. However, they 'had one very definite point of agreement ... As he himself had long recognized, they all seemed directed against himself.' But why did he wish to injure himself at all? Menninger came to the conclusion that the motives were sexual. It was significant, he felt, that in just one brief conversation the patient reported that his mother 'says I'm getting my desserts ... that I would never have gotten this way if I hadn't run around with girls so much!' While admitting there was little evidence of a connection between the patient's 'compulsive acts and the sense of guilt he betrayed by his boasting and the citation of his mother's threats', Menninger nonetheless assumed that there was one:

> I have since learned that this man, who is a member of a respectable family, has now for some time been living with a prostitute and also that in the course of a number of involuntary attacks upon himself he has nearly blinded himself. We see how inexorable the demands of the conscience may be.[56]

When separated into its parts, this statement is absurd by modern standards. Why should there be a direct link between a mechanic nearly blinding himself and living with a prostitute? What was the relevance of the 'respectable family'? As we have seen, sexual guilt and a moral understanding of self-injury had already been applied to male castration. The main difference between Menninger's outline of the 1930s mechanic and the reports of Isaac Brooks in the 1880s was the explicitly psychological phrasing of Menninger's article, which claimed a psychoanalytic 'significance' to self-mutilation.

It is important, then, not to overstate Menninger's contribution to writings on self-mutilation. Approaches to self-harm did not begin with

Menninger, and he certainly did not introduce the *term* 'self-mutilation' to psychiatry, as some have assumed.[57] Menninger's work was informed by categories developed in the late nineteenth and early twentieth century, in particular the notions of 'neurotic' mutilation and 'malingering', as well as the social and cultural ideals bound up in 'sexual' and 'hysterical' mutilation. However, *Man Against Himself* was important for a number of reasons. Menninger brought together a vast number of seemingly disparate cases, ranging well beyond the scale of self-mutilation outlined by Victorian psychiatrists. From 'purposive accidents' to 'polysurgery', from alcoholism and antisocial behaviour to religious asceticism, *Man Against Himself* vastly expanded the definition of self-mutilation. What's more, Menninger's Freudian view of human psychology informed a universal explanation of these acts: *all* self-damaging behaviour could be understood as representative of Freud's concept of the death instinct, a very different approach from Victorian psychiatrists.

Karl Augustus Menninger (1893–1990) was born in Topeka, Kansas, and followed his father into medicine, attending the Harvard Medical School. The young Karl did not, apparently, excel as a student. In 1915, however, he went to a lecture by Louville Emerson at the nearby Massachusetts General Hospital, outlining Freud's ideas. It was Emerson who sparked Menninger's interest in psychoanalysis, and he approached the analyst afterwards for a discussion on the topic. Soon after, in 1918, Menninger took a six-month residency at the Boston Psychopathic Hospital. Following this, at the suggestion of Psychopathic Hospital neurologist Elmer Southard, Menninger returned to Topeka to work in partnership with his father and, later, his younger brother William. The Menninger Diagnostic Clinic, which specialized in neuropsychiatry, was founded in 1919 and, in 1925, was expanded with the Menninger Sanitarium, a private inpatient hospital. However, the hospital did not achieve an international reputation as a mental health facility until 1951.[58]

Karl's reputation was forged earlier than that of the clinic, through his interest in popularizing psychiatry. His first volume, *The Human Mind* (1930), aimed to present a psychiatric concept of the human mind to 'the lay reader and the student'.[59] The book, Menninger claimed, represented (approximately) 'the younger group' in American psychiatry, who had a prevailing optimism not only about new methods of treatment, but also the wider place of psychiatry and psychology in the world.[60] His introduction built on interest in laboratory psychology in the early twentieth century to claim psychiatry as *the* science of the human mind, for, outside the restrictions of the laboratory, every human mind existed in constant interaction: a complex world that could only be understood through experience (as in psychiatry), and not sterile testing. Psychiatry, in Menninger's view, might just save the world. Indeed, Menninger appealed to a broad audience. *The Human Mind* became the best-selling psychology book of its time, and profits from its sale assured the expansion of the Menninger Clinic.[61] In the 1920s and '30s, Menninger also wrote regular columns for *Household Magazine* and then the *Ladies' Home Journal*, offering advice to parents and female readers. Using plain and straightforward language, with many a colourful turn of phrase, 'Dr Karl' (as he preferred to be known) refused to shy away from big issues. *Love Against Hate* was published midway through the Second World War, at a time when disillusionment with the erstwhile policy of passivity adopted by the Allied Powers towards Nazi Germany was immense. Menninger turned this broader concern into a rallying call for the future of psychiatry, promising solutions to the destructive tendencies of mankind that he had previously described in *Man Against Himself.* The psychiatrist's books were peppered with similar statements, his psychiatric cases mingled with narrative reports and newspaper cases, a style that some of his colleagues ridiculed but that certainly made his volumes readable and persuasive to a lay audience.

Menninger's work on self-mutilation needs to be understood in this context: intriguing cases and dramatic concepts became a method for presenting Freud's theories to a wider audience. Freud himself was hostile to the American psychoanalytic movement, which he thought had 'watered down' psychoanalysis, creating a pseudoscientific 'hodge podge' to appeal to lay audiences rather than being a serious scientific doctrine.[62] Despite being personally rebuffed by Freud, who 'did not treat me very nicely',

Menninger undertook a 'personal crusade' to prove his worth as an analyst and the value of Freud's ideas.[63] Indeed, *Man Against Himself* was a direct example of this commitment to Freudianism. Here, Menninger used the theory of the death instinct, which Freud had outlined in 1920, to explain self-damaging behaviour.[64] Following the devastating impact of the First World War, Freud had decided that human actions were governed by a constant conflict between the life and death instincts: the latter would invariably win out, for all human lives ended in death. Although some of Freud's followers were uncertain of this new direction, Menninger happily incorporated the concept into his understanding of human psychology. His psychoanalytic view of self-mutilation was thus quite different from Emerson's. For Emerson, the main factor behind self-inflicted injury was psychosexual trauma; for Menninger, self-damage was a form of sublimated aggression.

The death instinct meant that Menninger interpreted all forms of self-damaging behaviour in relation to suicide, an ethos that has since fallen from favour. *Man Against Himself* divided various acts up in the first instance by their link to suicide, starting with self-homicide itself. Then came the idea of 'chronic suicide', which Menninger described as the 'slow' destruction by addiction or religious self-denial; he also regarded psychosis as a form of ongoing self-destruction. This was followed by 'focal suicide', a concept that is the main focus of discussion here: a self-destructive desire focused on one part of the body in substitution for the whole. Focal suicide included self-mutilation, malingering and impotence. Finally, Menninger went so far as to describe physical disease of any kind as 'organic suicide': a psychological understanding of infection which viewed submission to pathogens as unconscious surrender to the death instinct. This enormously expanded the concept of self-injurious behaviour from nineteenth-century definitions.

Like Freud, Menninger saw the development of the life and death instincts as an important part of the evolution of the individual. In their early years, all humans were fixated on the 'intimate problems of the self'. As the personality developed, instincts would be properly directed outwards. If this development did not take place, self-destructive tendencies remained inwardly focused.[65] While Menninger largely avoided the thorny issue of responsibility by claiming that *no one* could be free of these instincts, others were more forthright on this front. A review in the *British Medical Journal* declared that the fundamental point of Menninger's work was to indicate that every man was ultimately responsible for his own self-destruction.[66] Menninger would certainly have disagreed with such a direct claim. Despite his tendency to emphasize individual responsibility, *Man Against Himself* emerged from Menninger's wider political and philosophical beliefs. If self-destruction could be considered a universal human tendency, it was a problem that affected nations as well as individuals. In a talk in October 1938, Menninger concluded that 'what suicide is for the individual, war is for the nation.' While he recognized the importance of politicians and arms manufacturers (who were 'impartially supplying both sides in order that the merry little game of tearing people apart can go on in all fairness'), his psychological understanding of conflict emphasized that it was the 'self-destructive impulses of the people at large who allow themselves to be manoeuvred into death and destruction.'[67]

It seems unlikely that Menninger, with all his world-changing zeal, intended *Man Against Himself* to be taken in the judgemental spirit of the *BMJ* review. However, his explicit focus on the individual nature of self-injury exacerbated the tendency to moralize seen in the Victorian era. His very explanation of the psychological mechanism of self-mutilation encouraged this view. Menninger described the 'suicidal wish' in three parts: 'the element of dying, the element of killing, and the element of being killed'. An individual first experienced the wish to be killed: an 'extreme form of submission', for 'in the end, death, is the essence of masochism.' This desire for death Menninger explained in terms of guilt and self-punishment. The basic ideas underlying this were little different from earlier concepts of self-mutilation as atonement for sin. This approach assumed that a sin existed, and therefore that the patient must feel guilty for it. While the mechanic described at the outset of this chapter, for example, may have been perfectly happy living with a prostitute, Menninger assumed that his socially incorrect behaviour *must* lead to this response.[68]

The element of dying was more complicated. It was this, perhaps, that inspired Menninger to consider all forms of self-damage in terms of the death instinct. Although Freud claimed that the death instinct was always disguised in an individual case, Menninger followed his former analyst Franz Alexander to conclude:

> nothing else can so well explain the pleasure in exposing one's self unnecessarily to great dangers – as do the mountain climbers, automobile racers, building scalers, or the popular interest in the antics of such movie actors as Harold Lloyd on the sides and tops of skyscrapers, etc.[69]

Lloyd was a well-known actor and stuntman. In his film *Safety Last!* (1923), one scene left Lloyd dangling from the hand of a clock on the side of a skyscraper: a stark illustration of risk. Menninger interpreted any and all risk – or rather, anything he *perceived* as more risky than average – as evidence of the death instinct. Despite the propensity of people to die on stairs, for example, he wasn't overly concerned about those cases. When a suicide attempt did not result in death it meant that the unconscious death instinct was not strong enough to result in fatality; conversely, if a minor self-inflicted wound led to infection and death, the death instinct must be stronger than initially anticipated.

The impetus that Menninger outlined first and foremost, however, was the desire to kill. According to Menninger, it was established that there were, 'beyond any question . . . murderous destructive wishes which arise in earliest infancy'. Again, these murderous wishes were 'naturally' turned outward during childhood, in response to a threat or challenge. If the individual did not fully develop, he would be unable to direct this aggression outwards. Thus, while he might have homicidal wishes against an external threat, he would act out those wishes by identifying with that hated person, and turning the aggression on himself: 'a person unconsciously hated may

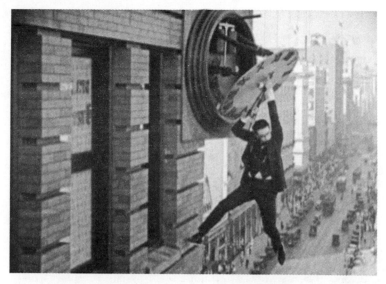

The famous clock scene in *Safety Last!*, showing the type of dangerous acts Menninger referred to as evidence of the universality of the death instinct.

be destroyed by identifying oneself with that person, or more accurately, identifying that person with the self, and destroying the self.' In this way, suicide became an act of aggression, and this concept of self-injurious behaviour as hostile has permeated many later depictions. In *Don't Monkey with Murder*, for example, Mrs Peach's self-inflicted injury was seen as stemming from the same motivations as the murder she committed.[70]

These same psychological explanations were incorporated into *Man Against Himself*, but presented with a more optimistic viewpoint. If man's life was a struggle between life and death instincts, Menninger suggested, then the vast majority of self-destructive acts might actually be attempts to *avoid* suicide: by instead destroying another, minor part of the self, the death instinct could be appeased. Menninger hoped that these sacrifices could be avoided by shining light on them, although sometimes he considered they might be necessary. This was how Menninger understood 'focal suicide' (which included self-mutilation):

the net result of a conflict between (1) the aggressive destructive
impulses . . . and (2) the will to live . . . whereby a partial or local
self-destruction serves the purpose of gratifying irresistible urges.[71]

Despite its necessity for protecting the individual, self-mutilation was
nonetheless seen as an aggressive act against others.

The contradictions arising from these conflicts led to an understanding of individual motivation that, contradictorily, absolved *and* increased
the blame applied to the self-harming person. This is particularly clear in
Menninger's approach to malingering, which he regarded as a form of focal
suicide when it incorporated self-injury. Although emphasizing the conscious input of the neurotic, who made secondary gains from their illness,
Menninger nonetheless pointed out the frequent imbalance between the
minor gains made by the patient and the extreme damage done to his or
her body. His first clinical example was a 29-year-old woman who was
thought to have a skull fracture (evidenced by her blood-soaked pillow
and the pain she suffered), for which she was given morphine. On observation, nurses discovered that the patient had been picking the skin of
her ear canal to cause profuse haemorrhaging. In the past, it was found
that she had gained insurance money as well as submitted to unnecessary
operations. Yet Menninger's view was not as simplistic as some pre-war
publications had been, pointing out that 'to say that the patient wanted
money, morphine, or attention, or all three, is to say the least, to disregard
the extraordinary means she used to obtain them.'[72]

While some of the dermatologists discussed in the previous chapter
had tended towards similar views, Menninger was newly interested in the
effects these patients had on those around them. He noted that, in this
particular case, the doctors and nurses had shifted their opinions rapidly
from extreme concern to hostility towards the patient, concluding that
this was a result of their feeling foolish and humiliated. Unlike other
psychological analyses of malingerers, Menninger decided that this was
an important element of the case. Hostility from others was a result the
patient unconsciously *desired*, from self-punishment and the wish to hurt

others. This attitude retained some of the stereotypical judgements made about the unconsciously manipulative hysteric. However, it increased the blame due to the patient, for enacting a 'provocative aggression'.[73] The primary drives in the act were both 'erotic and aggressive', with injuries 'strongly tinctured with the perverted erotic satisfaction incident to masochism and exhibitionism' – strongly reminiscent of the dangerously sexual female exemplified by the fictional Katharine Peach.

Karl Menninger's understanding of self-mutilation went further than any previous texts in allying normal and pathological acts. He claimed that this was new in the work of Freud and Jung, before which 'we still ignorantly believed that so-called insane behaviour had no meaning'.[74] As we have seen in previous chapters, this belief was certainly not new. However, the creation of a universal explanation *was* new to psychoanalysis, and this encouraged Menninger to go well beyond other writers in terms of what he considered to be self-damaging behaviour. In *Man Against Himself*, any act, no matter how minor, could be viewed as verging on the pathological, and this was nowhere more apparent than in Menninger's new category of 'purposive accidents'. Menninger had first written on this concept in one of several articles on focal self-destruction published in the run-up to *Man Against Himself*. A purposive accident was not, as in the case of malingering, a pretended accident, but a genuine mishap that served an unconscious purpose. To explain the concept, Menninger referred to an example in his own life. When seated next to someone he disliked at a dinner party, he spent the evening trying to be polite. All went well, until 'an unfortunate piece of clever clumsiness' caused him to knock a glass of water over the woman in question's lap. This accident served Menninger's unconscious wish to express his dislike of the woman, even though he had no intention of trying to spill something on her and was quite mortified to have done so.[75]

Clinical examples of purposive accidents were difficult to come by (although Menninger claimed Freud had described an 'indirect attempt at suicide' in the case of Dora).[76] The analyst resorted to a scrapbook of newspaper cuttings to prove his point. Over the course of a year (1931)

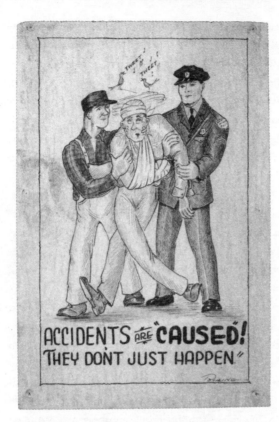

Poster produced by the U.S. Office for Emergency Management during the Second World War, suggesting that the idea of 'purposive accidents' was widespread beyond the realm of insurance; 1942–3.

he had gathered four newspaper clippings that all described the death or injury of a man in his own burglar trap. The regularity of this remarkable phenomenon, Menninger claimed, could not be chance, but was 'convincing evidence as to the unconscious intention and necessity for such individuals to kill themselves on account of their murderous wishes'.[77] In other words, these people desired to murder a thief or other threat, felt guilty on account of this, and unconsciously punished themselves. Menninger was criticized by colleagues for drawing conclusions from a handful of newspaper articles, and so he added further material from insurance companies and related organizations in *Man Against Himself*. The National Safety Council was founded in 1913, and from

1921 began to collect its own statistical material on injuries and accidents at home, work and on the road. From 1927, reporting of accident statistics became a regular feature of *National Safety News*. These reports highlighted the home and automobile as 'hazardous' locations, emphasizing that certain people were considerably more likely to have multiple similar accidents than others.[78] Their reports did not tend to draw any particular conclusions, suggesting merely that impulsiveness or carelessness might explain this. Menninger, of course, did not believe this defence, for,

> after all, if one permits himself to so far relinquish interest in his own personal safety in favor of contemplating the stock market or the purchase of a new dress, one is certainly paying self-destructive indifference to reality.[79]

This conclusion expanded the individual blame for any event: a person involved in an accident was no longer merely the victim but also the perpetrator. The 'purposive accident' became a national problem, of economics and medicine:

> The National Safety Council computes the economic cost of accidental deaths, injuries and motor vehicle damage to be approximately three and a half billion dollars a year. It would surprise many people to know that more men die daily in accidents than from any single disease except heart disease ... Every five minutes someone is killed in the United States in an accident and while one is being killed in an accident a hundred others are being injured.[80]

This statement was very much of its time. Statistical analysis of accidents was not possible before the growth of the insurance industry in the nineteenth century. In addition, it was only with the declining rate of infectious disease in the early twentieth century that the proportion of deaths through accidents became more visible. Menninger's concern over the cost was another factor of the insurance model, which enabled a price to be put on damage caused by accidents.

These factors (including ownership of motor cars) were still quite new in the 1930s, and thus it was an emerging concern that Karl Menninger quickly adopted as a cause for psychoanalysis. For, while plans were under way for 'reducing accidental hazards in industry, traffic, agricultural life, and in the home', none of these, according to Menninger, took into account the original self-destructive drive that lay behind 'purposive accidents'.[81] If policymakers and safety legislators did not take the death instinct into account, they would have no success in managing the problem. This, then, was the overall purpose of *Man Against Himself*. Social change, according to Menninger, should begin with the individual – just as treatment did in psychiatry. This gave psychiatrists an important role in the process. Psychiatrists and sociologists needed to work together to understand and solve social problems, approaching them from the psychological study of the individual as well as principles of mass action. This potential collaboration was highlighted, in *Man Against Himself*, by the looming threat of what became the Second World War. It was the shadow of war, Menninger concluded, that would prove psychiatry's worth in understanding the self-destructive nature of mankind. While today we might be sceptical of the breadth of Menninger's conception of self-destruction, we should recognize that in the final years of the interwar period, his arguments for self-mutilation as an illustration of a universal destructive tendency would have seemed far more compelling.

In conclusion, psychoanalytic approaches to self-mutilation uncritically incorporated various elements of Victorian and Edwardian ideas on the topic, including the relationship with hysteria, the concept of malingering, and the idea that exploring self-harm might shed greater light on the human condition more generally. American psychoanalysts also offered a new twist on Victorian concerns, reinterpreting the relationship of self-harm to sexuality. In addition, the psychoanalytic approach, in the work of Karl Menninger, vastly expanded the field of what could be understood as self-mutilation. Both Emerson and Menninger offered universal explanations for self-harm, couched in a Freudian framework: first of psychosexual trauma, and then of the death instinct. Unlike in Europe, where much psychoanalytic practice tended to focus on symbolic mutilations (the 'castration complex', for example), American analysts incorporated literal acts of bodily injury into their practice. The practical nature of U.S. psychiatry in this era suggested this extrapolation from the symbolic to the actual, moving self-harm from a psychiatric symptom to something that might explain human drives more generally, in particular sexuality and a desire for death.

These universal explanations for self-harm – in particular, Menninger's views – have been picked up unreflectively in later decades. However, they need to be viewed within the context of the period in which they were developed. Both explanations were dependent on American social and cultural values and wider concerns of the period in which they emerged. Emerson posited a social view of self-harm and female sexuality. For him, self-mutilation was the emergence in the adult of childhood psychosexual trauma, an explanation that influenced negative views of the family seen in later decades. The family increasingly became the focus of mental pathology, as described in the following chapter. However, the way Emerson understood psychosexual experiences was not the same as a modern understanding of trauma (see Chapter Seven). Instead, Emerson considered that early sexual experiences hastened and increased the sexualization of the individual, an acceptance of the prevailing social view of the dangerously hypersexual woman. Emerson was not alone in this view, which was widespread in early twentieth-century thinking about female hysteria, particularly but not only in the United States. However, by emphasizing the individual nature of these conflicts, his analyses also served to shift the focus from perpetrator to victim, making female sexuality (and not childhood sexual abuse) the defining factor behind self-inflicted injury. As in the case of Katharine Peach in *Don't Monkey with Murder*, self-harm was associated with individual taint and not wider social circumstances, suggesting the need for a pejorative approach.

Menninger offered an even more internalized view of self-harm, regarding the conflict between life and death instincts in the individual as responsible for a vast number of self-destructive behaviours. Here, outside experiences had almost no bearing, or only in so far as they exacerbated internal conflict. Indeed, Menninger even related major social and political events to individual conflicts. This served to promote psychoanalysis by emphasizing the importance of beginning with the psyche. However, it also sat within a contemporary American world view that laid responsibility for all life experiences with the individual. Menninger's view of self-harm as an aggressive act increased this censorious approach, assuming individual guilt without the need for evidence. While Menninger himself would certainly have argued that the patients he encountered – even those described as malingerers – were to be supported rather than vilified, his model was nonetheless a departure even from the loose social context in Emerson's cases. The cases of self-inflicted injury outlined in *Man Against Himself* became cast solely in terms of individual responsibility. There was certainly a wider political purpose to this claim. His anti-war articles and speeches suggest that Menninger genuinely saw recognition of the death instinct as the only possible way to improve an unpleasant and dangerous world. Nonetheless, the legacy of psychoanalysis has largely been that of an internalized and individual understanding of self-harm. This was adopted uncritically, alongside elements of both the hypersexual and aggressive explanations of self-injury, in the next model for discussion: delicate self-cutting.

SIX

DELICATE SELF-CUTTING
Schizophrenia and the 'Borderline' in Post-war North America

In 1948, aged just sixteen, the novelist Joanne Greenberg was admitted to Chestnut Lodge Hospital in Rockville, Maryland. Diagnosed with schizophrenia, Joanne spent the next three years in hospital, under the treatment of psychoanalyst Frieda Fromm-Reichmann. She remained an outpatient at Chestnut Lodge until 1955, continuing therapy with Fromm-Reichmann after her return to college. Greenberg was eventually discharged cured and, now in her eighties, has reported that she has remained in good mental health throughout her life. In 1964 she published a fictionalized account of her experiences, *I Never Promised You a Rose Garden*, under the pseudonym Hannah Green. The book was not intended as a case study or psychiatric profile, but as a 'hymn to reality': to depict the real experience of schizophrenia and the potential for recovery through a trusting relationship with a 'gifted therapist'.[1] *Rose Garden* suggested several ways of understanding self-injury from the viewpoint of patient, doctor and relative. In the novel, Esther Blau, the mother of Deborah (the Greenberg character), describes her daughter's actions as 'silly and theatrical wrist-cutting'. This 'childish attempt at suicide', the reader is told, had 'given all their [Deborah's parents'] nebulous feelings and vague fears weight', and led directly to Deborah's hospitalization.[2]

In the decade in which *Rose Garden* was published, 'wrist-cutting' underwent a significant shift in meaning in American psychiatry, contributed to by practitioners at Chestnut Lodge. In the later 1960s, these practitioners began to focus intently on this particular form of injury: cutting or scratching the skin. Self-cutting was not emphasized in any previous models of self-harm discussed in this book, although it was included in some of them, most notably the psychoanalytic approach outlined in the previous chapter. Most of those writing on self-cutting in the 1960s came from a psychoanalytic background, and they similarly attributed psychological meaning to physically damaging behaviours. Many claimed novelty for their approach, which distinguished 'delicate self-cutting' (as Chestnut Lodge's director, Ping-Nie Pao, labelled it in 1969) from suicidal behaviour.[3] They supported this argument with Erwin Stengel's contemporary work on attempted suicide, which claimed that it resulted from a very different psychological mindset from completed suicide. Stengel was working in Britain and thus, while I focus on North America in this chapter, I also highlight many transatlantic links. Psychiatrists working at this time tended to ignore or downplay cultural and political differences between Britain and the United States, and this meant that approaches were often transposed from one location to another, without questioning their applicability.

I begin with attempted suicide, which, in the work of Stengel and others, returned to prominence in this era. Self-harm was once again separated from suicidal behaviour but, in this instance, through a focus on attempted suicide. Self-poisoning became newly incorporated into definitions of self-harm, particularly in Britain. I contrast this approach with several autobiographical accounts of self-injurious behaviour from the 1940s and '50s. In these fictionalized accounts, self-destructive behaviour was presented as, often simultaneously, a suicidal gesture and a psychotic symptom. By 1967, medical writers had created a divide between these two concepts, and I go on to explore how this led to the category of 'delicate self-cutting'. Despite this shift in thinking, both the work of Sylvia Plath and Joanne Greenberg, whose fictionalized accounts are explored in the first part of this chapter, were used in support of this new 'syndrome'. The 1960s was the first time self-cutting had been singled out as a paradigm for self-harm. The North American medical writers who created this definition were mostly psychoanalysts. They viewed self-cutting as a psychotic symptom, associated either with schizophrenia or the emerging diagnosis of the 'borderline'. They admitted that their patients could 'pass' as normal between psychotic episodes, but nonetheless saw them as requiring intensive inpatient treatment.[4]

Borderline personality disorder was, in its early years as a diagnosis, closely linked to psychosis. However, the association of self-cutting with schizophrenia was fairly short-lived. The final section of this chapter explores the ways in which the definition of self-cutting shifted from being seen as evidence of psychosis to a symptom of a newly defined 'borderline personality' (no longer associated with schizophrenia) in the third edition of the American Psychiatric Association's *Diagnostic and Statistical Manual* (*DSM-III*). This view was the result of a struggle for dominance in American psychiatry in the 1960s and '70s, between psychoanalytically oriented practitioners and neo-Kraepelinian descriptive psychiatrists.[5] The neo-Kraepelinians tended to promote medication over psychotherapy and offered a biological (and frequently pessimistic) model of chronic mental illness. They appeared to win the struggle with the widespread acceptance of the *DSM-III*, in which self-harm became incorporated for the first time into a biomedical system. The complicated route by which this happened, however, as outlined below in this chapter, raises many questions about the relevance of this and later approaches to 'non-suicidal self-injury' in American psychiatry.

The suicidal gesture: 'I don't care whether I live or die'

In the summer of 1953, Sylvia Plath's mother took her twenty-year-old daughter to the family doctor, after noticing several partially healed cuts on her legs. When she asked her daughter about them, the young poet informed her mother that she 'just wanted to see if she had the guts' and that she wished to die.[6] In her semi-autobiographical novel *The Bell Jar*, Plath described the infliction of a similar cut wound as a kind of rehearsal for suicide:

Then I thought, maybe I ought to spill a little blood for practice . . .
I felt nothing. Then I felt a small, deep thrill, and a bright seam of
red welled up at the lip of the slash. The blood gathered darkly, like
fruit, and rolled down my ankle into the cup of my black patent
leather shoe.[7]

The Bell Jar was published just a few weeks before Plath's death by suicide at
the age of thirty. Like Greenberg, she used a pseudonym (Victoria Lucas).
Because of the poet's death, as well as a previous near-fatal suicide attempt
that led to her admission to a psychiatric hospital in 1953 (described in the
novel), readers had no trouble interpreting Plath's self-injurious behaviour
as part of an inexorable path towards suicide.

This was also the case before the poet's death, despite the emergence in
the 1950s of a new concept of attempted suicide as a 'cry for help'. Plath
herself explicitly rejected the view of attempted suicide as communication.
The suicide attempt in *The Bell Jar* is explained in painstaking detail: 'I
knew just how to go about it,' the protagonist declares, describing how she
took a glass of water and a bottle of sleeping pills into a neglected crawl
space in the cellar of the family home, blocking herself in with rotting
fireplace logs.[8] In real life, it was three days before Plath was found, by
accident, when her groans were overheard by her brother.[9] The literary
critic Al Alvarez, whose study of suicide *The Savage God* began with an
account of his friendship with Plath in her final years, noted that the poet
was wryly detached when she spoke of suicide: 'It was obviously a matter
of self-respect that her first attempt had been serious and nearly successful,
instead of a mere hysterical gesture.'[10] Like Sylvia herself, Alvarez rejected
the notion that Plath's suicide attempt was a cry for help. His words also
reflected the gendered notions found in the early twentieth-century
assumption that 'hysterical' women were emotionally manipulative and
deceitful, an idea he wished to disassociate from Plath. Despite this,
Alvarez considered Plath's later suicide as at least partly a cry for help that
tragically backfired, as well as 'a last desperate attempt to exorcize the death
she had summoned up in her poems'.[11]

The association of the term 'cry for help' with Plath's attempted and final suicide, whether as a rejected concept or partial explanation, reflected a new approach to suicide advanced in this era. It is impossible to explain the concept of 'delicate self-cutting' without understanding the background in shifting approaches to suicide. As we have seen in Chapter Two, debate on the social, economic, religious and cultural implications of suicide has a long history. In the 1950s, however, suicide was still a crime in Britain (it was not decriminalized until 1961). In London, psychiatrist Erwin Stengel began to study attempted suicide as a topic in itself, rather than viewing it as a means of gathering information about the possible causes of suicide. Stengel defined suicide attempts as a specific behaviour pattern. Given that only about one in eight resulted in death, he decided that death was not necessarily the 'purpose' of a suicide attempt, and that many were carried out instead 'in the mood "I don't care whether I live or die"'.[12]

It is not, of course, the case that all psychologists, psychiatrists or sociologists before Stengel read attempted suicides solely as 'failed' attempts at death: indeed, Freud and his circle had discussed many potential reasons for suicide, only one of which was the individual's desire to die. One important distinction made by Stengel, however, was that *survival* made the suicide attempt, whatever the motivation, 'a different behaviour pattern from suicide and a meaningful and often momentous event in a person's life'.[13] Al Alvarez considered his attempted suicide a pivotal moment in his existence. For years, he had thought that suicide would be some kind of 'answer' to the ongoing struggles of his life:

> I had expected death not merely to end it [despair] but also to explain it. Then, when death let me down, I gradually saw that I had been using the wrong language ... I no longer thought of myself as unhappy; instead I had 'problems'. Which is an optimistic way of putting it, since problems imply solutions ... Once I had accepted that there weren't ever going to be any answers, even in death, I found to my surprise that I didn't much care whether I was happy or unhappy.

Alvarez blamed 'Americanization' for his way of looking at suicide: an internalized, psychotherapeutic view of the world caused by 'too many movies, too many novels, too many trips to the States'.[14]

This cultural view of psychoanalysis in which psychotherapy became a lifestyle has certainly become associated with 1960s and '70s America – epitomized in film by the work of Woody Allen. However, this psychological view of suicide was not necessarily peculiarly American. Indeed, in this chapter we shall see an increasing overlap in transatlantic views of self-inflicted injury, despite certain national differences. British writers, including Stengel, tended towards a wider, psycho-social view of suicide than their American counterparts. Nonetheless, they also emphasized the individual patient's immediate social interactions (in particular, romantic and family relationships), rather than environmental or political circumstances. Specific social relationships were viewed, perhaps for the first time, as the most significant indicators of a person's mental health. Indeed, this interest in interpersonal relationships in psychiatric circles was a necessary precursor to the understanding of attempted suicide as a form of communication. In his work on the 'forgotten cry for help', Chris Millard has

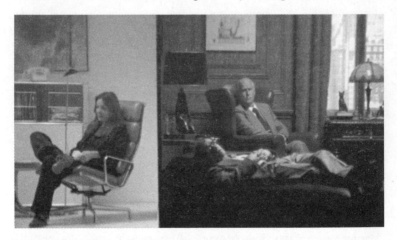

Psychoanalysis was famously portrayed throughout Woody Allen's film *Annie Hall* (1977). In this scene, the protagonists Annie and Alvy simultaneously visit their therapists and discuss differing perspectives on their relationship.

explained how an 'epidemic' of attempted suicide in Britain in the years after 1945 was interpreted in this manner. This 'cry for help' was associated with self-poisoning and overdosing, particularly when carried out by young people, most often women. Millard traces two reasons for the emergence of the concept at this time: first, in Britain, the incorporation of mental health care into a National Health Service, which increased the psychological scrutiny on general hospital patients. Second, he acknowledged a shift in psychiatric thought, with an increasing emphasis on socially focused models of mental health: in particular, a view of mental illness as caused by interpersonal relations. This was supported by a new system of psychiatric social work, set up in Britain in the late 1920s and early 1930s to emulate the American system described in the previous chapter.

Millard's work has focused on overdosing and cutting. He described a significant shift from the view of self-poisoning as communicative in the post-war years to an individualized, regulatory model of self-harm focused on cutting, which emerged in the 1980s in Britain. In addition to the changes in health care outlined above, Millard viewed these two models as more broadly representative of a shift in political emphasis. This changed from a 'collective, communicative and socially embedded' model, epitomized by the welfare state and nationalized industry in post-war Britain, to the rise of an 'individualised understanding of human beings as competitive and market-driven' in the 1980s. Thus, between the 1950s and the 1980s, the 'archetypal meaning' of self-harm shifted from 'self-poisoning as communication, to self-cutting (and burning) as emotional control'.[15] In Millard's view, this was indicated by the removal of overdosing or self-poisoning from late twentieth-century definitions of self-harm or self-injury. Most recently, *DSM-5* described non-suicidal self-injury (NSSI) as intentional damage to the surface of the body, emphasizing cutting and burning over overdosing. Armando Favazza, author of one of the most influential works on self-harm in the 1980s, has commented, 'the definition of NSSI is problematic: the Brits include overdoses but the Americans don't.'[16] Favazza views this as a lack of clarity in defining the syndrome; however, the history of self-harm in Britain indicates a more complex reason for this difference. This also suggests that the shift in focus may not have been neat or decisive; instead several models continued to function alongside each other in later twentieth-century Britain, and even the United States.

Plath did not describe any of Esther's self-injurious acts in *The Bell Jar* as communicative. However, the responses to Esther's (and Plath's own) suicide attempt – evaluation in general hospital before transfer to the psychiatric wing, and then to a private psychiatric hospital – followed a similar pattern to that described by Millard in a British context. In her novel, Plath described Esther's self-cutting as a rehearsal for her overdose. Indeed, the omission of Plath's real-life encounter with her mother over the wounds on her legs served to diminish the presentation of self-injury as a socially embedded behaviour, even though, to the reader, the overdose might appear to have served such a purpose. Esther's suicide attempt seems to have precipitated her recovery from a breakdown, as she finally receives the recognition and help her mother had repeatedly refused to believe she needed. Previously, Mrs Greenwood could not believe her daughter was like 'those awful dead people at that hospital' (a psychiatric facility).[17] Indeed, despite this shift in emphasis, textbooks and studies continued to regard overdosing and other forms of self-injury as a comparable 'form of language' into the 1980s.[18]

Deborah's self-inflicted injuries in *Rose Garden*, meanwhile, indicate even further the complexity of regarding self-inflicted injury as, first and foremost, a communicative practice. As in *The Bell Jar*, Deborah has been perceived not as sick but 'just unhappy' by her parents until she cuts her wrists.[19] Yet, within the hospital, Deborah's self-mutilation (cutting and burning her arms with cigarettes) is regarded as the outward sign of a worsening mental condition; a psychotic break that twice leads directly to the teenager's transfer to the 'Disturbed Ward'. On the first occasion, she draws the top of a tin can down her upper arm, 'until the inside of the arm was a gory swath'. The nurses ponder this act with interest, viewing it as evidence that the 'kid was really sick' after all, and not just a 'spoiled little rich kid'.[20] Deborah's mother also sees her burns as a sign of worsening

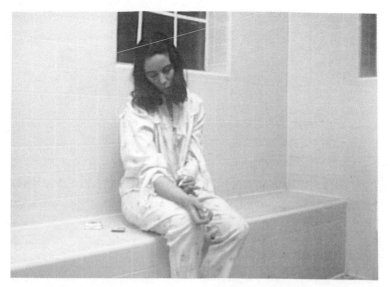

One of several depictions of Deborah Blau's self-injurious acts in the film of
I Never Promised You a Rose Garden (1977).

illness, showing that, in hospital, Deborah only 'gets sicker and more violent all the time'.

In *Rose Garden*, self-cutting is not singled out for particular relevance,
although the later burning is explained in much more detail. Here, Dr
Fried, Deborah's psychoanalyst, suggests an explanation cast in shared
understanding. Since Deborah burned herself during Dr Fried's absence
on vacation, the psychiatrist suggests that 'maybe you got in this bad shape
to tell me how angry you are that I went off and left you.'[21] In Dr Fried's
view, Deborah's burning is an attempt to punish another (the therapist)
and to communicate anger and betrayal – it is rooted in psychoanalytic
understandings of separation anxiety. The suggestion focuses on the psychoanalytic approach to self-mutilation and suicidal behaviour as rooted
in interpersonal conflict. This is related to Menninger's view, outlined in
the previous chapter, that the desire to kill is the most important drive to
suicide: the individual identifies himself with a person who has thwarted or
disappointed him and attempts to destroy that person by harming himself.

In real life, Frieda Fromm-Reichmann (the model for Dr Fried) believed that cultural forces shaped the lives of people experiencing psychosis just as much as anyone else. When Freud developed his ideas, the repression of sexuality had been an important cultural problem, she thought, but in mid-century America, where people were much more able to talk openly about sexual issues, it was the shadow cast by two world wars that was of far greater importance. 'Hostility, antagonism and malevolence', she wrote in her textbook, *Principles of Intensive Psychotherapy* (1953), are 'more subject to disapproval in our Western culture, therefore to more repression, than any other unacceptable brand of human behaviour'. In Fromm-Reichmann's view, people in the 1950s were much more likely to turn their anger and hatred inward than had been the case previously: 'an attempt to counterbalance' the destruction of war.[22] One of these examples appeared in *Rose Garden*, perhaps a case Greenberg had discussed with Fromm-Reichmann. Dr Fried recounted 'a patient who used to practice the most horrible tortures on himself', pre-empting the things he expected the world to do to him. This, he told his doctor, made him 'master of my own destruction'. Yet the world, it seemed, was worse even than the imaginings of the mentally ill. The patient got well, and 'then the Nazis came and they put him into Dachau and he died there.'[23]

This post-war sense of the futility of aggression appears to have been a shared one between doctor, patient and relative. However, describing Deborah's self-harm as an effort to communicate her anger and frustration could not convey the complexity of her world. As she puts it, 'Furii [Dr Fried] was wrong about the reason for the burning and the need for it, and most wrong about its seriousness.'[24] If Deborah regards her self-burning as a means of communication, it is not to her doctors that she is trying to speak but the gods of Yr, the kingdom whose rules she believes she is bound to follow. The first time she burns herself, the act is suggested to her by 'Idat, the Dissembler' as a way of easing her pain and anger:

Deborah perceived that by burning she could set a backfire that would assuage the burning kiln of the volcano, all the doors and vents of which were closed and barricaded. And by this same burning she could prove to herself finally whether or not she was truly made of human substance. Her senses offered no proof; vision was a gray blur; hearing merely muffled roars and groans, meaningless half the time; feeling was blunted, too.[25]

Here, self-harm becomes a response to the fear induced by the symptoms of illness: a proof she is alive, as well as a way to communicate with Yr. Deborah is nonetheless scared by the escalating burning. When offered a return to B ward, she fears that the increased freedom will give her the opportunity to burn herself to death, and so she reveals her hidden self-harm as a way of remaining on D ward. Interestingly, communicating through self-inflicted injury is described as a two-way process. It is a new doctor, unaware of Deborah's wounds, who notes that her improvement will mean a quick return to B ward. Deborah interprets this as his giving her permission to die, an opinion confirmed by his leaving a burning cigarette behind on his departure: an apparent hypocrisy between his words and actions.

The context of Sylvia Plath's and Joanne Greenberg's fictionalized accounts of self-inflicted injury and suicidal behaviour differed considerably from those described by Millard. Unlike the new British National Health Service, founded in 1948 with the intention of providing equal access to health care for every citizen, both Plath and Greenberg received treatment in private American hospitals, in a system dominated (at that time) by the internalized individualized approach of psychoanalysis. Yet there were also certain similarities between the British and American models that led to a broadly shared understanding of self-inflicted injury in the medical realm as communicative. Thus, while the institutional model in the United States in the 1950s was not identical to that in Britain, certain elements that emphasized suicidal 'gestures' as part of a socially embedded model of mental illness were present. In the next section, we see how this understanding was incorporated into and altered by the new view of 'delicate self-cutting' in the 1960s.

Wrist-cutting: the meaning of a gesture

If Plath and Greenberg fitted only loosely within the concept of the 'cry for help', some patients were more explicit about their efforts to communicate through self-harm. In 1952, the young artist William Kurelek arrived at the Maudsley Hospital in south London. The Ukrainian-Canadian had, he later reported, gone to London with two specific purposes: to finish art school, and to find a cure for his chronic depression. A day after arriving from Canada, the 25-year-old turned up at the Maudsley, where he was almost immediately interviewed by a doctor, found temporary lodgings nearby and given a date to be moved into hospital for observation. Nevertheless, a short stay at the Maudsley didn't give Kurelek the resolution he longed for. After being discharged to the outpatient service, he travelled in Europe and briefly worked as a labourer, continuing his psychotherapy and trying to realize himself as an artist. Bitter and angry with his doctor, the young artist wrote demanding letters, some of which were later reproduced in his autobiography: 'It's not enough just to *know* what my problem is,' he declared, frustrated by the long psychotherapy; '*SOMETHING HAS TO BE DONE.*'[26]

Kurelek returned to Canada after his psychiatric treatment in Britain, where he found recognition as an artist and wrote his autobiography many years later. Thus, while his experiences with British psychiatry were in some ways quite different from the psychoanalytic views on the other side of the Atlantic, his story provides an interesting bridge between British and North American approaches to self-harm. When his 'smiling, serene' psychiatrist Dr Cormier refused to react to his frustration, Kurelek described his efforts to 'break this stalemate' himself:

> In the loneliness of my room, I decided that violence against myself was the only way I could attract attention. Having planned it all carefully beforehand, I exposed my arm up to my elbow on the evening before the next interview and, with a new razor blade, made a series of cuts from the wrist up. Then I reverently bound up the arm

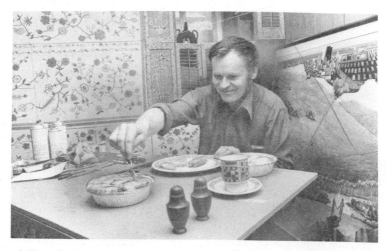

William Kurelek in Canada, 1972, serving himself traditional Ukrainian cabbage rolls and surrounded by art materials.

with bandages to soak up what blood came out of these cuts, which were actually superficial . . . Now at last I had something concrete and obviously serious to show Dr Cormier. And I did. He blanched, but showed little or no evidence of panic, enquiring instead into the circumstances of my deed. A day or so later I was invited by the hospital to re-enter as an in-patient.[27]

This account, written some years later, reads with surprising frankness. Starkly different from Plath's and Alvarez's determination not to have their suicide attempts interpreted as 'hysterical gestures', Kurelek was open about his conscious decision to manipulate his doctors in order to receive the treatment he required. The account was, of course, written retrospectively; the logical, careful process may or may not have been quite so considered at the time. There was also no particular indication, in Britain, that Kurelek's injuries were seen as holding any deeper meaning. What was clear, however, was that Kurelek – and, seemingly, his doctors – considered self-harm as a clear, external indicator of the seriousness of his mental state, even though the wounds themselves were 'superficial'.

The word superficial brings to mind the 'delicate self-cutting' articles referred to earlier. Many of these used the same term to describe the injuries observed in psychiatric inpatients: as Ping-Nie Pao put it, wounds were often 'superficial, delicate, carefully designed incisions'.[28] Kurelek's act pre-dated this model; his autobiography did not, however, and may well have been interpreted in light of later attention to 'wrist-cutting' in the 1960s. In 1967, at least six studies were published on the topic and a symposium was held at Chestnut Lodge Hospital.[29] The terms used to describe self-injuring patients varied, from 'wrist-cutter' to 'wrist-slasher', and descriptions were often blunt and even derogatory. Harold Graff and Richard Mallin, for example (taking their lead from Stengel's differentiation between suicide and attempted suicide), distinguished 'the person who makes an isolated suicidal gesture from the chronic "cutter" . . . Cutters slash themselves at the slightest provocation, stirring the hospital into a turmoil.'[30] This phrasing immediately marked out 'cutters' as problem patients, having a serious impact not only on their own bodies but also on those around them – staff and other patients alike. Menninger's earlier contention, of course, had been that 'malingerers' desired the hostility of those around them as part of their self-punishment. In the 'delicate cutting' articles, however, this element appears to have been lost from the discussion. Self-cutting hospital patients became simply troublesome.

Critiques of these articles have emerged in recent years on a variety of levels. Armando Favazza initially reported them as 'pioneering studies [that] helped to shed light on the characteristics of cutters and the reasons for their behavior', although more recently he has noted that the number of reports was too limited for 'delicate self-cutting' to be considered a model and it 'totally ignored all the other types of self-harm'.[31] Indeed, these articles emphasized 'self-cutting' as the primary form of self-inflicted injury, despite reporting many other types of self-harm, and the words 'cutting' and 'slashing' were used interchangeably with 'mutilation'.[32] However, we also cannot assume that this new 'identity' was imposed from above: the label of 'cutter', 'slasher', 'slicer' or 'scratcher' was claimed to have been adopted by patients and staff alike.[33] This identification was picked up on the jacket

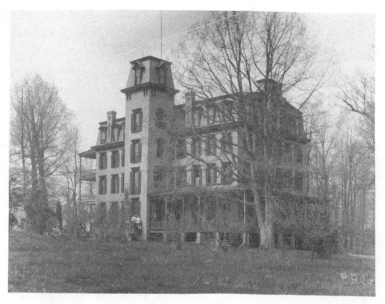

Woodlawn Hotel, Rockville, Maryland, c. 1900. In 1910, this building became Chestnut Lodge Hospital.

of journalist Marilee Strong's influential *A Bright Red Scream*, published in 1998: 'They call themselves "cutters" – and this book is their story.'[34]

It was in the 1960s, then, that 'self-cutting' emerged as the primary form of self-inflicted injury. Even where other behaviours were described (as in almost all the 'delicate cutting' articles), they were nonetheless used to support conclusions drawn about cutting. In one of his articles from 1967, Harold Graff, psychiatrist at the private Institute of Pennsylvania Hospital, even referred to what was then believed to be a fictional example in *I Never Promised You a Rose Garden* to support his theory. In the novel, 'Deborah would burn herself repeatedly with cigarettes and matches, feeling no pain, and would seek opportunities to burn herself. *The slasher does exactly the same thing*.'[35] Here, Graff reinterpreted the fictional Deborah Blau as evidence of his findings about 'wrist-slashers', emphasizing self-cutting as the 'primary' example of multiple forms of self-harm (even though, as Graff's phrasing indicates, cutting was *not* emphasized over and above other forms of self-injury in *Rose Garden*). Pao used the same example to support the retrospective interpretation of Emerson's 'Miss A' (discussed in the previous chapter) as a delicate cutter.[36] Similarly, Sylvia Plath's poem 'Cut' was used in other articles on the 'syndrome', although it appeared to describe a quite different circumstance.

Why did the reports emphasize this particular behaviour, to the exclusion of all others? The number of clinicians writing about 'delicate cutting' was fairly small and psychoanalytically orientated. Most worked in private psychiatric facilities on the East Coast of the United States: in New York, Pennsylvania and Massachusetts, as well as Maryland. This was a focus of psychoanalytic thought in the u.s. at this time, with the New York and Washington–Baltimore schools vying for dominance. As we shall see in the next section, psychoanalysis in America in the 1960s and '70s was also battling against a resurgence of descriptive psychiatry, taking its lead from turn-of-the-century German clinician Emil Kraepelin (neo-Kraepelinian thought) and the advent of medication and somatic therapies. Self-cutting was an example of a 'gesture' that was externally and dramatically visible, but could be interpreted as having internal psychoanalytic significance. The 'wrist-cutting' emphasis associated these articles with contemporary literature on suicide, while blood and pain had particular psychodynamic meaning.[37] Thus, the articles in this period repeatedly stressed the 'syndrome' as characterized by 'wrist-slashing', despite supporting these arguments with case studies showing a variety of very different self-injurious behaviours (only some of which involved cutting) on almost every part of the body.

In addition, these studies portrayed a very specific, gendered model of self-harm. This is particularly surprising if we take, as has often been assumed, a 1960 article by Daniel Offer and Peter Barglow as the start of the self-cutting literature. Offer and Barglow described an 'epidemic' of self-mutilation in an adolescent and young adult hospital setting.[38] This involved twelve patients, most of whom lacerated themselves with razor blades, and was regarded as unusual in comparison to the occasional cases of self-inflicted injury encountered in previous years. The article focused on the best way of managing the problem (preventing self-injury), through therapy, group meetings, increased activities and controls, including the transfer of patients with a history of self-mutilation. The Offer and Barglow report, however, is remarkable in that it did *not* make any claim towards a gendered model of self-cutting – quite unlike the later, 'delicate cutting' reports. Of the twelve patients involved in the episode, four were male and eight female, and the number and types of injuries were not described as varying by gender. Although two-thirds of the small sample were female, Offer and Barglow did not consider this of wider relevance, and concentrated on diagnosis rather than gender. In stark contrast, Graff and Mallin (1967) declared:

> the typical cutter was an attractive young woman, age 23, usually quite intelligent. More than half had attended college. Three-quarters were unmarried, although most of them were old enough to be married.

The sample of 21 patients included one man, 'a 56-year-old dentist, [who] was excluded from the study because we felt he was atypical'. The oldest female patient, at 42, might equally have been considered atypical – she was by no means a young woman, after all. However, as gender was considered the primary emphasis by the authors, she remained included, despite diverging from the profile.

In the vast majority of self-cutting articles in this period, men were excluded from populations under study because they were not considered 'typical', thus creating a self-fulfilling prophecy. In one paper, from 1972, almost a third of the small sample under study was ignored for this reason: 'We also interviewed 11 male patients who were hospitalized during this period and who had histories of wrist cutting, but the findings were so different from those of the women that they will be presented in a separate paper.'[39] The separate study was not published, further emphasizing self-cutting as a 'female' behaviour. The samples discussed in these studies were almost all from private psychiatric hospitals, in which female patients predominated.[40] Pao's sample from Chestnut Lodge included 24 female patients (75 per cent of the group studied) and eight male (25 per cent). At first glance this seems like a significant difference, despite the small size of the sample. However, in a study on therapy at Chestnut Lodge published a decade earlier, 66 per cent of patients at the hospital were female (182 out of 275).[41] With such an overall gender ratio, we would expect 21 or 22 of Pao's group of 'cutters' to be female anyway. The small size of the sample means that the slightly higher proportion found by Pao could easily be put down to chance.

Pao used another strategy to emphasize the 'female' nature of cutting: he divided his group into 'delicate' and 'coarse' cutters. The latter, he claimed, made single, deep and life-threatening incisions, while the wounds of the former were superficial. Neither group were necessarily suicidal. However, 'of the five coarse cutters, four were male and one female, whereas 23 of the 27 delicate cutters were female' (85 per cent).[42] The use of the term 'delicate' was another means of gendering the act of cutting, and the adoption of Pao's term elsewhere served to perpetuate the notion of cutting as feminine.[43] This depiction of 'delicate cutting' as female relied on prior notions of female pathology: indeed, we encountered this very idea in the early twentieth-century reports on 'hysterical mutilations' and 'motiveless malingering' in Chapter Four. This suggests that many of the notions supporting the 1960s model of self-harm as specifically *female* self-cutting relied on prior male assumptions about female behaviour. While most articles criticized assumptions made by staff that cutters were solely or primarily 'attention-seeking', they continued to use the same language to describe the acts.[44]

Similarly, the 'normal feminine masochism' outlined in early psycho-analytic approaches to self-harm also reappeared as explanation. Robert C. Burnham, at the Chestnut Lodge Symposium on Impulsive Self-mutilation, assumed this 'natural' masochism to be a factor behind 'delicate self-cutting' as a syndrome, despite acknowledging that it didn't explain 'why it fails to have more appeal for masochistic males'.[45] This idea of the 'naturally' passive and masochistic female, a staple of Victorian medicine, has been extensively critiqued in feminist literature, yet it is remarkable how much currency the notion still has, particularly in modern understandings of self-harm. Psychiatrists in the 1960s often gave short shrift to their female patients' efforts to locate their distress in wider social or political disadvantage. When Miss B complained to Pao that she had been turned down for certain roles due to being female and spoke of 'job disadvantage', he declared that this was 'not a reality'.[46] The United States government implemented an Equal Pay Act in 1963 (followed by the UK in 1970), while the Civil Rights Act of 1964 aimed to protect employees against discrimination on the basis of gender, race or religion. This legislation did not, of course, end discrimination: a 2005 estimate reported that women's wages had risen from 62 per cent of men's in 1979 to 80 per cent in 2004, while informal discrimination still occurs today.[47]

Pao's situating of Miss B's frustration purely in an internal struggle with her own sexuality was very much a part of the psychoanalytic realm in which he worked. As we have seen in the previous chapter, psychology was already emphasized over and above sociological and environmental influences in the United States in the 1920s and '30s. By the 1960s, this might be to the complete exclusion of wider influences or reinterpretation of them as evidence of the patient's behaviour or state of mind. While this approach emerged from a psychoanalytic and psychological context, an even more blinkered view was adopted within a neo-Kraepelinian framework, which regarded unusual or deviant acts first and foremost as evidence of biological disease, and their content as largely meaningless. This shift in American psychiatry, from a psychoanalytic to a neo-Kraepelinian view of self-harm, can be seen most strongly in the concept of the 'borderline', the topic of the final part of this chapter.

First, I want to return to William Kurelek, whose story conflicted with many of the assumptions in the 'delicate cutting' literature. Most notably, of course, Kurelek was male but, rather than being suicidal or one of Pao's 'coarse cutters', he inflicted superficial injuries on himself. He also claimed that these had been for a specific purpose at a time he felt he had been failed by mental health care. His experiences were a world away from those of the psychoanalytic inpatient 'cutters' in North America. A few months after his first reported episode of self-harm, the artist was transferred to Netherne Psychiatric Hospital, near Croydon. Netherne had almost two thousand patients and, 'isolated out there in the country' with its 'fenced-in

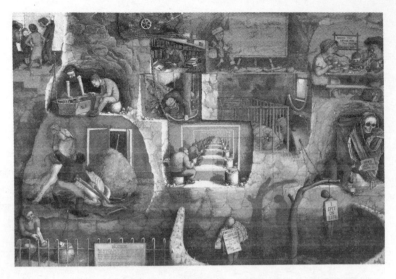

William Kurelek, *I Spit On Life*, c. 1956. Painted while at Netherne Hospital, this is one of Kurelek's bleakest works. The artist can be seen cutting into his own arm in the bottom left of the painting, beside a mocking sign noting that 'these animals have self-pitying suicidal tendancies [sic], visitors are requested not to humour their egoism'.

villas' but 'the security of an indefinite stay', it was a very different place from the forward-thinking Maudsley Hospital.[48] Yet the placid immovability of the psychiatric system and its staff continued to frustrate Kurelek, spurring him on to further acts of self-injury, including cross-hatching the inside of his arm with a razor blade. Kurelek described his self-injury openly as a desperate plea, founded in his long-held belief in the potential efficacy of psychiatry: one of the first paintings he completed after arriving at Netherne was called simply *HELP ME PLEASE HELP ME PLEASE HELP ME – PLEASE HELP*. A few days after his doctor failed to respond to his new injuries, the young artist took eight sleeping pills and lacerated his face and arms. In retrospect, he was

> no longer [able to] remember how much of my 'suicide' was a form of protest and how much real conviction. The self-mutilation that went with it would suggest it was a mixed-up brew of the two motives.[49]

A mixture of protest, despair and appeal, Kurelek's acts were not quite the 'cry for help' outlined by British psychiatrists in the 1960s, but nor was this the depersonalized, aggressive and semi-manipulative 'delicate self-cutting' described by their American counterparts.

Borderline personalities: sensation-seeking but 'nearly normal'

In 1967, the year that the first 'delicate cutting' articles were published, eighteen-year-old Susanna Kaysen was admitted to McLean Hospital in Belmont, Massachusetts, for eighteen months, following a half-hour interview with a psychiatrist.[50] Twenty-five years later she published a memoir of her experiences, *Girl, Interrupted*. Bleakly humorous, and often thought-provoking and insightful, the book was made into a well-received film in 1999. Those familiar with the film will probably remember a number of references to self-harm, specifically cutting. In one memorable scene, Susanna and her friend Lisa run away from the hospital to visit Daisy, a former patient, on their way to Florida. During an altercation with Lisa, half-healed cuts and scars on Daisy's forearms are revealed. When challenged, Daisy retorts that Lisa should look at her own arm, suggesting to the viewer that self-injurious behaviour is widespread.[51] Lisa's response highlights several assumptions about self-cutting: 'I'm *sick*, Daisy, we know that. But here you are in so-called recovery playing Betty Crocker cut up like a goddamn Virginia ham.' Daisy's cutting, then, is intended to represent her ongoing mental distress, even though she's been discharged from hospital. Lisa also suggests that Daisy is too cowardly to commit suicide. The next morning, the friends find Daisy hanging in her bathroom, dead, blood from her arms on her hands and dressing gown.

These scenes were added for the film. In Kaysen's account, Daisy does not cut herself, and her suicide after discharge is reported to the patients by a nurse. The visit presumably never happened. While episodes of self-injurious behaviour *were* described in the memoir, Kaysen did not emphasize or label them. On one occasion, for example, Lisa was described as burning her arm briefly with a cigarette (without attracting comment from anyone)

...nile on another Susanna banged open her hand, fearing she had no ...ones. The only explicit references to self-mutilation were retrospective. Unlike in the film, in which the girls break into the psychiatrist's office to read their medical notes, Kaysen did not discover her diagnosis until 25 years later. After making a legal request for her case files she discovered that the 'established diagnosis' was that of 'borderline personality'. When the author looked this up in the *DSM-IIIR*, she was particularly struck by the description of 'self-mutilating behavior (e.g., wrist-scratching)'.[52] Kaysen reinterpreted her own past actions in this light: 'Wrist-scratching! I thought I'd invented it. Wrist-banging, to be precise.'[53] Although the novelist's description of her own former behaviour reads nothing like the 'delicate self-cutting' articles of the same era, Kaysen nonetheless interpreted her regular, repeated bruising of her wrists as the same practice.

This reminds us that it was (and is) not only psychiatrists who perpetuate labels. For patients and former patients, putting a name to something troubling might serve to make it appear more tangible, less threatening and perhaps more manageable.[54] It can, of course, equally be the reverse: a

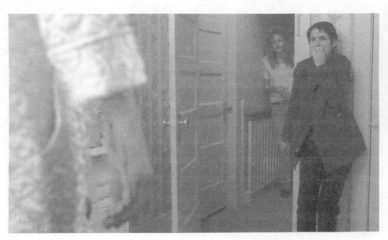

Daisy's suicide in the film of *Girl, Interrupted* (1999). Daisy's hand, streaked with blood, presumably from cutting her arm, can be seen in the foreground. A horrified Susanna (Winona Ryder), who has just found her friend hanging in the bathroom, is on the right.

stigma or a self-fulfilling prophecy. Kaysen's acceptance of certain elements of the 'borderline' label did not make her uncritical of the gendered nature of the diagnosis, with concepts such as promiscuity applied very differently to men and women. She assumed, nonetheless, that the 1987 description of 'borderline personality disorder' was directly equivalent to the 'borderline personality' she was diagnosed with in 1967. This could not be further from the truth. Within psychoanalysis, the 'borderline' shifted considerably from the 1940s to the 1980s,

> transformed from a severely disturbed near-schizophrenic to a rather milder and far more common type and, in the hands of many, from a stock male to a paradigmatically female figure.[55]

The 'delicate cutting' literature formed part of this shift. For some practitioners at least, this was a concerted effort to shift diagnostic boundaries in an era of increasingly biomedical neo-Kraepelinian psychiatry. Indeed, self-injurious behaviour – in particular, 'wrist-slashing' or 'delicate cutting' – led to a particular characterization of 'borderlines' in *DSM-III*.

Across the 'delicate self-cutting' articles and before, patients were given a range of diagnoses. In Offer and Barglow's early study (1960), for example, this included 'borderline state', 'severe character disorder', 'schizo-affective reaction', 'schizoid personality' and 'schizophrenic reaction'. Most had been hospitalized on multiple occasions, and were considered 'seriously and chronically ill'.[56] Graff and Mallin, meanwhile, claimed that 'wrist slashers have become the new chronic patients in mental hospitals, replacing the schizophrenics.'[57] This did not mean that the two labels were mutually exclusive: 40 per cent of Graff and Mallin's patients were diagnosed with schizophrenia (the most common diagnosis), as were a fifth of Robert Goldwyn and John Cahill's patients. Pao noted that his patients had mostly been diagnosed with 'schizophrenic reaction' because of episodic periods of psychosis marked by 'perceptual distortion, hallucinations, [and] tenuously formulated delusional systems'. In retrospect, however, he diagnosed them as 'severe borderline states'.[58] Henry Grunebaum and

Gerald Klerman preferred the label 'a syndrome in the borderline group', while noting that diagnosis of 'wrist slashers' was often a cause of staff conflict, with some staff favouring schizophrenia and others hysteria or psychopathy.[59]

It is clear, then, that many of the 1960s studies were extremely uncertain about how to categorize 'wrist-slashing' patients, despite being confident that they presented as a specific syndrome. Most agreed that patients experienced psychosis at times but were also able 'when not psychotic' to 'pass as being "normal" and were capable of responsible work'.[60] So what did these clinicians mean when they spoke of the 'borderline'? Some referenced Robert Knight in support of their diagnosis. Knight's 1953 paper 'Borderline States' discussed the complications around the use of a borderline diagnosis which 'conveys no diagnostic illumination of a case other than the implication that the patient is quite sick but not frankly psychotic'. In other words, these patients fell somewhere between psychosis and neurosis – too ill for the latter diagnosis, but not yet quite as unwell as the former. Self-mutilation remained a psychotic symptom, 'evidence of implicit loss of reality sense.'[61] The psychoanalyst Otto Kernberg, meanwhile, proposed to incorporate *all* the so-called 'borderline states' under the term 'borderline personality organization'. The similarity between conditions was, Kernberg declared, a marked similarity in 'ego pathology', which supported the idea that 'these patients must be considered to occupy a borderline area between neurosis and psychosis.'[62] In both instances, as well as the 'delicate cutting' articles, the diagnosis of borderline personality disorder thus emerged from the concept of schizophrenia.[63]

Later texts have rewritten this history as a deterministic picture of the 'discovery' of borderline personality disorder as a curable form of schizophrenia, before becoming an entity in its own right. This has been seen as optimistic: a diagnosis created when 'psychiatrists began to develop more hope about the ultimate outcome for the schizophrenic patient.'[64] Yet the concept of the borderline has a deeply fragmented and contentious history, and has *never* been accepted outright by clinicians, even in the United States, its apparent birthplace. This makes borderline personality disorder today a very different category from diagnoses like schizophrenia or bipolar disorder, which are usually accepted by clinicians, if not always by patients, as diagnostic labels. The coherence of the standard psychiatric history of borderline personality disorder (and, indeed, the category itself) 'is imposed, achieved through a process of after-the-fact exclusions . . . and held together in places by the term borderline and little else'.[65]

Retrospective interpretation of borderline cases was an important element of its incorporation into *DSM-III*. Hannah Decker, in her comprehensive text on the formation of *DSM-III*, took some of the claims of its architects (a task force with Robert Spitzer at the helm) at face value. In the 1970s she wrote, 'schizophrenia was being overdiagnosed in the United States, a fact recently acknowledged as the result of an important study.'[66] The study, the U.S./UK Diagnostic Project, began in 1965 to compare diagnosis of psychiatric patients in the United States and England and Wales (specifically New York and London). The project stemmed from the notion that psychiatric diagnosis was 'an unreliable procedure', and included some interesting statistical massaging to ensure that it supported the notion that diagnosis rates of schizophrenia were considerably higher in New York than in London and that this was 'largely, but not entirely, due to differences in the diagnostic criteria used by the staffs of the two hospitals'. Whether or not one agrees with the findings of the original study, which stemmed from the belief that diagnostic rates ought to be equivalent (despite finding differences in symptom prevalence), the assumption that this 'over-diagnosis' must apply to the entirety of the United States seems something of a leap. Indeed, the study even concluded that 'we do not know whether the differences revealed here between London and New York provide an accurate picture of overall Anglo-American differences'; they had already admitted that Brooklyn State Hospital was chosen for 'practical reasons', and not because it was close to the average diagnostic rates in New York. However, it has subsequently become, as Decker's wording indicates, accepted as 'proof' that over-diagnosis occurred.[67]

Around the publication of *DSM-III*, then, an increasing number of studies considered the effects of this 'over-diagnosis' of schizophrenia, and re-evaluated historical patients accordingly. Remi Cadoret and Carol North even argued for a retrospective diagnosis of many well-known autobiographical or fictionalized accounts of mental illness. Among the patients they re-diagnosed was 'Deborah Blau' (still not openly identified as Joanne Greenberg). According to Cadoret and North, Deborah suffered not from schizophrenia but from 'somatization disorder': physical symptoms not connected to a lesion or other physical cause. The authors had a bleak outlook on schizophrenia, which they considered a long-term and debilitating disorder. Popular books, they felt, raised 'false hopes [of recovery] ... in people who have real schizophrenia or who have loved ones with it'.[68] Strangely, six years later Carol North published her *own* account of personal recovery from schizophrenia.[69] Yet, in a climate in which this view of schizophrenia was becoming increasingly pessimistic, this seems to have had rather less impact than the article. Other clinicians were suggesting that the concept of the borderline had led to the 'broadening of the concept of schizophrenia', which resulted in differing diagnostic tendencies between American and British psychiatrists.[70] One of Robert Spitzer's goals in *DSM-III*, then, was explicitly to *reduce* the diagnosis of schizophrenia in the United States, and the definitions of both schizophrenia and borderline personality disorder reflected this aim.[71]

To create a sharper contrast between schizophrenia and 'the borderline', Spitzer and his colleagues reviewed the borderline literature and decided that the term was applied in two ways: first, to 'a constellation of relatively enduring personality features of instability and vulnerability' and second to 'psychopathological characteristics ... assumed to be genetically related to a spectrum of disorders including chronic schizophrenia'. This resulted in two new diagnoses for *DSM-III*: borderline personality disorder and schizotypal disorder, separating the former borderline in two. The separation does not appear to have been particularly neat. When the new criteria were tested, over half of borderline patients (54 per cent) met the criteria for *both* personality disorders, yet the two were nonetheless separated. Interestingly, while *both* types of borderline had been associated with self-harm in the 'delicate cutting' articles, only the diagnostic criteria for borderline personality disorder included 'impulsive and self-damaging behaviour'. This continued the depiction of self-harm as a female behaviour, for in the sample there was a slightly higher proportion of female to male patients in the 'borderline' category (81 per cent of female patients and 64 per cent of male). *DSM-III* further asserted that borderline personality disorder was more commonly diagnosed in women, underlining the association between self-injurious behaviour and female psychiatric patients.[72]

DSM-III was published in 1980. A five-hundred-page volume listing 265 diagnoses, it was an enormous expansion on the slim texts of *DSM-I* and *II*. Five new personality disorders were included, borderline and schizotypal among them. The *DSM* definition explicitly separated 'the borderline' from psychosis for the first time. Although personality disorders remained controversial, borderline personality disorder was a prominent backdrop for understandings of self-harm for at least the next two decades. Despite increasing criticism, this connection remains strong even today and, until the publication of *DSM-5* in 2013, this diagnosis was the only place where self-injury was found in the *DSM*. It has often been suggested that diagnosis has been made on the basis of this one symptom alone. The label of borderline personality disorder has thus been a problematic one. Patients considered 'difficult' long-term users of psychiatric services were characterized as 'resistant' to therapeutic intervention, and thus blamed for their failure to recover. Kernberg, whose psychoanalytic descriptions of borderline conditions were influential in early descriptions, felt that the 'self-destructiveness' of the borderline patient was an 'ominous prognostic sign for treatment'. This, in Kernberg's view, was due to the impact on forming a psychotherapeutic relationship with the practitioner. While many tendencies could be described as self-destructive, Kernberg declared that 'perhaps only in cases of chronic tendency toward physical self-mutilation does one have sufficient certainty for considering this symptom as a serious prognostic sign.'[73] This notion, along with the description of the borderline as a 'personality disorder' (implying that a pathology is deep-rooted in an individual) has proliferated the view that self-mutilating psychiatric patients are difficult to treat. When Susanna Kaysen wrote herself into the category of borderline personality disorder, she emphasized certain characteristics of her teenage behaviour as self-injurious. The film version of *Girl, Interrupted* went even further in depicting a connection between self-cutting and mental disorder in young women. Yet just as self-harm became a symptom of borderline personality disorder, so too the borderline shifted. Self-harm moved from being regarded as a psychotic symptom that was evidence of the severity of a near-psychotic condition, to a 'nearly normal' but manipulative response to the pressures of modern life.

Taking *DSM-III* as a starting point, self-harm in the 1980s became enshrined in a new condition of borderline personality disorder and widely associated with young women with mild to moderate mental illness. As I have shown, this was not the way it was understood in the 1940s and 1950s. Dr Fried in Joanne Greenberg's account made none of these assumptions. Deborah's self-injury was depicted as a desperate attempt to communicate through and with severe psychosis. In Sylvia Plath's case, self-injury was primarily associated with suicide. It was only in the 1960s that self-harm became regarded as a sign of a particular syndrome, first associated equally with psychosis and 'borderline states' and later intentionally reinterpreted as a non-psychotic but severe 'personality disorder'. Both delicate self-cutting and borderline personality disorder were characterized as inherently 'female', despite the existence of male psychiatric patients, like William Kurelek, who engaged in exactly the same behaviours.

In this chapter I have shown the complexity of this change in views, impacted by wider social and cultural shifts in both Britain and the United States. In Britain, the social and political impact of the post-war welfare state promoted a view of self-harm as a socially embedded, communicative behaviour. In the United States, psychoanalytic models of self-injury after the Second World War also emphasized a social context. Self-harm became a sign of the futility of the aggression that had been earlier described by Menninger, characterized by the devastation caused by two world wars. It was also in this period that self-cutting became singled out as the paradigm for self-harm. The institutional model depicted self-cutting as a social behaviour. It was communicative but troublesome, drawing comments from staff and other patients. The gendering of the behaviour continued to draw attention to the supposed manipulative nature of women. Nonetheless, self-injury was still seen as a psychotic symptom, requiring inpatient treatment. This remained the case when self-injury was incorporated into definitions of borderline personality disorder. The framing of the borderline in the United States, intentionally drawn away from its previous associations with schizophrenia, gradually diminished this view. The borderline patient became a chronic, but less disturbed, figure, a process that served to increase the level of responsibility the patient was assumed to have, and thus the attribution of blame for acts of self-harm.

This reinterpretation of self-injury did not take place solely within psychiatry. In the 1970s and early 1980s, further studies explored self-harm in prisons and reform schools.[74] However, the psychiatric assumptions have proven particularly hard to shake. On the surface, many of these reports seem reasonable and it is easy to read into them, as later clinicians have done, modern experiences and views of self-harm. However, to do this is to miss the significant changes in the characterization of self-injury in relation to mental disorder, as well as the often deliberate way in which self-cutting and the characteristics of 'the cutter' were presented as a specific gendered entity. In particular, we should be acutely aware of the way in which generalizations made on very small samples of inpatients in private American institutions (in which women formed a large proportion of the population) were subsequently assumed to apply to anyone and everyone who self-harmed. The incorporation of self-harm into a biomedical system (in *DSM-III*) is also surprising given that, as we have seen, self-inflicted injury had previously been viewed from psychological or psychoanalytic perspectives. In the later twentieth century, an increased focus on a pathological understanding of superficial self-injury sat uncomfortably alongside the view of those who self-harm as 'nearly normal' and a sociological approach that cast self-injury as an indictment of modern Western life. It is this complexity that makes it especially important to view 'delicate self-cutting' through a historical lens. Questioning the foundations of this universal model has important consequences for understanding self-harm in the twenty-first century.

SEVEN

TRIGGER HAPPY
Culture, Contagion and Trauma
in the Internet Age

In the early 2000s, like many other twenty-somethings, I was a member of various online clubs and forums. The Internet seemed new and exciting. Many of us had not had access to it until at least the age of eighteen. The Internet made most sense as an extension of our daily lives. While we recognized that online anonymity could make it easier to say things one wouldn't necessarily say in real life, we didn't treat Internet conversation as particularly different from everyday chat; nor were we overly concerned about the potential for other users to lie and manipulate their identities. Most of us wrote under our real names. We used accounts and email addresses (and even postal addresses) that were easily searchable. Our forums were policed in the same way we managed real-life situations: no one appeared outwardly concerned about something difficult or troubling until it happened. When upsetting situations arose we supported each other and dealt with it as best we could. Some forums had rules; others didn't. No one ever added warnings to their posts.

More than a decade later, this description sounds like a rose-tinted exercise in nostalgia. In many ways, it is. The World Wide Web can be an unpleasant and even threatening place, and scare stories abounded even in the 1990s. Forums fractured over internal arguments all the time. Splinter groups formed new fan communities where members cemented their identities by insulting their former associates. Trolling (anonymous abuse for the sake of causing trouble) and cyber stalking were not uncommon.

Nonetheless, my memory of Internet communities is still of a place where people talked openly and acceptingly and where friendships began that frequently and often rapidly shifted into the 'real' world through face-to-face meetings. Many people I met then are still among my closest friends.

I begin with this reflection because 'the Internet' (if there can ever be such a discrete entity) has been viewed with unease where self-harm is concerned. This is not just the case in clinical circles, but is an issue that has infiltrated the wider public sphere. In 2012, the blogging website Tumblr made the decision to ban pro-self-harm and pro-anorexia-nervosa (pro-ana) blogs.[1] Facebook's 'community standards' include a section on self-injury, stating that the social networking site 'prohibit[s] content that promotes or encourages suicide or any other type of self-injury, including self-mutilation and eating disorders'.[2] Fear that the Internet might promote undesired activities is not, of course, limited to self-harm and suicide. This concern has also covered paedophilia and 'online grooming', as well as extremist religious views and incitement to terrorism (usually termed 'radicalization'). In many instances this focuses on young people. As represented by adults, they are cast as both susceptible victims *and* dangerous influencers. Take, for example, news stories in 2015 about British teenagers who planned to leave, or left, home to join Islamic State in Syria. The attribution of terms like 'fanatic' and 'terrorist' to young people attempts to draw a divide between those who are vulnerable and those who are a threat, without ever identifying where exactly this line might be.[3]

While this approach to young people as a group is not new, it has become more prevalent with the increased visibility of youth culture online. In this chapter, I explore the emergence of these ideas about self-harm around the millennium, as the medical focus moved away from the institution. First, I look at the so-called normalization of self-harm as a response to the pressures of modern life. The modern view of self-harm as a coping mechanism sits awkwardly alongside the paternalistic, protective model applied to self-injurious behaviour in youth culture. Today this has become especially associated with online communities. However, the idea of 'peer contagion' in self-harm emerged from studies of institutionalized teenagers and young adults in the 1980s and '90s. This model was quickly applied to the wider world, and adopted by researchers and journalists alike to explain what appeared to be an increase in self-harm.[4] Self-inflicted injury was portrayed as a reaction to modern preoccupations and, paradoxically, also a *product* of modern culture. Film, television and media coverage all reflected and shaped this picture, but perhaps no area of youth culture has received as much attention as music, here illustrated by the media attention paid to Richey James Edwards, the former Manic Street Preachers guitarist. From grunge to heavy metal to goth, as each genre has come to the forefront in a particular generation it has been analysed by researchers searching for a solution to the spread of self-harm.

It is the Internet, however, that has encapsulated modern preoccupations with self-harm. A seemingly limitless and largely un-moderated resource, the Internet can represent information and confusion; a source of support and a threat of disorder. Medical professionals and mental health service users alike have contributed to efforts to police this continuous flow of online information. I will go on to look at this through the spread of the 'trigger warning'. Ten years ago, this phrase was barely seen. Today, the Internet is littered with warnings for content from self-harm and suicide to sexual abuse and racism. These warnings have also sometimes been considered in an educational setting, stamping university course outlines with content that might prove traumatic to students.[5] But where did the concept of the 'trigger' and its associated warning come from? Here, I look at the notion as it pertains to self-harm in particular, highlighting the contradictions inherent in the idea. On the one hand, the modern concept of self-injury depicts the behaviour as a private, personal act related to individual inner turmoil; on the other, the 'trigger' is embedded in a neurobiological model of conditioning, based on reflex responses. Where does one begin and the other end? The modern, individual, internalized model of self-harm can ultimately appear as confused and confusing as the social and cultural implications of self-mutilation in the Victorian era.

Away from the institution: the normalization of self-harm

In February 1975, twelve-year-old Caroline Kettlewell tried to saw into her arm with the blade of a Swiss Army knife in the toilets of her school in rural Virginia. She 'managed to wear no more than a raw, angry, two-inch abrasion' before she was discovered by a teacher.[6] In her memoir, *Skin Game*, published nearly a quarter of a century later, Kettlewell recalled the subsequent conversation with her mother: a quick, awkward dismissal by both parties that the act had any meaning whatsoever. This was Kettlewell's first attempt to injure herself but she soon began cutting her arms regularly with a blade prised from a disposable razor. Billed as 'the first former cutter to tell her own story', Kettlewell's book was published the year after Marilee Strong's *A Bright Red Scream* achieved widespread acclaim and captured the imagination of the American public. Kettlewell's account was very different from the 'delicate self-cutting' reports of previous decades. Unlike the 'borderline' patients in psychiatric hospitals, her self-harm was secret for most of her life. Caroline injured herself only where she could hide the scars: 'high on my arms and hips and legs'.[7] Apart from her self-injury and an unrelenting sense of misery, which coloured every recollection of her childhood, 'every other feature of my life was utterly, ordinary twelve'.[8] It wasn't until she was in her mid-twenties that Kettlewell entered the fringes of the mental health system, with six years spent in and out of therapy, later taking antidepressants.

Skin Game was less about psychiatry than a psychological approach to self-harm, the same approach followed by Strong, who interviewed large numbers of 'cutters' to tell their stories. The text focused almost entirely around an internal monologue. Other characters made an occasional appearance – Caroline's family, a few boys at school and, later, her two husbands – but only where their words or actions impacted on her self-injurious behaviour in some way. Antidepressants, quickly followed by the birth of a child, marked the end of Kettlewell's story of self-harm. This rather neat solution – medication ending decades of turmoil – was not an unusual claim in the late 1990s, and says more about the optimistic assertions made for SSRIs at that point than anything else. A relatively new type of antidepressant, the SSRI (selective serotonin reuptake inhibitor), was actively marketed in the United States and Britain in the 1990s, and chemical models of depression and mental health gained increasing public acceptance.[9] This put self-injury in a very different context: associated with mild to moderate anxiety and depression, rather than the 'borderline' inpatients of earlier decades.

Kettlewell cast self-harm as an expression of her inner turmoil. This way of understanding self-injury was growing increasingly popular. It was often contrasted in fiction with a protagonist who, on the surface, appeared to be successful. In Steven Levenkron's teen novel *The Luckiest Girl in the World* (published two years before Kettlewell's memoir), the main character Katie Roskova is similarly presented as hiding her distress from the outside world, using self-inflicted injury to keep the mask from

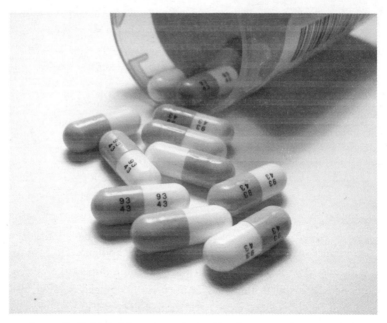

Prozac pills (fluoxetine). Prozac, manufactured by pharmaceutical company Eli Lilly, became the most well-known brand of antidepressant in the 1990s.

slipping. The very title of the novel indicates that Katie has no obvious reason to harm herself. As Caroline Kettlewell similarly put it, 'I could never get past the conviction that life had not entitled me to fall apart.'[10] In the late 1990s and early 2000s, in both Britain and America, self-harm increasingly appeared in media and popular culture as a common, albeit unusual, survival strategy, usually of young, white, middle-class women.[11] These girls had much in common with the 'borderline' patients of the 1960s, with one important difference: most were not institutionalized, and frequently those around them knew nothing of their acts. Unlike the 'delicate cutters', they were not recognizable as psychiatric patients. How, then, were they understood?

One of the key writers on self-mutilation in this era was Armando Favazza, who challenged contemporary views of self-harm as a pathology or sign of mental illness. His major study, *Bodies Under Siege*, was first published in 1987 and did much to normalize self-harm as a coping mechanism. Favazza originally studied anthropology; after completing his medical training, this background led him first to community psychiatry and later to cultural psychiatry. In a 1978 article he explained the relevance of the latter approach, a form of psychiatry that took account of findings in anthropology and social psychology. This emphasized cross-cultural themes and ethnography as well as specific cultural contexts, such as family and social relationships, sexual behaviour and roles and methods of communication.[12] In the preface to the second edition of *Bodies Under Siege*, Favazza described the lack of interest in viewing self-mutilation from a cultural perspective when he began his research. To his surprise, the 'standard anthropological sources did not even include mutilation as a topic.' In his search for cross-cultural information, Favazza found both historical psychiatric reports and accounts of religious and cultural rituals of self-mutilation around the world. It was the breadth of this material that made him 'intrigued by the possibility that some forms of self-mutilation represent an attempt at self-healing'.[13] This was not a popular view in the 1980s, when many students and practitioners 'considered self-harm as a senseless behavior that in some way represented a type of semi-suicidal act'.[14] Favazza

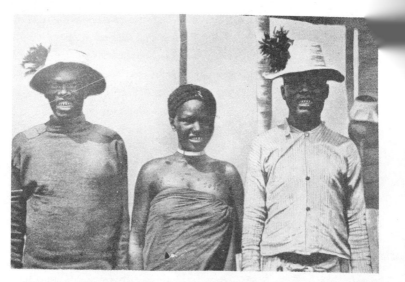

This photograph of a group of Azande (Nyam-Nyam), an ethnic group of north-central Africa, was taken by the Wellcome Tropical Research Labs in 1911. The picture is posed to show the Azande's sharpened teeth, indicating the ongoing Western fascination with body modification in non-Western cultures.

sought to challenge this by combining descriptions of culturally sanctioned mutilations (often, but not always, ritual and healing practices) with what was deemed pathological, setting self-mutilation within a broader cultural and psychological context.

Favazza was not the first to use anthropological studies to support wider conclusions about self-mutilation, a technique that was common in the late nineteenth century. Unlike Favazza, these writers used the comparison with so-called 'savages' to confirm self-mutilation as a pathological behaviour. As Charles Darwin saw it, the face 'with us is chiefly admired for its beauty, so with savages it is the chief seat of mutilation', drawing a distinction between primitive and civilized nations.[15] The nineteenth-century American physicians George Gould and Walter Pyle, meanwhile, described non-Western body modification to highlight a potentially worrying decline of civilization in the West: 'the ludicrous custom of piercing the ears for the wearing of ornaments, typical of savagery and

...und in all indigenous African tribes, is universally prevalent among our own people.'[16] The starkly different set of associations made in the late nineteenth century indicates that the 'normalization' of self-harm was by no means the only or obvious outcome of exploring socially accepted self-mutilation. To view self-injurious acts as 'normal' required a prior understanding of cultural relativism (the notion that acts or beliefs should be evaluated in relation to the culture they occur in, not through ideals in other cultures). This did not become widespread in anthropology until the 1940s. Outside anthropological circles, practices of body modification and tattooing had to be accepted as something other than 'primitive' by medical practitioners (who were usually white, male and Western) for self-harm to similarly be viewed in a positive, socially beneficial light.[17]

In the late 1980s and '90s, the increasing prevalence of this view outside anthropology circles helped self-harm to become accepted as a cultural phenomenon in the Western world. Certainly, Favazza's teaching and lecturing in the wake of *Bodies Under Siege* informed a shift in views, as did the work of other educators and public speakers. This included Favazza's collaborator Karen Conterio, who set up 'SAFE Alternatives' in 1985, described as the 'first outpatient support group for those who engage in repetitive self harm behavior'.[18] By the 1990s, self-harm was no longer necessarily associated with 'the other'. The borderline inpatient of the 1960s became the 'white, suburban, attractive teenage girl' presented in popular reports in the late twentieth century, epitomized by Caroline Kettlewell and the fictional Katie Roskova.[19] Fiction, film and television representations emphasized this, with at least half of the films depicting self-injury between 1980 and 2005 popularizing the profile of the white female 'cutter'.[20] Some, such as *Fatal Attraction* (1987), in which Glenn Close plays a successful, professional woman who cuts her wrists (and, later, her leg) in a manipulative act of obsessive jealousy, reinforced negative stereotypes.[21] In other films, self-injury was connected to contemporary culture more broadly. In David Cronenberg's *Videodrome* (1983), Debbie Harry's character Nicki Brand is shown burning herself with a cigarette. This act, along with her request to be cut by her lover, Max Renn, relates

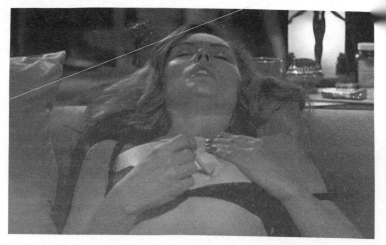

Videodrome (1983): Nicki Brand (Debbie Harry) burns herself with a cigarette in the pursuit of erotic pleasure.

self-injury to the pursuit of pleasure in a sensationalist televised world: a sign of a hedonistic Western culture, lost to 'normal' desires through the pursuit of a consumerist ideal.[22]

Fictional and autobiographical accounts of self-harm in the 1980s and 1990s were often tied to a late twentieth-century white, middle-class lifestyle. Self-injury became 'part' of Western life, and thus 'normalized' (when viewed outside clinical pathology). Both Caroline Kettlewell and Katie Roskova had no clear 'reason' to injure themselves. Kettlewell's account presented the fractured relationships and internal focus associated with a modern psychological 'self'. For Katie it was the pressures of a busy and successful modern life that drove her to self-harm. In both instances, self-mutilation was a product of the modern world. Despite similarities between fiction and memoir, however, the external world was presented quite differently in the two books. Katie Roskova's salvation was not medication but therapy (perhaps unsurprisingly, given that Levenkron, the author, was a psychotherapist).[23] For Levenkron, Katie's main need as an isolated teen was to belong to a social group, and her acceptance into a circle of friendly, albeit dysfunctional, teenagers in group therapy brought her out of her shell. For Kettlewell, however, other people were presented as challenges, not least the fifteen-year-old schoolboy whose self-cutting sparked her own interest in razor blades.[24] Admittedly, Kettlewell did *not* consider her acts to be imitative: the book begins with her first attempt well before she encountered anyone else who injured themselves, situating self-harm as something discovered alone and quite by chance. These two books, however, presented both aspects of youth culture, well before the Internet age: peers can be protective *and* dangerous; self-harm is a response to the pressures of modernity *and* created by modern culture. In the next section, I explore this further through British media attention to self-injury through youth (music) culture.

This is yesterday: music, culture and peer contagion

On 1 February 1995, Richard James Edwards (then usually known as Richey James), guitarist with the British rock band Manic Street Preachers, left the Embassy Hotel in London. He drove to his home in Cardiff Bay, Wales, where he left his antidepressants, credit cards and passport. On 15 February, the story was made public. Two days later, Edwards's car was found at a service station by the Severn Bridge. The widespread assumption was that he had committed suicide, although his body was never found. In the weeks following Edwards's disappearance, the letters pages of the music press filled with missives from fans. These were 'unusual in their quantity and their anguish' as 'distraught fans wrote of their own experiences of desolation and even self-mutilation.'[25] In early April 1995, *Melody Maker* dedicated two special issues to the topic, inviting medical, health and charity representatives to offer advice, and publishing reader letters.[26] As the music paper's editor Allan Jones put it in an accompanying article in *The Guardian*, 'the question, really, is this: are our rock stars more vulnerable these days, and is that vulnerability a reflection of the vulnerability of their audience?'[27]

This concept of 'vulnerability' focused primarily on depression and self-harm. I begin with this example because, unlike many American examples

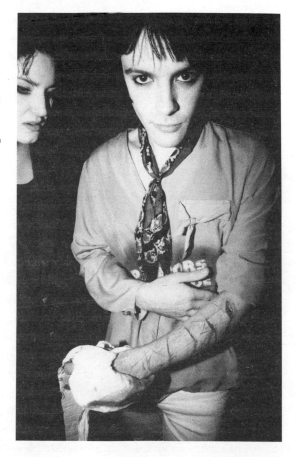

This photograph of Richey Edwards's self-harm in 1991 has become an iconographic image of rock history despite its disturbing nature, emphasizing the complicated relationship between culture, psychiatry and self-injury.

of celebrity self-injury, the Manic Street Preachers story was played out before the mass availability of the Internet.[28] Moreover, reporting was much more specifically focused on self-harm, with multiple interviews and features about the band emphasizing the topic. Edwards was well known to have injured himself for some time before his disappearance, often by cutting himself with a razor blade. This became very public in 1991 when, after a gig in Norwich, *New Musical Express* (*NME*) journalist Steve Lamacq interviewed the band. Lamacq suggested that some people might think their political sloganeering was a sham. Edwards's response was to carve the words '4 REAL' into his arm; 'He had 17 stitches, apparently. What a dumb way to end an evening.'[29] Although Lamacq described the episode as 'dumb', the NME's photographer nonetheless took a picture, leading to some debate in the paper's office as to whether the photograph could be printed. Some journalists saw the episode as artistic expression or epitomizing the destructive nature of rock 'n' roll; others thought it 'horrible', 'disgusting' or 'childish' and feared that printing the picture would encourage fans to copy their idol. Yet the NME *did* print the image, in full colour, and the photograph became an iconic moment in 1990s music history, reproduced countless times over the following years.[30]

It was not until after Edwards's disappearance, however, that the media began to pay significant attention to the impact he had on the band's followers. The Manic Street Preachers were 'one of the last bands to break before the internet arrived', which meant that many public reactions were printed in the letters pages of the music press (in NME this page was appropriately called 'Angst'), giving journalists a key role in facilitating or focusing discussion.[31] It was the NME and *Melody Maker* that decided what to print and when, and how public to make the story:

> Bands hadn't really written about anorexia, bulimia and self-harming before this . . . And so these fan letters piled in to NME, some written in blood, others chopped together from beauty mags and problem pages . . . the writers felt an intense empathy with Richey. They too had suffered some of those problems with self-image and with internal pain. And they were pleased that he was airing these issues, making it less secretive. The other person to go into this area was Princess Diana, although she probably had a different fanbase.[32]

The comparison to Diana, Princess of Wales – known as 'the people's princess' – might seem surprising. Widely adored for her perceived vulnerability, Diana's death in a car accident in 1997 provoked a huge outpouring of grief across Britain: a reported 31.5 million people watched her funeral, while thousands thronged the streets of Westminster.

As in the case of Edwards, Princess Diana's public battles with self-harm and bulimia nervosa were seen as the expression of a private, inner turmoil. That the two figures could be compared despite their very different lives and circumstances is revealing of the new understanding of self-harm as a product of white, Western culture, as applied in Britain as well as the United States. Interestingly, gender appears less of a defining factor here (although the music papers were quick to point out that Edwards's fan-base was largely female, and his actions were often described in gendered terms). In very different ways, Richey Edwards and Princess Diana were seen as an indictment of modernity, epitomizing a hopeless, lost, alienated generation. Yet this internalized despair seemed, to some observers, to be oddly formless, even apolitical. While this received little comment in the American examples outlined above, it was more glaring in Britain, where older writers expected rock and indie music to be rooted in social and political criticism. In the 1970s and '80s, 'indie angst could be more tangibly rooted in social woes', claimed *Melody Maker*, citing Joy Division's music as a response to the poverty of recession and the threat of nuclear war. In

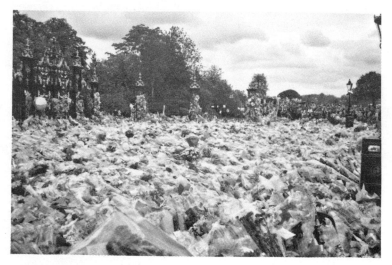

Flowers and tributes left at Kensington Palace soon after the death of Diana, Princess of Wales on 31 August 1997.

contrast, 'the letters we received [following Edwards's disappearance] never referred to outside social ills, talked instead in intransitive terms of grief, despair, a sort of existential isolation.'[33]

Yet Edwards *was* openly political. Like his fellow band members, his views were shaped by the political theory and social activism of Situationism, and hugely affected by the Welsh miners' strikes of his youth. Much of the Manic Street Preachers' early music consisted of apocalyptic rants, from the anti-capitalist fury of 'NatWest-Barclays-Midlands-Lloyds' to 'REPEAT', which damned the monarchy and nationalist sentiment.[34] Even on 1994's *The Holy Bible*, widely regarded even at the time as evidence of Edwards's fragile mental state, many tracks looked out rather than inwards, criticizing Western social and political ideals: 'IfWhiteAmericaToldTheTruthForOneDayItsWorldWouldFallApart', declared one song title.[35] When Edwards spoke of his depression and acts of violence towards his body, his interviews were nonetheless interspersed with references to political hunger strikes and historical events.[36] He was unhappy, certainly, and often introspective, but even after his discharge from a private psychiatric hospital in the summer of 1994, when interviewers tended to focus entirely on his mental state, he still spoke in terms of wider cultural references and talked about the need for changing the economic infrastructure.[37] So how exactly did Richey Edwards become the British poster boy for a newly internalized medical and popular understanding of self-harm? Largely, it seems, this was due to the perceived effect he had on young fans of the band.

While the self-harm of public figures, including Edwards and Princess Diana, tended to be presented in the media as a response to modernity, similar acts among their fans and followers were viewed as a *product* of the modern culture represented by their idols. *Melody Maker* wrote scathingly of the response in the general press to their Samaritans special issue:

> What the mainstream media wanted, however, was a Story. They wanted to hear that Britain's youth, that gullible and homogeneous entity, were being 'swept' by a wrist-slashing cult inspired by sexy,

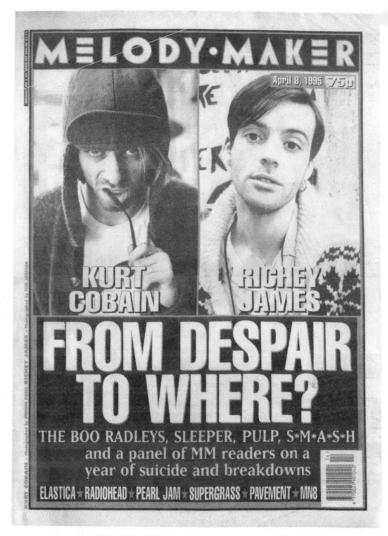

The cover of a special issue of *Melody Maker*, in which the music paper responded to an outpouring of angst in their reader letters following the disappearance of Richey Edwards with a panel discussion on depression and self-harm and advice from the Samaritans.

wasted, missing pop star Richey. The tabloids reprinted distraught letters from past Backlashes [*Melody Maker* letters page], even made up letters when we refused to show them the ones we had received, in an attempt to sensationalise the misery of the minority.[38]

Even in the broadsheets, articles sat under headlines like 'Is This Music to Die For?', seeking to examine the 'dangerous, unprecedented trend of young pop music fans identifying closely with the torment of their heroes'.[39] Not that the suddenly pious music press had never been guilty of sensationalizing the topic: headlines like 'the scarred revival: back from the brink', 'Richey in new slashing drama' and 'Manic's depressive' were all a dramatic way of drawing attention to stories that were rarely as salacious as the headlines suggested. And the *NME*, after all, had printed the '4 REAL' photograph despite the misgivings of some journalists. It was the mainstream press, however, that obsessed over a 'culture of despair' in modern music, fearing for the effects it might have on young people. This notion has remained strong, even though styles of music have altered: over the years, despair and alienation has been associated with grunge, heavy metal and goth music in particular. Most studies do state that they have found no causal link between music and self-harm. However, the general assumption was, and remains, that certain groups are more 'at risk' of self-harm than others due to their cultural preferences; interestingly, the alternative – that young people might join cultural groups in response to a sense of alienation or depression – is often added only as an afterthought.[40] What *has* shifted is the way this risk is conceptualized. Studies have moved from fearing that young people might be emulating their idols (as was claimed in 1995) to a model that emphasizes the role of peer contagion.

The general idea of contagion in self-harm was not a new one, although it has changed considerably. While it has often been connected with studies of imitation in suicide, there are important differences between the two fields. Most of the early self-harm research focused on intensive, inpatient settings and viewed the structures of the hospital, and not the media or wider culture, as responsible for this spread. A 1960 paper by Daniel Offer and Peter Barglow was prompted by an 'epidemic' of self-mutilation in the ward for adolescents and young adults in the psychiatric section of Michael Reese Hospital, Chicago. The authors concluded that 'self-mutilation incidents had a contagious quality with widespread imitation and identification' and that the behaviour could be 'learned and propagated in the highly structured setting of a general psychiatric hospital'.[41] Other writers suggested that, within a hospital setting, self-mutilation might become an 'identity', which 'confine[s] the patient to the level of his symptom, yet confirm[s] for him a distinctive and functional role in the hospital'.[42] One of the most comprehensive studies in this area was Ross and McKay's *Self-mutilation* (1979). This was the result of ten years of research by a team of psychologists at a correctional institution in Ontario, Canada. Grandview School catered for twelve- to seventeen-year-old girls, admitted after a long history of delinquent behaviour. Hugh Bryan McKay and Robert Robertson Ross, both criminologists at the University of Ottawa, were 'appalled' and 'dismayed' by the stark environment and the harsh discipline of the institution. The appearance of the girls was their most immediate cause for concern: in particular, the fact that 'almost every girl had ugly cuts and scars on her legs, her hands, and her arms . . . Otherwise attractive, pretty teenagers grossly disfigured by permanent lesions.'[43]

As in the 'delicate cutting' articles, it was this contrast between the young, attractive female population and the 'disfiguring' nature of their wounds that was especially distressing. Had this been a facility for adult male offenders, the language used by the authors and the reader's emotional response might have been very different. 'Carving', as the girls called it, was a long-running practice in the institution:

When the university began its affiliation with the training school there were 136 girls in the institution, 117 had carved at least once. Eighty-six percent of the population had mutilated themselves. Many girls had carved themselves on multiple occasions. The average girl had lacerated her skin eight times. The same figures describe almost any period in the thirty or so years of the institution's history. It was a perennial problem.[44]

Ross and McKay's book outlined their repeated efforts to deal with this problem, which they resolved at first by accident and, later, when the practice recurred, intentionally. The resolutions were invariably temporary.

Although Ross and McKay's book has been referred to as a study of contagion, the authors actually had very little to say about the way in which self-harm spread at Grandview. Indeed, they noted that 'in spite of the frequency of references in the literature to epidemics of self-mutilation there is really very little concrete evidence of such phenomena.' While pointing to a number of ways in which self-injurious behaviour might be communicated and copied – as a mark of status, an initiation rite, anti-establishment behaviour, to emphasize group membership and as a result of peer coercion – they felt the epidemic might ultimately be 'more meta-phorical than actual'.[45] The 'contagion', then, did not follow a set pattern or process, and it was the size of the problem rather than the means of its spread that resulted in the term 'epidemic'. Similarly, one of the papers they cited – a study from an adolescent unit in Plymouth, England, in the late 1960s – showed the difficulty of studying contagion in outbreaks of self-mutilation: a systematic analysis of the communication process in a small group of young people indicated some clear lines of imitative or shared behaviour, as well as others that were not obviously related.[46] Some adolescents, moreover, were not involved at all, despite appearing just as potentially vulnerable as those who were.

In the mid-1980s, the psychologists Barent Walsh and Paul Rosen designed an empirical test to explore whether a contagion effect could, in fact, be proven for self-injurious behaviour. Their test involved 25 adolescents, all patients at a Community Treatment Centre in Worcester, Massachusetts. The investigators gathered data on nine categories of behaviour (one of which was self-injury) to compare the effects of contagion. Of these categories, they found that only self-mutilation occurred in clusters throughout the year, with a total of 73 instances of self-injury recorded.

Their definition of self-mutilation contagion involved just 'two or more acts of self-mutilation that involved two or more individuals and occurred on the same day or consecutive days'.[47] The young people mostly attended the centre only during the day, and there was no record of whether those injuring themselves had prolonged or indeed any contact with each other. The study design also excluded those who had never previously mutilated themselves, thus beginning with a group more potentially receptive to self-injurious behaviour. Nonetheless, Walsh and Rosen concluded that 'the adolescents were triggering the behavior in each other,' although they admitted that replication studies were needed to explore whether or not the results of their extremely small sample could be generalized.[48]

Small studies like this were incorporated into later papers, which took for granted the existence of a contagion effect in self-harm, despite the uncertain conclusions of these experiments. These later articles also ignored the specific context of this work in the 1970s and '80s, which was almost entirely limited to institutional settings. The locations tended to be intensive, with rigid structures and enforced discipline, and were often closed to outside influences. Ross and McKay found that the environment itself provoked outbreaks of self-injurious behaviour at Grandview:

> When, for example, institutional security measures were tightened following a high incidence of abscondance (as happened very frequently) the girls, having less of an opportunity to escape, would carve instead.[49]

In the early 1990s, the acknowledgement that restrictive settings might play a more important role in increased self-injurious behaviour than social or cultural 'contagion' led to some new approaches to inpatient mental health care in Britain. Mental health nurse Jane Bunclark, who pioneered one of these approaches, reflected on changing attitudes to self-harm through her career. In the 1980s, efforts had been made to extinguish self-harm. This often led to detention under the Mental Health Act, with patients on fairly intense levels of supervision, removal of implements which were considered ones that they could possibly use to harm themselves – and of course we totally failed to stop people injuring themselves!

Even flecks of paint, Bunclark recalled, were used for self-injurious purposes 'and I think we got caught in the dynamic in which the staff and the patients were both monitoring the environment to see what could be used'.[50] According to Bunclark, this constant monitoring encouraged patients to take up any opportunity to injure themselves, without pausing to consider other ways of managing their symptoms or emotions. This view has been supported by mental health service users, reflecting on inpatient care in this period: restrictive intervention, some claimed, increased both the frequency and severity of their injuries.[51]

In 1992, Bunclark co-founded the Crisis Recovery Unit (CRU) at London's Maudsley Hospital with Dr Michael Crowe. This was a national inpatient unit for people who self-harmed, and functioned on the same framework as a therapeutic community – residents (as they were known) were not prevented from injuring themselves but were set boundaries and expected to work with staff on their recovery. This approach was designed to equip patients with the skills to take responsibility for their own self-harm, 're-learning how to be responsible about their lives when they'd had many years in mental health services of staff being terribly responsible for them'.[52] In later years, this type of practice was incorporated into the concept of 'harm minimization'. In 2006, this received wider attention through media responses to a debate on 'safe self-harm' at the Royal College of Nursing (RCN) Annual Congress, raised by nurse-consultant Chris Holley (who sadly died a few years later). RCN professional lead for mental health, Ian Hulatt, found it a challenging time: the 'press were all over it like a rash' and 'good' media coverage sat alongside ideas like 'nurses putting razor blades on the drug trolley' and 'razor blades on prescription'.[53] A similar emphasis on cutting – and sensationalized responses to it – emerged in Bunclark's recollection of the 'bizarre reputation' the CRU had at the Maudsley:

Junior doctors who might get called . . . would come along imagining that blood was flowing everywhere and it was sort of chaotic and stuff and [were] always surprised about how quiet and calm it was.[54]

Hulatt regarded comparisons made between safe self-harm and the provision of clean needles to drug addicts as proof of the medical efficacy of minimization approaches. For journalists, however, the link was more sinister. Self-harm was popularly viewed as repetitive and potentially addictive. Debates over harm minimization in mental health care sat alongside the view of self-harm as contagious: tolerance and endorsement seemed uncomfortably close for anyone who feared that the normalization of self-harm was likely to increase its prevalence. Most importantly, however, *both* of the models cited above (self-harm contagion and harm minimization) were almost entirely developed and used in small, controlled inpatient settings. One (contagion) is widely accepted, while the other (harm minimization) is still regarded as dubious: neither the RCN nor the NMC (Nursing and Midwifery Council) offers clear guidance on harm reduction, and NICE (National Institute for Health and Care Excellence) guidelines barely acknowledge the issue. The CRU, meanwhile, closed in 2012 due to funding problems.

It is the emergence of the World Wide Web that has led to greater emphasis on contagion as a model for understanding self-harm. While we should not assume that inpatient studies on contagion apply to self-harm within a community setting, this is just what studies in the Internet era have done. One American psychological study of the Internet and adolescent self-injury, for example, suggested that the

tendency for self-injurious behavior to follow epidemic-like patterns in institutional settings such as hospitals and detention facilities suggests that the behavior may be socially contagious in other settings and, therefore, through the Internet as well.[55]

...is is a gross assumption, given the extremely different circumstances within a rigid, rule-bound 'total institution' and the haphazard and often casual nature of social Internet use. However, this example *does* highlight the spread of views about self-harm, which is the wider focus of this chapter. While contagion and epidemics of self-harm were initially assumed to be an institutional problem, from the 1990s this was expanded to include a wider population of so-called 'self-harmers', many of whom had never come into contact with mental health services at all. Findings about the meaning and mechanisms of self-harm in inpatient studies were largely transferred unquestioningly onto a general, particularly adolescent, population. Conversely, studies in which staff worked with service users to develop models like harm minimization or peer support services were not. This led to a framing of Internet activity that emphasized peer contagion over peer support, an approach that will be explored in the final part of this chapter.

Trigger warning: self-harm, PTSD and the Internet

'My body comes with a trigger warning,' wrote Seaneen Molloy-Vaughan, a writer and activist in her early thirties, in a blog post for the British mental health awareness charity Mind in 2015. Molloy-Vaughan described the scars on her arms (the result of twelve years of severe self-harm) and reactions to them, criticizing wider concern about visual images of self-inflicted injury:

> How do you say people who self harm should be treated with kindness when their bodies are seen as attacks on others, to say that self harm shouldn't be a problem hidden in the dark, when we do exactly that by not allowing representations of self harm?[56]

Molloy-Vaughan's post referred to the increasing prevalence of 'trigger warnings' accompanying representations of self-harm online. Self-inflicted injury is just one of many things that, in recent years, have been thought to require a warning to reduce the risk of 'triggering' trauma in a reader or viewer. However, certain associations apply to triggers in relation to self-harm that are not always the case in other areas, such as sexual assault, discrimination and gendered and racial violence. One is reflected in Molloy-Vaughan's statement: a self-harm survivor can *themselves* be a visible trigger in a way that a rape survivor, for example, is not.[57] Alongside this lies the ongoing notion of contagion. While a trigger warning for domestic violence is made to help prevent the re-emergence of traumatic memories (rather than stopping an outbreak of copycat abuse), trigger warnings for self-harm assume that viewing images or reading detailed descriptions of a particular act may cause others to replicate it. In this section, I explore these two emphases within the wider context of trigger warnings online.

A trigger warning is a caveat used in blogs, message boards and on social media (and sometimes in mainstream media) to warn readers of specific content. Warnings can be detailed, and are often required by a particular website or forum. Journalists have located the origin of the trigger warning on feminist message boards and blogs in 'the early days of the internet' (the late 1990s).[58] An article in *The Atlantic*, tellingly entitled 'The Coddling of the American Mind', claimed that 'search-engine trends indicate that the phrase broke into mainstream use online around 2011, spiked in 2014, and reached an all-time high in 2015.'[59] Authors Greg Lukianoff and Jonathan Haidt assumed that trigger warnings were part of a sinister trend, designed to crush free-thinking and diversity. Conversely, Laurie Penny in the *New Statesman* saw trigger warnings as evidence of alternative ways of reading culture: 'Trigger warnings are not about censorship – they are about openness, and that's what's really threatening.'[60] For Penny, the origin of the trigger warning in lived experience and empowerment made it a feminist, and overtly left-wing, plea for empathy and openness. The fact that the trigger warning emerged at a grass-roots level before being adopted in mainstream media and clinical contexts partly supports this notion. Even those reporters critical of triggers have suggested that trigger warnings reached the Internet from women's support groups at crisis centres for rape and sexual assault.[61] The terminology, however, suggests the neuro-biological context of modern psychiatry. The 'trigger' in trigger warning is a shortening of 'trauma trigger': the notion that a sight, sound, smell or other stimulus can set off a flashback of a past traumatic experience in an individual.

This does not, of course, mean that the trigger warning cannot be critiqued. For some people, the very concept opposes free speech. Feminist writers have also questioned the spread of the term, in particular its adoption in social media since the advent of Tumblr in 2007: trigger warnings now appear so frequently as to seem meaningless. These warnings may also be useless in the face of past trauma – an 'illusion of safety', as Roxane Gay put it. The things that have triggered her memories of rape have mostly been experiences that cannot be warned about in advance:

> When I see men who look like him or his friends. When I smell beer on a man's breath. When I smell Polo cologne. When I hear a harsh laugh. When I walk by a group of men, clustered together, and there's no one else around. When I see a woman being attacked in a movie or on television. When I am in the woods or driving through a heavily wooded area. When I read about experiences that are all too familiar. When I go through security at the airport and am pulled aside for extra screening, which seems to happen every single time I travel. When I'm having sex and my wrists are unexpectedly pinned over my head. When I see a young girl of a certain age.[62]

Everything, Gay pointed out, can be a trigger for someone, and she questioned the use of trigger warnings in online communities to imply a safe space to discuss trauma, which gives users the 'illusion they *can* be protected'. The writer and historian Tim Smith also critiqued his own use of trigger warnings as 'No Go' signs, suggesting that avoiding reading material on bereavement after the loss of his child enabled, rather than sheltered him from, his pain.[63] Smith raised an interesting point about power: a trigger warning makes the writer of a piece the arbiter of what is or is not traumatic, taking the decision away from the reader. The expectation of trauma can silence as well as empower.

Given the complexity of this debate, it is hard to define just what it is about certain topics that suggests they might be particularly triggering. Moreover, what, exactly, are they supposed to trigger? The vast majority of modern articles have situated triggers in the history of trauma, generally dating it back to the notion of shell shock during the First World War. Triggers, we are told, are external events which cause an intense, psychologically painful reaction, often a flashback of a past traumatic experience. Flashback in the *DSM-5* description of post-traumatic stress disorder (PTSD) is a popular term for 'dissociative states' that include recurrent memories with 'sensory, emotional, or physiological behavioural components'. These occur when a person 'is exposed to triggering events that resemble or symbolize an aspect of the traumatic event (e.g., windy days after a hurricane; seeing someone who resembles one's perpetrator).[64] Yet the flashback as we currently understand it is a recent phenomenon, first included in the *DSM* in 1987 in the description of PTSD. Before this time, the term was used to describe altered states of awareness from the use of hallucinogenic drugs. From the late 1980s, however, flashbacks became viewed as specific memories of real-life events.[65] Prior to this, we can't even assume that the modern idea of flashbacks was even commonly experienced as a symptom of trauma-related disorders. One retrospective study of ex-servicemen across a variety of wars concluded that flashbacks were not reported at all in Boer War records, and rarely in the First and Second World Wars (0.5 per cent and 1.4 per cent of the samples respectively). The reporting of flashbacks was significantly greater in the most recent soldiers, who had served in 1991.[66]

If we look at personal accounts or literary representations of war neurosis from the First or Second World War, nightmares and dreams were more frequently described than waking flashbacks. Many of the symptoms of shell shock in the First World War were physical: muteness, paralysis, contractures and blindness that had no obvious somatic cause. Even where a psychological origin was assumed, there was no specific connection to the assumption that symptoms could be triggered by reminders of trauma that took place in the real world. Yet the existence of trigger warnings today assumes this cause-and-effect model, despite indications that the creation

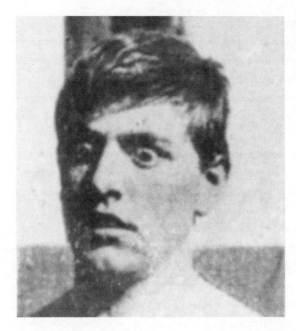

Private E, suffering from war neurosis 'resulting from prolonged terror', from Arthur Hurst's *Medical Diseases of the War*, 2nd edn (1918).

and later reshaping of the diagnosis of PTSD was politically and culturally driven. Included in the DSM in 1980 as a direct response to widespread opposition to the Vietnam War in the United States, the criteria for PTSD have since been widened significantly, such that trauma can today refer to almost any unpleasant or distressing experience – or simply the threat of it. While this shifting of boundaries is not unusual in psychiatric diagnoses (as we have seen in the case of borderline personality disorder), it is certainly an important factor to bear in mind when considering attention to triggers today. The very idea that there is a 'universal trauma reaction', 'by which terrifying experiences are permanently and accurately preserved by being encoded in the brain in the manner of skills, habit and reflex reactions', is questionable to say the least.[67]

But if trauma, and the experience of PTSD, is less universal than we might have supposed, what does this suggest for the value of trigger warnings in relation to self-harm? Self-harm and triggers have a complex relationship. A large number of studies (including many of the 'borderline' papers presented in the previous chapter) have posited a link between self-injury and past experiences of trauma, particularly sexual abuse.[68] Yet triggers tend to be more directly associated with descriptions of self-injurious acts. LifeSIGNS, a British online user support forum set up in 2002, is just one of the online communities that have absorbed these ideas about triggering into their rules, in order to create a safe space for users:

> We do not allow images of self-injury, graphic descriptions, or discussions about specific methodology or severity. Instead we ask our members to focus on talking about their emotional distress and the reasons behind their self-injury, not the self-injury itself.[69]

While the sentiment behind this statement is clearly intended to be supportive, it also indicates the complex relationship between self-harm and the trigger. If trauma triggers include reliving painful experiences, then how can hearing about the distress of others be presented as 'safer' than viewing an image of self-harm?

This raises a challenge in terms of censorship, with the potential to become a form of internal policing. Trigger warnings might be required on 'off-topic' threads that simply include photographs of users carrying out everyday activities (if they show visible injuries), discouraging some from participating. They can also serve to make such a thread 'about' self-harm, even when the topic is ostensibly about something very different, perpetuating the label of 'self-harmer' as an identity that permeates all areas of someone's life. Indeed, when the same happens in a clinical context we think about it as 'objectification, it's reduction of an individual'.[70] The guidelines for the National Self-Harm Network Forum (another user support group) state that:

> The posting of images showing recent self harm is not allowed. NSHN promotes a reduction in the stigma associated with self harm and pictures with historical scars that are incidental to the main focus of the image will be allowed. Moderators will exercise their discretion.[71]

The edges of this boundary cannot be other than blurred. For those who take on the concept of triggers, any image that appears to depict self-harm may be perceived as one. For others, the notion that their own bodies are triggering – that they possess the capacity to harm other people simply by being looked at – may prove equally distressing. Trigger warnings, then, sit at a strange boundary between empowerment and silencing; between freedom and stigma. As the self-harm consultant Clare Shaw reflected, 'I want to be able to talk about who I am and why I am who I am, and I don't want to have to label my life with a trigger warning.'[72]

While there have been efforts in mental health services and general practice in recent years to express a more compassionate and user-led approach to self-injury, medical professionals nonetheless retain power over what is and is not considered healthy. Peer support forum moderators, despite their lived experience, may need to adopt elements of a medical viewpoint in order to be seen as legitimate, avoiding being demonized as 'pro-self-harm'. The rules and regulations in user communities become an outward-facing badge of responsibility as much as a protection for members; a sign to medical professionals that peer groups are just as responsible as the medical community. This does not, of course, mean that peer support forum members never question medical authority – often it is quite the reverse. But they are only able to challenge it through a strongly regulated group identity.[73] The prevalence of the idea of the trigger, however, may lead medical professionals to downplay certain elements of Internet communities, such as the availability of ongoing, 24/7 support and the creation of interpersonal relationships, and emphasize others through a belief in the negative nature of 'pro-self-harm' sites. Clare Shaw commented that she regularly heard about the influence of such sites on young people during her training programmes, usually from staff or parents. However, most often she found that these concerned adults hadn't accessed the sites in question: her personal opinion was that many described safer practices, rather than being pro-self-harm per se.[74] Recent studies have suggested that a prohibition on pro-ana blogs on Tumblr has not affected what is available to readers, but has merely pushed such communities further away from health care providers.[75] There is, after all, a fine line between peer support and promotion: what might look like glorification to an outsider might be much needed help for someone else. Shutting sites down is

> quite a paternalistic approach . . . it's something about what we consider to be dangerous for the public and dangerous for consumption and it might trick people into more risky behaviour, so I think it's an attitude that's quite pervasive in that respect.[76]

This paternalistic approach has built on assumptions about peer contagion adopted wholesale from mental health institutions. Social media sites and peer group forums, we are told, have become breeding grounds for self-harm, suicide and anorexia nervosa: the idea that the Internet *must* have amplified the concerns seen in institutional settings is rarely questioned. A recent *Washington Post* article pointed to a study connecting newspaper reports on suicide to clusters of teen suicides between 1988 and 1996: 'of course', the journalist concluded, on the Internet 'each of those factors is magnified tenfold.'[77] Favazza, meanwhile, stated that:

> Since then [1989] . . . the overwhelming majority of self-injurers now report that they were turned on to NSSI because of stories in newspapers and magazines, television shows, movies, and the Internet. In 2004, Rideout et al. reported that persons from 8 to 18 years old are exposed to more than eight hours a day of media messages.[78]

These two statements are linked solely by the assumption that the more media we consume or are exposed to, the more likely we are to view something relating to self-harm. Yet this assumes that everyone who browses the Internet is entirely passive, and that their use of it is not guided by beliefs and ideas they already hold. Such a supposition is led by the concern of adults about the effects of the Internet on young people generally, alongside the widespread view that 'cutting and other forms of self-mutilation have reached epidemic proportions among our youth.'[79] The Internet, it is widely assumed, *must* have increased this incidence, and not simply its visibility. Yet whether or not there is a causal link does not appear to have been proved to date.

The trigger warning became news primarily when it moved beyond the Internet. In May 2015, in the wake of several calls for trigger warnings on American university syllabuses, the Organization of American Historians hosted a discussion on trauma and trigger warnings in the history classroom. Six academic historians, at different stages of their career, debated the need to be aware of the potential for difficult historical material to 'trigger' a traumatic response in their students, and whether trigger warnings on classroom material were the best way to protect vulnerable young people.[80] Most of those involved regarded trigger warnings as an important and responsible aspect of their course materials. Some thought that potentially traumatic material was clearly identifiable; others that *anything* could be a 'trigger' for memories of past trauma, and that general warnings were most appropriate. Nonetheless, teaching these traumatic materials remained a vital element of education for all the professors concerned; warnings in no way impinged on their own free speech or the potential of their students to develop critical skills and awareness.

Yet trigger warnings *can* be both protective and silencing. Here, I have explored the way the trigger warning became associated with self-harm through two particular approaches to self-injury: normalization and contagion. In the 1990s, self-inflicted injury increasingly became viewed as Western, white and middle class, and was no longer primarily associated with psychiatric inpatients. Alongside anthropological and historical approaches to self-injury, this meant that the topic was viewed more in cultural terms than in relation to clinical pathology; however, it also meant that those who did not fit the profile for reasons of race or gender might face an even greater struggle for recognition and support.[81] The increased visibility of self-injury encouraged greater attention to its spread, although whether or not there has been an actual increase in incidence remains debatable, albeit often assumed. The topic of contagion had previously been explored largely in relation to inpatient communities. Many of the conclusions drawn from these studies were assumed also to apply to broader populations: adolescents generally, and particularly within Internet communities. These broader studies shifted in their focus, however, from 'copycat' behaviour (in relation to cultural icons or media stories) to emphasizing the importance of peers in the spread of behaviour. It was in response to this focus on peer contagion that the trigger warning emerged, initially from user support groups and peer communities, as a badge of outward respectability as much as the sign of a safe space for users.

Today it is a widespread understanding that triggers and their associated flashbacks are, and have always been, an important symptom of trauma. Yet we cannot assume that post-traumatic stress disorder has been a constant state throughout history. The notion that painful flashbacks can be set off by external events is a recent one that assumes an individualized and internalized concept of trauma, similar to the way that self-harm has increasingly been viewed as an individual, psychological phenomenon. Despite modern preoccupations with contemporary culture (particularly youth culture), the examples in this chapter tend to show an emphasis on internal psychology over and above broad social and political concerns. It is not culture that has been emphasized in peer contagion, but the purported influence of one individual or group of individuals on another. Young people are removed from their social and environmental circumstances to become either victims or aggressors, often both at the same time. This paternalistic approach may be oppressive and patronizing rather than supportive; silencing rather than communicative. Moreover, it fails to recognize the important role that peer support plays for many people through difficult periods in their life. The role of the Internet in this is particularly complex. The myriad worlds that people inhabit and the different ways they represent themselves – through social media, online communities, blogs and newsrooms – demand an entirely different way of thinking about people and their interactions with one another. Rather than shifting conclusions from one field to another, we must acknowledge that an entirely new set of rules may apply.

THREE NARRATIVES OF
BODILY HARM

C lare Shaw is a poet and self-harm consultant. The two things are interconnected: the very visual language of poetry can perform some of the same functions as self-injury. Poetry is

> a distillation of everything in language. So it's about rhythm and texture and meaning and context and it's about history and personal history, social history . . . It's shape and sound and silence.[1]

In her early and mid-twenties, Clare was deeply embedded in mental health services. She spent six years in and out of hospital or living in supported accommodation. Clare was injuring herself by the age of ten, often by cutting. She found that hospitalization was still the main response to self-harm in the 1990s. In hospital, she spent most of her time on the 'chaotic, bewildering, dirty, threatening' wards: in six years she recalled going to occupational therapy just twice. It was through reading accounts by survivors of the mental health system that, she says, 'my world changed'; 'these women saved my life.'[2] Some of these were accounts of self-harm, which may be

> the strategy that someone uses to deal with the multiple pains of being abused, including the despair of being unheard. It may also be the most powerful language someone has.

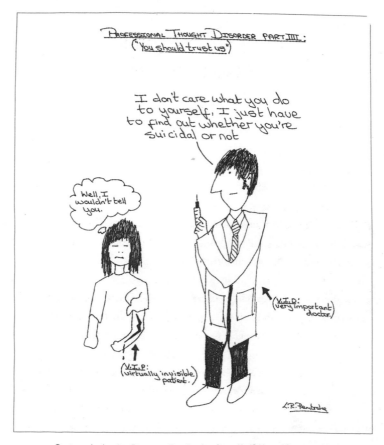

Cartoon by Louise Roxanne Pembroke, from 'Self-Harm: Perspectives
from Personal Experience', produced by Survivors Speak Out, one of the
first organizations to hold a user-led conference on self-harm, in 1989.

To draw a dividing line between accepted artistic practice and self-injury is to make a false distinction. Clare sees both as communication; the metaphor in poetry 'allows us to create our own language'. What's most important is the way these metaphors demand effort of the reader as well as the writer. 'We have to engage,' Clare says, 'we have to be willing to go with it, to see beyond the surface. That's the challenge of listening to self-harm.'[3]

Liz Atkin is a visual artist. Through much of her work she uses her skin as a canvas, often painting directly onto her body. In 2013, she performed at the Anxiety Festival in London, an 'intense and cathartic' experience in which she travelled from the top to the bottom of an arts venue, ending up crouching and covered in black paint. 'I was really trying to express how I felt my body changed when I got ill,' she says. When she revisited the performance some six months later, she was in a very different place; in a similar dance she ended up covered in multicoloured pigments. Liz has been picking her skin since she was six or seven years old. Her compulsive skin-picking (which she describes by using psychiatric terms) was often unconscious. In modern medicine, skin-picking is often considered quite separately from self-harm; in the early twentieth century, in contrast, it was seen as exemplary of it. This change in boundaries is associated with a broader shift in approaches to self-injury, based on assumptions about motivation and purpose that may be questionable in themselves. At its worst, Liz recalls, she would pick in her sleep and wake up with blood on her sheets, or zone out in the bathroom, later discovering she had spent six or seven hours picking at her skin. It was a master's degree in dance that forced her to confront her skin-picking. Within the first week, students were told to take a video camera and record their daily movements, exploring how their bodies naturally moved:

So I set the camera up on a tripod and I did the exercise but, of course, there it was. There was my *dance*! There's my hands moving across my skin, and the skin picking happening.

Liz decided to 'leap into the Lion's den' and explore her experiences in her work:

If this is the thing that my body has done since it was a child, then it's the movement pattern I know better than anything else. So like a ballet dancer repeatedly moves their feet, or a contemporary dancer works out how to work with gravity, my fingers have done this thing all this time. So what happens if I work with it rather than against it? What happens if I'm not hiding it any longer? What happens if I start making something from it? What if the scars are actually important, valuable, rather than the things that no one needs to see?

Art, Liz says, is

absolutely central to what I think human beings can do to express things that don't have words, to express feelings that are challenging or frightening or complicated. And it also liberates the individual.[4]

I am a writer and historian. Recently, I had to complete an occupational health questionnaire. One question rather intrusively asked if I had ever seen a psychiatrist and, if so, what was the outcome. My first impulse was to answer: 'The outcome was that I became a historian.' Between the ages of eighteen and 29, I was in and out of various parts of the mental health service. I took antidepressants continuously through my twenties – at least five different kinds over the years. Twice I was referred to psychiatric services (and once more to a university psychiatrist); I had three different counsellors and one course of cognitive behavioural therapy. I learned to avoid talking about self-harm as far as possible, because I quickly became aware that scars seemed to speak louder than anything else I had to say. I didn't want to be the awkward, troublesome person one GP described in a psychiatric referral: 'I just don't know what to do with her!' Little of this journey helped me make sense of my life and experiences, although some of it eased the pain for a little while. The history of medicine has been a solution for me in the way medicine itself never was. History invites critical thinking and analysis; it may not always provide answers but sometimes that isn't the point. Education empowers in a way that psychiatry, with its rigid frameworks and imposed stereotypes, will always struggle to. It invites questions, rather than imposing answers. It ties the personal with the political, the individual into the broader cultural framework. Unlike psychiatry, it is also not primarily a temporary solution to crisis.

Language – whether written or visual, spoken or dance – allows us to create our own narratives. Psychiatry as a discipline, as described in this book, has largely suggested narratives framed in clinical, biomedical or individual terms. Often, this ignores the things that happen to people or the environments they live in. Poverty, homelessness, abuse, racism, oppression – all these things become internalized as symptoms of either biomedical failing or internal conflict. This is not to say that psychiatry cannot be helpful in making sense of our narratives or that medical services may not serve a valuable purpose. But it can never be the *only* thing that shapes us. To view self-harm as a symptom of borderline personality disorder, schizophrenia or depression is not to explain it. The same can be said of many other psychiatric symptoms. Eleanor Longden, for example, has spoken articulately of the way in which mental health services dismissed her voice-hearing as a symptom of severe illness. Yet it was only when she *listened* to the voices and tried to understand them that she could escape the hold they had over her.[5] While the descriptive terms of a diagnosis may help people to make sense of past experiences, they can also trap us in the reverse, imprisoning us within a rigid, neurobiological framework we have no hope of escaping. Indeed, the very idea of 'recovery' itself can be and has been used for social or political ends: medicine's failure to help the 'borderline' patient, for example, became characterized as his or her 'resistance' to treatment. The twenty-first-century 'recovery agenda', meanwhile, initially seemed to suggest that recovery was relative, encouraging self-determined goals that might or might not meet earlier clinical definitions. Yet these goals are often created in relation to specific medical and cultural criteria (such as the assumptions of a middle-class professional as to what *must* be healthy), and, if they are not met, for whatever reason, treatment and social or financial support might be withheld. 'Recovery' (however defined) may be possible, but it is by no means inevitable.[6]

As I have shown in this book, psychiatric narratives are just as constructed as historical, literary or artistic narratives of self-injury. The creation of self-harm as a psychiatric category has in no way been self-evident. Yet modern studies tend to begin with that assumption, referring to self-harm or non-suicidal self-injury (NSSI) as if either were a natural, stable category, which has simply only recently been recognized by clinicians. Even today many texts differ as to what acts they include in definitions. The 2011 NICE guidelines in the UK explicitly excluded anorexia nervosa, but the mental health charity Mind included eating disorders in their remit by deeming them a 'coping strategy'.[7] Both, however, claimed self-poisoning to be a means of self-harm, while Armando Favazza, among others, adamantly asserted that it is very different.[8] This conceptual confusion should lead to a questioning of the category and yet it does not, because the assumption behind grouping diverse acts under one heading is that they are all ways 'of expressing very deep distress . . . a means of communicating what can't be put into words or even into thoughts'.[9] In a circular manner, this understanding alters the population described by the term, encouraging the exclusion of any act considered to have been carried out for another purpose.[10] Self-harm, it is widely believed, is a *private* act that provides a physical vent for *inner* turmoil. Such an explanation, as historical sources reveal, is by no means obvious. Certainly, many people would consider their self-inflicted injuries to be communicative. But to impose one general meaning or form of language across a set of behaviours has its dangers, which have emerged time and again across this book. When we see people in terms of one particular act, judgements and stereotypes are not far behind, and this stigma haunts many people who self-injure to this day. Sometimes these judgements and stereotypes have much broader consequences. If women are thought to self-injure because they are manipulative (as in the early 1900s) or sexually aggressive (a decade or two later), then this may be used as ammunition for the notion that *all* women are 'naturally' deceitful or hypersexual.

The attribution of psychiatric meaning to self-inflicted injury has thus emerged from a variety of other concerns and frameworks for understanding human identity. The creation of a category of self-mutilation, self-injury or self-harm, however, has directly contributed to a broader shift from a social and environmental model of human functioning to one that offers an internalized view of the individual, couched either in biological or psychological terms. Chris Millard suggested that this was the most significant shift in views of self-harm in Britain during the twentieth century, from a socially embedded, communicative model of self-poisoning after 1945 to an individualized understanding of self-cutting (and human beings in general) in later years, associated with the rise of neoliberal economics.[11] Should this matter? Of course it should. If we assume that the story of Richey Edwards, for example, is 'about' self-harm, then we ignore all the social and political factors about which he spoke so eloquently. The broader picture becomes peripheral to the focus on an individual; poverty, education, class, race, gender – a multitude of other factors are swept away or ignored. Yet how can we ever hope to 'heal' someone living in poverty if we ignore their circumstances? Imposing a psychiatric meaning onto a behaviour exacerbates this tendency; it can also increase the stigma attached to a topic by depersonalizing the person associated with it. An individual becomes a symptom or diagnosis – an object of scientific inquiry; we speak of them 'in the species mode', as Ian Hacking has termed it.[12]

In 1906, the psychiatrist George Savage followed the 'species mode' when he warned his fellow doctors about 'the self-mutilator', one of a number of psychiatric cases that could not be certified as insane, but nonetheless presented a social and moral problem, on the 'borderland of insanity'.[13] One hundred years later, in 2006, the noun 'self-harmer' was added to the *Oxford English Dictionary*.[14] Savage had little to say about self-mutilators, whose acts were 'allied to the hysterical'. These cases were mysterious:

> one can hardly understand the girl who introduced pins between the upper and lower eyelids and accused others of doing it, or the girl ... who had for months produced the most extraordinary worm-like sloughs ... by means of the application of liquor potassae.

Indeed, Savage and his colleagues rarely *did* try to understand these patients: most of their explanations were couched in broad ideas and theories of their time.

Despite examples of people who *have* tried to explore self-harm in other terms, Savage's approach has not been uncommon in the period covered in this book. It is only by looking beyond this psychiatric framework that we can attempt to understand self-harm. My conclusions here are in no way intended to be dismissive of mental health care as a vital service. I fully accept that, in some cases, a psychiatric model offers a useful and potentially therapeutic model of self-harm, and that there are workers across today's mental health system who are genuinely trying to make a difference in people's lives. Yet if psychiatry has one major failing, it is that it tries to function *outside* of all the other narratives, remaining separate from other ways of understanding self-harm, or mental illness more generally:

> The medical model is so rigid and it sits at the centre of the system and . . . it sort of blocks all the other stuff that we're learning – art therapy, recovery, they're actually sideshows. And they will remain sideshows as long as the wards, or the places where we go when we're in crisis remain medically driven. Because that's where the power is – the power's in the doctor.[15]

This power-based model is in part an economic one. Since the medical elements of psychiatry tend to be emphasized in state and research funding of health services, it is invariably those services on the periphery (including social and community services, day centres and arts programmes) that are seen as the legitimate target of cuts. Yet if there is one thing that the history of self-mutilation teaches us, it is that no one meaning of self-harm can be considered more 'true' or genuine than any other, and that medical, social and artistic solutions to mental distress can only function in conjunction with each other.

REFERENCES

Locations and full bibliographic details for references to archival material can be found in the Bibliography under Archives and Unpublished Material.

Introduction

1 See John Collie, 'Fraud and Skin Eruptions', *Lancet*, CLXXXVIII/4868 (1916), pp. 1008–10; Frederick Parkes Weber, 'The Association of Hysteria with Malingering', *Lancet*, CLXXVIII/4605 (1911), pp. 1542–3. Weber nonetheless considered that these patients should be 'pitied', as can be seen in his subject collection of 'Self-mutilations for various purposes' in the Wellcome Institute Library; e.g. letter from P. Milligan to Weber, 9 December 1929, in Wellcome Library, London (WLL), papers of Frederick Parkes Weber, PP/FPW/B163/3.

2 Sarah Chaney, 'Useful Members of Society or Motiveless Malingerers? Occupation and Malingering in British Asylum Psychiatry, 1870–1914', in *Work, Psychiatry and Society, c. 1750–2010*, ed. Waltraud Ernst (Manchester, 2016), pp. 277–97.

3 Articulately argued in Mark Cresswell and Zulfia Karimova, 'Self-harm and Medicine's Moral Code: A Historical Perspective, 1950–2000', *Ethical Human Psychology and Psychiatry*, XII/2 (August 2010), pp. 158–75.

4 A history of these groups can be found in Mark Cresswell, 'Self-harm "Survivors" and Psychiatry in England, 1988–1996', *Social Theory & Health*, III/4 (November 2005), pp. 259–85. Other groups include the International Hearing Voices Network (www.hearing-voices.org) and the Service User Research Enterprise at King's College London, which highlights personal experience as an important qualification for research, alongside traditional academic training. Diana Rose, '"Having a Diagnosis is a Qualification for the Job"', *BMJ (Clinical Research Edition)*, CCCXXVI/7402 (14 June 2003), p. 1331. Bristol Crisis Service for Women is now known as Self-injury Support.

5 Charley Baker, Clare Shaw and Fran Biley, eds, *Our Encounters with Self-harm* (Ross-on-Wye, 2013). See also Louise Roxanne Pembroke, ed., *Self-harm: Perspectives from Personal Experience* (London, 2009).

6 For the former, see Rose, "'Having a Diagnosis is a Qualification for the Job'". For an alternative, user-led definition of self-harm, see Pembroke, ed., *Self-harm*, pp. 2–3.

7 American Psychiatric Association, *DSM-5: Diagnostic and Statistical Manual of Mental Disorders* (Arlington, VA, 2013), pp. 803–6.

8 Armando Favazza recently described his efforts to have self-injury included in *DSM-IV*, published in 1994, as a 'Disorder of Impulse Control'. This was refused because the committee saw self-harm as solely a symptom of borderline personality disorder. Armando Favazza, interview by Sarah Chaney, 6 August 2015.

9 Favazza, in particular, was one of the most vocal advocates of this approach. He nonetheless supports the inclusion of NSSI in a biomedical/descriptive psychiatric classification system. Armando R. Favazza, *Bodies Under Siege: Self-mutilation, Nonsuicidal Self-injury, and Body Modification in Culture and Psychiatry*, 3rd edn (Baltimore, MD, 2011), pp. xiii–xiv.

10 Although this may sometimes simply mean that they were not informed of a documented diagnosis until later; for example, Baker, Shaw and Biley, eds, *Our Encounters with Self-harm*, p. 97.

11 A point well made by Sander Gilman. Sander L. Gilman, 'From Psychiatric Symptom to Diagnostic Category: Self-harm from the Victorians to DSM-5', *History of Psychiatry*, XXIV/2 (2013), p. 162.

12 Musafar revised the epilogue for the 2011 edition, describing his 'great satisfaction' that he had played a part in changing culture and understandings of body modification as a transformative experience. Favazza, *Bodies Under Siege*, pp. 281–95.

13 This was based on important scholarship in the field that nonetheless made sweeping statements about the period, often inspired by criticism of the place and state of psychiatry when these histories were written. For example Andrew T. Scull, *Museums of Madness: The Social Organization of Insanity in Nineteenth-century England* (London, 1979); Michel Foucault, *Madness and Civilization: A History of Insanity in the Age of Reason*, trans. Richard Howard (London, 1989); Gerald N. Grob, 'Mental Institutions in America: Social Policy to 1875' (New York, 1973).

14 Most clearly drawn out in George Savage, 'The Influence of Surroundings on the Production of Insanity', *Journal of Mental Science*, XXXVII/159 (1891), pp. 529–35; George Savage, 'Presidential Address, Delivered at the Annual Meeting of the Medico-Psychological Association', *Journal of Mental Science*, XXXII/139 (1886), pp. 313–31. The term 'survival of the fittest' was coined by psychologist Herbert Spencer to describe Charles Darwin's evolutionary theory of natural selection.

15 A particularly troubling example of this is Cara Angelotta, 'Defining and Refining Self-harm: A Historical Perspective on Nonsuicidal Self-injury',

Journal of Nervous and Mental Disease, CCIII/2 (2015). If the author had read
the primary sources, rather than taking all her quotes from secondary texts, she
would have found a great deal that contradicted her argument that historical
texts prove NSSI to be universal.

16 Savage, 'Presidential Address', p. 317.

17 For some interesting historical reflections on this, see Charles E. Rosenberg
and Janet Golden, eds, *Framing Disease: Studies in Cultural History* (New
Brunswick, NJ, 1992).

18 This was one of the most important contributions of Armando Favazza, *Bodies
Under Siege*, especially in the second edition with the inclusion of text by Fakir
Musafar (2nd edn, Baltimore, MD, 1996).

19 Chris Millard, 'Making the Cut: The Production of "Self-harm" in Post-1945
Anglo-Saxon Psychiatry', *History of the Human Sciences*, XXVI/2 (2013),
pp. 126–50.

20 Interestingly, the *DSM* definition does *not* claim this. *DSM-5*, p. 804.

21 Favazza, *Bodies Under Siege* (1996), p. 232; Barent W. Walsh and Paul M. Rosen,
Self-mutilation: Theory, Research, and Treatment (New York and London, 1988);
Patricia A. Adler and Peter Adler, *The Tender Cut: Inside the Hidden World of
Self-injury* (New York and London, 2011), p. 14. Favazza reduced his emphasis
on Menninger in the third edition of *Bodies Under Siege* (2011), and the
psychoanalyst no longer appears in the index (although *Man Against Himself*
is still cited in the references).

22 Karl A. Menninger, *Man Against Himself* [1938] (San Diego, New York and
London, 1985).

23 One only has to look at books and journal articles to see this. For example
Adler and Adler, *The Tender Cut*; Janis Whitlock, Jane L. Powers and John
Eckenrode, 'The Virtual Cutting Edge: The Internet and Adolescent Self-injury',
Developmental Psychology, XXXXII/3 (2006), pp. 407–17; Marilee Strong,
A Bright Red Scream: Self-mutilation and the Language of Pain (London, 2000).

24 Self-mutilation was the phrase most widely used in the Victorian era; today,
some clinicians only use this term for severe, permanent alteration of the body,
such as amputation or castration. The lack of clarity in all three terms does
not indicate any one specific use. Favazza, *Bodies Under Siege* (2011), p. 197.
Interestingly, the term 'nonsuicidal self-injury' was not included in the title of
editions of Favazza's book before 2011, in which self-mutilation was assumed to
describe all self-injurious tissue damage, superficial or permanently damaging.

1   The Pre-history of Self-harm: From Ancient Castration to
Medicinal Bloodletting

1 Eusebius, *The History of the Church from Christ to Constantine*, ed. G. A.
Williamson and Andrew Louth (Harmondsworth and New York, 1989),
sec. 6.8, p. 186.

2 Ibid.

3 Peter Robert Lamont Brown, *The Body and Society: Men, Women, and Sexual Renunciation in Early Christianity* (New York, 2008), p. 140.

4 Eusebius, *The History of the Church*, sec. 6.6, p. 186.

5 *The Bible: Authorized King James Version*, ed. Robert P. Carroll and Stephen Prickett (Oxford, 1998), p. 27.

6 Gary Taylor, *Castration: An Abbreviated History of Western Manhood* (New York and London, 2000), pp. 68–70.

7 There are a few unique cases of eunuch memoirs, all significantly later – the castrato Filippo Balatri, the Chinese imperial eunuch Liu Ruoyu and some twentieth-century Skoptsy and *hijra* reports. Shaun Tougher, *The Eunuch in Byzantine History and Society* (Abingdon, Oxon, 2008), p. 24.

8 Gender dysphoria replaced gender identity disorder in the DSM-5. It is applied as a diagnosis to people who express significant distress in response to the gender assigned at birth. Gender identity disorder, in contrast, could be applied to *anyone* who questioned their birth gender, whether or not they were in distress. Genderqueer has been adopted by many people who do not identify as exclusively male or female, but any combination of both or neither.

9 Tougher, *The Eunuch in Byzantine History and Society*, pp. 11–12.

10 The Assyrian Empire (1260–612 BCE) contained parts of Iraq, Syria and Turkey, while the Persian Empire (from around 550 BCE) was centred in modern-day Iran. For a useful overview of eunuchs from the ancient world to voluntary castration in the modern world, see Tougher, *The Eunuch in Byzantine History and Society*, pp. 7–13.

11 Ibid., pp. 26–9.

12 Maria Grazia Lancellotti, *Attis, Between Myth and History: King, Priest, and God* (Leiden, 2002), p. 103.

13 James Frazer, *The Golden Bough: A Study of Magic and Religion* [1890] (London, 1993), p. 347.

14 James Adam, 'Self-mutilation', in *Dictionary of Psychological Medicine*, vol. II, ed. Daniel Hack Tuke (London, 1892), p. 1147.

15 Phrygia was located in central Anatolia – now part of Turkey. Ovid (Publius Ovidius Naso) wrote about the myth in *Metamorphoses* (*c.* 8 CE). Gaius Valerius Catullus, writing in the first century BCE, described the myth in more detail in his 63rd poem.

16 Later Roman writers tended to see these as local variations on the same story or theme. Mathew Kuefler, *The Manly Eunuch: Masculinity, Gender Ambiguity, and Christian Ideology in Late Antiquity* (London, 2001), pp. 246–7.

17 For more detailed discussion of the variations of the myth see Jaime Alvar, *Romanising Oriental Gods: Myth, Salvation and Ethics in the Cults of Cybele, Isis and Mithras*, trans. Richard Gordon (Leiden, 2008), pp. 63–8; Lancellotti, *Attis, Between Myth and History*, pp. 91–6; Kuefler, *The Manly Eunuch*, pp. 246–7.

18 Gaius Valerius Catullus, *The Poems of Catullus: An Annotated Translation*, trans. Jeannine Diddle Uzzi (Cambridge, 2015), p. 101.

19 Ibid., p. 101.

20 Kuefler, *The Manly Eunuch*, p. 98.

21 Ibid., p. 379 n. 15.

22 Alvar, *Romanising Oriental Gods*, p. 259.

23 Ibid., p. 255.

24 Ibid., p. 266.

25 Aline Rousselle, *Porneia: On Desire and the Body in Antiquity*, trans. Felicia Pheasant (Oxford, 1988), p. 122. Martijn Icks reports that this story came from Cassius Dio, who had little interest in portraying Elagabalus' religious practices accurately. Martijn Icks, *The Crimes of Elagabalus: The Life and Legacy of Rome's Decadent Boy Emperor* (Cambridge, MA, 2012), p. 52.

26 Kuefler, *The Manly Eunuch*, pp. 250–52; Rousselle, *Porneia*, p. 123.

27 Kuefler, *The Manly Eunuch*, pp. 97–8; Tougher, *The Eunuch in Byzantine History and Society*, pp. 33–4.

28 Luc Brisson, *Sexual Ambivalence: Androgyny and Hermaphroditism in Graeco-Roman Antiquity*, trans. Janet Lloyd (London, 2002), p. 147.

29 Kuefler, *The Manly Eunuch*, pp. 101–2. Kuefler claims that other historians interpret the law of 342 CE as applying to men who married other men. However, he considers that the language is more specific, suggesting it applied to eunuchs in particular. A man who wished to ensure that an intimate male partner (not a eunuch) could inherit from him could use a ceremony of fraternal adoption, rather than marriage.

30 Ovid described the festival in Rome *c.* 8 CE, although he did not go into detail about the rituals. Ovid, *Fasti*, Book IV, trans. G. P. Goold (Cambridge, MA, 2014), pp. 201–15.

31 Rousselle sees this as the major purpose of castration in antiquity. Rousselle, *Porneia*, p. 122.

32 Lancellotti, *Attis, Between Myth and History*, p. 114.

33 Ibid., p. 101.

34 Justin, *Apologies*, trans. Denis Minns and P. M. Parvis (Oxford, 2009), p. 161 (29.2).

35 Ibid., p. 156 (27.4).

36 Adam, 'Self-mutilation', p. 1147.

37 Taylor, *Castration*, pp. 68–70; Kuefler, *The Manly Eunuch*, p. 267.

38 Brown, *The Body and Society*, p. 168. For more detail on the relevant aspects of Origen's theology, see pp. 163–72.

39 Kuefler, *The Manly Eunuch*, p. 221.

40 Ibid., p. 226.

41 Kathryn M. Ringrose, *The Perfect Servant: Eunuchs and the Social Construction of Gender in Byzantium* (London, 2003), p. 11.

42 For more on the Skoptsy, see Chapter Three and Laura Engelstein, *Castration and the Heavenly Kingdom: A Russian Folktale* (Ithaca, NY, and London, 1999).

43 Thomas Laqueur, *Making Sex: Body and Gender from the Greeks to Freud* (Cambridge, MA, and London, 1990), pp. 144–53.

44 Alvar, *Romanising Oriental Gods*, p. 250.

45 English translation of the Nordhausen Inquisition taken from Niklaus Largier, *In Praise of the Whip: A Cultural History of Arousal*, trans. Graham Harman (New York, 2007), pp. 149–50.

46 Jeremy Bentham, *An Introduction to the Principles of Morals and Legislation*, ed. Benjamin Giles King (London, 1823), p. 1.

47 Roselyne Rey, *The History of Pain*, trans. Louise Elliott Wallace, J. A. Cadden and S. W. Cadden (Paris, 1993), pp. 105–7.

48 *Curious Cases of Flagellation in France: Considered from a Legal, Medical and Historical Standpoint with Reference to Analogous Cases in England, Germany, Italy, America, Australia and the Soudan* (London, 1901), p. 102.

49 Jacques Boileau, *History of Flagellation Among Different Nations* (London, 1888), p. 25.

50 Largier, *In Praise of the Whip*, pp. 79, 60.

51 Peter Damian, letter 56, cited ibid., p. 90.

52 James Glass Bertram, *Flagellation and the Flagellants: A History of the Rod in All Countries, from the Earliest Period to the Present Time* (London, 1877), p. 65.

53 Ibid., p. 70.

54 Marla Carlson, *Performing Bodies in Pain: Medieval and Post-modern Martyrs, Mystics, and Artists* (New York, 2010), p. 108; Largier, *In Praise of the Whip*, pp. 131–2.

55 Largier, *In Praise of the Whip*, pp. 104–9; Carlson, *Performing Bodies in Pain*, p. 109; Patrick Vandermeersch, 'Self-flagellation in the Early Modern Era', in *The Sense of Suffering: Constructions of Physical Pain in Early Modern Culture*, ed. Karl A. E. Dijkhuizen and Jan Frans van Enenkel (Boston, MA, 2009), p. 255.

56 Largier, *In Praise of the Whip*, p. 104.

57 Caroline Walker Bynum, 'Fast, Feast and Flesh: The Religious Significance of Food to Medieval Women', *Representations*, XI (1985), pp. 1–25.

58 Bethlem Royal Hospital Archives (BRHA), Bethlem Female Patient Casebook 1860 (CB/77–39).

59 Some bloodletting continued well into the twentieth century, however. Shigehisa Kuriyama, 'Interpreting the History of Bloodletting', *Journal of the History of Medicine and Allied Sciences*, L (1995), pp. 11–46; Kay Codell Carter, *The Decline of Therapeutic Bloodletting and the Collapse of Traditional Medicine* (New Brunswick, NJ, 2012).

60 Isabella Beeton, *The Book of Household Management* (London, 1868), p. 1065.

61 A religious model was suggested by Jonathan Barry, 'Piety and the Patient: Medicine and Religion in Eighteenth-century Bristol', in *Patients and Practitioners: Lay Perceptions of Medicine in Pre-industrial Society*, ed. Roy Porter (Cambridge and New York, 1985), p. 173. For more on bloodletting as placebo, see Carter, *The Decline of Therapeutic Bloodletting*, pp. 18–19; David Wootton, *Bad Medicine: Doctors Doing Harm Since Hippocrates* (Oxford, 2006), pp. 67–70.

62 It is now widely agreed that the sixty or more Hippocratic texts were written by a variety of people. It is even arguable as to whether Hippocrates himself even

practised humoral theory. Vivian Nutton, *Ancient Medicine* (London and New York, 2005), pp. 53–71.

63 Peter Brain, *Galen on Bloodletting: A Study of the Origins, Development, and Validity of his Opinions, with a Translation of the Three Works* (Cambridge and New York, 1986), pp. 112–13.

64 George Thomson, *Galeno-pale; or, A Chymical Trial of the Galenists . . .* (London, 1665), title page.

65 For more on Galen's life and practice, see Nutton, *Ancient Medicine*, pp. 216–29. In 'On Anatomical Procedures', Galen referred to his demonstrations: 'You have seen me demonstrate all these things both privately and publicly, using pigs because there is no advantage in having an ape in such experiments and the spectacle is hideous.' Galen, *On Anatomical Procedures*, trans. Charles Singer (London, 1956), p. 218.

66 Kuriyama, 'Interpreting the History of Bloodletting', p. 16; Nutton, *Ancient Medicine*, p. 240.

67 Aulus Cornelius Celsus, *De Medicina*, trans. W. G. Spencer (London, 1938), book II, 10.1.

68 Brain, *Galen on Bloodletting*, pp. 122–34.

69 Peter Heuer Niebyl, 'Venesection and the Concept of the Foreign Body: A Historical Study in the Therapeutic Consequences of Humoral and Traumatic Concepts of Disease', PhD thesis, Yale University, 1970, p. 143.

70 Bernard de Mandeville, *A Treatise of the Hypochondriack and Hysterick Passions* (London, 1711), p. 55.

71 Thomas Willis, *The London Practice of Physick* (London, 1689), p. 113. The location of bleeding in pleurisy was at the centre of the earlier bloodletting controversy.

72 William Harvey, *The Works of William Harvey*, trans. Robert Willis (Philadelphia, PA, 1989), p. 70.

73 Ibid., p. 59.

74 Willis, *The London Practice of Physick*, p. 184.

75 William Charles Ellis, *A Treatise on the Nature, Symptoms, Causes and Treatment of Insanity* (London, 1838), p. 163; James Cowles Prichard, *A Treatise on Insanity and Other Disorders Affecting the Mind* (London, 1835), p. 255.

76 Barbara T. Gates, *Victorian Suicide: Mad Crimes and Sad Histories* (Princeton, NJ, 1988), p. 15.

77 For the former, see Annie P., BRHA, Bethlem Female Patient Casebook 1899 (CB/161–51). For an example of the latter, George J., BRHA, Bethlem Male Patient Casebook, 1880 (CB/116–70).

78 BRHA, Bethlem Male Patient Casebook, 1900 (CB/163–50).

79 Armando R. Favazza, *Bodies Under Siege: Self-mutilation, Nonsuicidal Self-injury, and Body Modification in Culture and Psychiatry*, 3rd edn (Baltimore, MD, 2011), p. 189.

2 **Morbid Impulse and Moral Insanity:** The Emergence
of Self-mutilation in Late Nineteenth-century Psychiatry

1 'Domestic News', *Cornwall Royal Gazette, Falmouth Packet and Plymouth Journal*, January 1845.

2 William Llywelyn Parry-Jones, *The Trade in Lunacy: A Study of Private Madhouses in England in the Eighteenth and Nineteenth Centuries* (London, 1972), p. 55.

3 There were exceptions to this. The ancient charitable institution of Bethlem, for example, first employed a physician in 1634, while in France, physicians such as Philippe Pinel and Jean-Étienne Esquirol were heavily involved in Paris hospitals in the late 1700s and early 1800s.

4 Today, this is the *British Journal of Psychiatry* (the journal of the Royal College of Psychiatrists, which the MPA became in 1971).

5 There continued to be many non-medical personnel in asylums, key to their functioning and therapeutics, including attendants (as untrained nurses were known), hospital chaplains and even families of the medical officers.

6 Daniel Hack Tuke, *Reform in the Treatment of the Insane: Early History of the Retreat, York: Its Objects and Influence, with a Report of the Celebrations of its Centenary* (London, 1892), p. 36.

7 For the former view, see Michel Foucault, *Madness and Civilization: A History of Insanity in the Age of Reason*, trans. Richard Howard (London, 1989); Andrew T. Scull, 'Psychiatry and Social Control in the Nineteenth and Twentieth Centuries', in *The Insanity of Place / The Place of Insanity* (London and New York, 2006), pp. 107–28. For the reverse, see Jan Goldstein, *Console and Classify: The French Psychiatric Profession in the Nineteenth Century* (Chicago, IL, and London, 2001); Sonu Shamdasani, '"Psychotherapy": The Invention of a Word', *History of the Human Sciences*, XVIII/1 (2005), pp. 1–22.

8 Tuke, *Reform in the Treatment of the Insane*, p. 37; John Charles Bucknill and Daniel Hack Tuke, *A Manual of Psychological Medicine*, 4th edn (London, 1879), p. 663.

9 The movement was specific to England and Wales, although influential in the separate Scottish system, in particular due to the movement of alienists back and forth across the border. Non-restraint received some criticism on the Continent, despite the evangelical efforts of a number of alienists, including Daniel Hack Tuke, to preach non-restraint around the globe. Daniel Hack Tuke, 'American Retrospect: The Insane in the United States', *Journal of Mental Science*, XXXI/133 (April 1885), pp. 89–116.

10 By 'mechanical restraint', Hill included chains, handcuffs, strait-waistcoats, straps, collars or other garments. The term did not apply to confinement in a padded or other room, which was increasingly used in the later nineteenth century. Robert Gardiner Hill, *A Concise History of the Entire Abolition of Mechanical Restraint in the Treatment of the Insane* (London, 1857), p. 11; John Conolly, *The Treatment of the Insane without Mechanical Restraint* (London, 1856).

11 Francis Pritchard Davies, 'Chemical Restraint and Alcohol', *Journal of Mental Science*, XXVI/116 (1881), pp. 526–30.

12 This interest was intensified by evolutionary debate, which saw man as part of a natural hierarchy, particularly following Wallace's application of Darwin's theory of evolution by natural selection to mankind. Alfred Russel Wallace, 'The Origin of Human Races and the Antiquity of Man Deduced from the Theory of "Natural Selection"', *Journal of the Anthropological Society of London* (1864), pp. clviii–clxxxvii.

13 George Savage, 'Presidential Address, Delivered at the Annual Meeting of the Medico-Psychological Assosication', *Journal of Mental Science*, XXXII/139 (1886), pp. 314–15.

14 Bethlem Royal Hospital Archives (BRHA), Bethlem Female Patient Casebook 1900 (CB/136–118).

15 This question was not altered until Bethlem belatedly became incorporated under the Lunacy Acts in 1853, and the reception order from the 1845 Act (which referred only to suicide) was adopted. See BRHA, Patient Casebooks 1844–1852 (CB/030–CB/059).

16 BRHA, Male Patient Casebook, 1853 (CB/060–25), and Female Patient Casebook, 1853 (CB/06–33).

17 P. Maury Deas, 'The Uses and Limitations of Mechanical Restraint as a Means of Treatment of the Insane', *Journal of Mental Science*, XXXII (1896), p. 104; James Shaw, *Epitome of Mental Diseases* . . . (Bristol and London, 1892), p. 31.

18 Maury Deas, 'The Uses and Limitations of Mechanical Restraint', p. 102; James Adam, 'Self-mutilation', in *Dictionary of Psychological Medicine*, vol. II, ed. Daniel Hack Tuke (London, 1892).

19 Samuel Johnson, *Dictionary of the English Language* (London, 1755).

20 J.A.H Murray, ed., *The Oxford English Dictionary* (Oxford, 1933). The discarded slips sent in by volunteer readers for the first edition do include a quotation for 'self-mutilation' in the first edition, which was not used. Oxford University Press Archive (OUPA), un-numbered (discarded) slips for 'self' from first edition.

21 At least one of the major contributors was *in* an asylum – William Chester Minor, an American army surgeon, contributed to the dictionary from Broadmoor Hospital. Simon Winchester, *The Surgeon of Crowthorne: A Tale of Murder, Madness and the Love of Words* (London, 1998).

22 Henry Rayner, 'Melancholia and Hypochondriasis', in *A System of Medicine*, vol. VIII, ed. T. Clifford Allbutt (London, 1899), p. 371.

23 Michael MacDonald puts this between about 1500 and 1660. Michael MacDonald, 'The Medicalization of Suicide in England: Laymen, Physicians, and Cultural Change, 1500–1870', in *Framing Disease: Studies in Cultural History* (New Brunswick, NJ, 1992), ed. Charles Rosenberg and Janet Golden, p. 86.

24 For example, E. J. Seymour, 'Thoughts on the Nature and Treatment of Several Severe Diseases of the Human Body', in *Three Hundred Years of Psychiatry, 1535–1860*, ed. Richard Alfred Hunter and Ida Macalpine (London and New York, 1847), pp. 960–62; Conolly, *The Treatment of the Insane*, p. 82.

25 'Asylum Reports for 1871', *Journal of Mental Science*, XVIII/82 (1872), p. 274.

26 George Savage, 'The Mechanical Restraint of the Insane', *The Lancet*, CXXXII/3398 (1888), p. 738. The same justification was made in Maury Deas, 'The Uses and Limitations of Mechanical Restraint'.

27 This was associated in London with the efforts of the new Metropolitan Police to maintain public order (from 1829), and a little later with police efforts elsewhere. See Olive Anderson, *Suicide in Victorian and Edwardian England* (Oxford and New York, 1987), p. 283. Suicide remained a criminal offence in England and Wales until 1961.

28 BRHA, Female Patient Casebook, 1900 (CB/136–118).

29 Thomas N. Brushfield, 'On Medical Certificates of Insanity', *The Lancet*, CXV/2958, pp. 711–13.

30 'James Adam (Obituary)', *Journal of Mental Science*, 55 (1909), pp. 208–9.

31 Adam, 'Self-mutilation', p. 1147.

32 Ibid., p. 1148. The notion of the 'borderlands of insanity' became increasingly popular following Andrew Wynter, *The Borderlands of Insanity* (London, 1877).

33 Adam related this particularly to criminals, but the idea also became connected with hysteria, as we shall see in Chapter Four.

34 This total includes only behaviours not specified as suicidal by alienists (strangulation, cut-throat, suffocation or shooting), in addition to excluding individuals who refused food, which was usually considered quite separately from self-mutilation in this period.

35 P. S. Abraham, 'Self-mutilation of a Lioness', *Medical Press and Circular*, 1 (1885), pp. 211–12.

36 P. S. Abraham, 'Self-mutilation in a Lioness', *Journal of Mental Science*, XXXII/137 (1886), p. 50.

37 W. Griesinger, 'German Psychiatrie; An Introductory Lecture, Read at the Opening of the Psychiatric Clinique, in Zürich', *Journal of Mental Science*, IX/48 (1864), p. 539.

38 Richard von Krafft-Ebing, *Text-book of Insanity: Based on Clinical Observations for Practitioners and Students of Medicine*, trans. Charles Gilbert Chaddock (Philadelphia, PA, 1904), p. 120. The book was first published in German in 1875.

39 William Carmichael McIntosh, 'On Some of the Varieties of Morbid Impulse and Perverted Instinct', *Journal of Mental Science*, XI/56 (1866), pp. 512–33. McIntosh also wrote several earlier articles on the topic in *The Medical Critic and Psychological Journal* (1863).

40 Laycock was an important contributor to mid-nineteenth-century physiological psychology, in particular for his application of reflex theory to the brain and mental processes. Herbert Spencer is best-known today for applying Darwin's theories to psychology, as well as promoting the French philosopher Auguste Comte in Britain.

41 McIntosh, 'On Some of the Varieties of Morbid Impulse and Perverted Instinct', p. 512.

42 Theo Hyslop, *Mental Physiology: Especially in its Relations to Mental Disorders* (London, 1895), pp. 444–53.

43 George M. Gould and Walter L. Pyle, *Anomalies and Curiosities of Medicine* (London and Philadelphia, PA, 1897), pp. 743–58.

44 McIntosh, 'On Some of the Varieties of Morbid Impulse and Perverted Instinct', p. 528.

45 William Carmichael McIntosh, 'On Morbid Impulse', *The Medical Critic and Psychological Journal*, III (1863), p. 103.

46 Adam, 'Self-mutilation', p. 1151; George Fielding Blandford, *Insanity and its Treatment: Lectures on the Treatment, Medical and Legal, of Insane Patients* (Edinburgh and London, 1871), pp. 194–5.

47 BRHA, Female Patient Casebook, 1895 (CB/152–14).

48 Shaw, *Epitome of Mental Diseases*, p. 31.

49 When the confession was published, it did not include the latter admission, although this explanation was assumed by all involved. See 'The Extraordinary Death-bed Confession', *Sheffield and Rotherham Independent*, 7 January 1882, p. 3.

50 'The Case of the Farmer Brooks', *The Lancet*, CXIX/3046 (1882), p. 73.

51 'The Case of Isaac Brooks', *Journal of Mental Science*, XXVIII (1882), p. 73.

52 This was complicated by the use of two very similar terms in French medical texts: *le moral* (the psychological functions) and *la morale* (morality). See Eva Yampolsky, 'La Perversion du suicide, entre la pathologie et la morale', *Criminocorpus: Revue hypermédia* (forthcoming, Autumn 2016).

53 Daniel Hack Tuke, *Prichard and Symonds in Especial Relation to Mental Science: With Chapters on Moral Insanity* (London, 1891). Tuke added additional notes to this version of the case, pp. 105–7.

54 Daniel Hack Tuke, 'Case of Moral Insanity or Congenital Moral Defect, with Commentary', *Journal of Mental Science*, XXXI/135 (1885), p. 363.

55 'The Extraordinary Confession at Leek', *Manchester Times* (14 January 1882), p. 7.

56 Tuke, 'Case of Moral Insanity', p. 363.

57 George Savage, 'Moral Insanity', *Journal of Mental Science*, XXVII/118 (1881), p. 147; Henry Maudsley, 'The Genesis of Mind (II)', *Journal of Mental Science*, VIII (1862), p. 90.

58 George Savage and Charles Arthur Mercier, 'Insanity of Conduct', *Journal of Mental Science*, XXXXII/176 (1896), p. 2.

59 George Savage, 'The Influence of Surroundings on the Production of Insanity', *Journal of Mental Science*, XXXVII/159 (1891), pp. 533–5. There was a complicated tension between 'self-help' and 'self-sacrifice' in the Victorian era, in which the individual pursuit of commercial gain for the good of all was pitted against commitment to new secular notions, such as altruism.

60 'The Case of Isaac Brooks', *Journal of Mental Science*, p. 72.

61 'The Extraordinary Confession of Perjury Near Leek', London, *The Guardian* (7 January 1882), p. 7.

62 'The Extraordinary Death-bed Confession', *Sheffield and Rotherham Independent.*

63 Judith R. Walkowitz, *City of Dreadful Delight: Narratives of Sexual Danger in Late-Victorian London* (London, 1992), pp. 81–120.

64 'The Case of Isaac Brooks', *Journal of Mental Science*, p. 73.

65 Charles Darwin, *The Descent of Man* [1871], ed. James H. Birx (Amherst, NY, 1998), pp. 596–7.

66 Savage, 'The Influence of Surroundings', p. 533.

3 **Sexual Self-mutilation:** Masturbation, Masculinity and Self-control in Late Victorian Britain

1 'Annotations', *The Lancet*, CXIX/3047 (1882), p. 118.

2 George M. Gould and Walter L. Pyle, *Anomalies and Curiosities of Medicine* (London and Philadelphia, PA, 1897), p. 732.

3 'Index-catalogue of the Library of the Surgeon-General's Office, United States Army', 2nd series (Washington, DC, 1910), pp. 394–5.

4 These two examples have very different connotations, the first emphasizing the relation of castration to sterility and the second to sexual pleasure. Much has been written about Isaac Baker Brown's controversial practice of clitoridectomy to 'cure' madness and hysteria in women. Andrew T. Scull, '"A Chance to Cut is a Chance to Cure": Sexual Surgery for Psychosis in Three Nineteenth-century Societies', in *The Insanity of Place / The Place of Insanity* (London and New York, 2006), pp. 151–71; Ornella Moscucci, *The Science of Woman: Gynaecology and Gender in England, 1800–1929* (Cambridge and New York, 1993).

5 For more on this topic, see Chandak Sengoopta, *The Most Secret Quintessence of Life: Sex, Glands, and Hormones, 1850–1950* (Chicago, IL, and London, 2006).

6 For an interesting account of the relation of vasectomy to castration, see the introduction to Gary Taylor, *Castration: An Abbreviated History of Western Manhood* (New York and London, 2000), pp. 10–11.

7 Peter Robert Lamont Brown, *The Body and Society: Men, Women, and Sexual Renunciation in Early Christianity* (New York, 2008), pp. 19, 168–9.

8 Robert Darby, *A Surgical Temptation: The Demonization of the Foreskin and the Rise of Circumcision in Britain* (Chicago, IL, 2005); Robert Darby, 'The Masturbation Taboo and the Rise of Routine Male Circumcision: A Review of the Historiography', *Journal of Social History*, XXXVI/3 (2003), pp. 737–57.

9 James Adam, 'Cases of Self-mutilation by the Insane', *Journal of Mental Science*, XXIX/126 (1883), p. 214.

10 James Adam, 'Self-mutilation', in *Dictionary of Psychological Medicine*, vol. II, ed. Daniel Hack Tuke (London, 1892), p. 1150.

11 Adam, 'Cases of Self-mutilation by the Insane', p. 217.

12 Ibid.

13 John Marten, *Onania; or, The Heinous Sin of Self-pollution, and All its Frightful Consequences in Both Sexes, Considered* (London, 1716). For more on shifting medical views of masturbation, see Thomas Laqueur, *Solitary Sex: A Cultural History of Masturbation* (New York, 2003).

14 Laqueur, *Solitary Sex*, pp. 267–78.

15 Michael Mason, *The Making of Victorian Sexual Attitudes* (Oxford and New York, 1994), p. 194.

16 Lesley Hall, '"It was Affecting the Medical Profession": The History of Masturbatory Insanity Revisited', *Paedagogica Historica*, XXXIX/6 (2003), pp. 685–99.

17 Robert Ritchie, 'An Inquiry Into a Frequent Cause of Insanity in Young Men', *The Lancet*, LXXVII/1955–60 (1861), p. 185.

18 Ibid., p. 235.

19 Carol Anne Reeves, 'Insanity and Nervous Diseases Amongst Jewish Immigrants to the East End of London, 1880–1920', PhD thesis, University of London, 2001, pp. 166–7. See also David Yellowlees, 'Masturbation', *Journal of Mental Science*, XXII/98 (1876), pp. 336–7; David Yellowlees, 'Masturbation', in *Dictionary of Psychological Medicine*, vol. I, ed. Daniel Hack Tuke (London, 1892), p. 785.

20 Bethlem Royal Hospital Archives (BRHA), Male Patient Casebook 1886, CB/128–112.

21 Adam, 'Cases of Self-mutilation by the Insane', p. 217.

22 Kent County Archives (KCA), West Malling Place Case Histories (Visitors), 1877–1893 (Ch84/Mc3), p. 200.

23 William Hepworth Dixon, *Spiritual Wives* (London, 1868).

24 Mason, *The Making of Victorian Sexual Attitudes*, p. 17.

25 Adam, 'Self-mutilation', p. 1150.

26 For more on the *hijda*, see John Shortt, 'The Kojahs of Southern India', *Journal of the Anthropological Institute of Great Britain and Ireland*, II (1873), pp. 402–7; Laurence W. Preston, 'A Right to Exist: Eunuchs and the State in Nineteenth-century India', *Modern Asian Studies*, XXI/2 (1987), pp. 371–87.

27 Adam, 'Self-mutilation', p. 1147.

28 KCA, Case Histories (Visitors), 1877–1893 (Ch84/Mc3), p. 201.

29 William J. Brown, 'Notes of a Case of Monomania with Self-mutilation and a Suicidal Tendency', *Journal of Mental Science*, XXIII/102 (1877), pp. 242–8.

30 Ibid., p. 243.

31 The so-called repression hypothesis was strongly refuted in Steven Marcus, *The Other Victorians: A Study of Sexuality and Pornography in Mid-Nineteenth-century England* (London, 1966).

32 This was powerfully argued by Foucault, and many studies of sexuality still rely on Foucault's premise. Michel Foucault, *The History of Sexuality*, vol. I: *The Will to Knowledge*, trans. Robert Hurley (London, 1998).

33 Criminal Law Amendment Bill, 300 *H.C. Deb.* 1397–8, 7 August 1885.

34 Charles Upchurch, 'Forgetting the Unthinkable: Cross-dressers and British Society in the Case of the Queen vs. Boulton and Others', *Gender & History*, XII/1 (2000), pp. 127–57.

35 Lesley Hall, *Hidden Anxieties: Male Sexuality, 1900–1950* (Cambridge, 1991); Timothy H. O'Neill, 'The Invisible Man? Problematising Gender and Male Medicine in Britain and America, 1800–1950', PhD thesis, University of Manchester, 2003.

36 William Winwood Reade, *The Martyrdom of Man* (London, 1884), p. 454.

37 Arthur Conan Doyle, *The Adventures of Sherlock Holmes* [1892] (London, 1994), p. 281.

38 Ibid., p. 284.

39 BRHA, Female Patient Casebook, 1893 (CB/146–26).

40 As described in Judith R. Walkowitz, *City of Dreadful Delight: Narratives of Sexual Danger in Late-Victorian London* (London, 1992), pp. 61–5.

41 BRHA, Female Patient Casebook, 1896 (CB/154–88).

42 BRHA, Female Patient Casebook, 1895 (CB/152–33).

43 BRHA, Female Patient Casebook, 1891 (CB/140–36).

44 Judith R. Walkowitz, *Prostitution and Victorian Society: Women, Class and the State* (Cambridge, 1980), p. 87.

45 Judith R. Walkowitz, 'Jack the Ripper and the Myth of Male Violence', *Feminist Studies*, VIII/3 (1982), pp. 542–74.

46 BRHA, Female Patient Casebook 1889 (CB/137–38).

47 The classic in the history of psychiatry is Elaine Showalter, *The Female Malady: Women, Madness, and English Culture, 1830–1980* (London, 1987).

48 The new Victorian emphasis on altruism as a secular emotion is explained in Thomas Dixon, 'The Invention of Altruism: Auguste Comte's Positive Polity and Respectable Unbelief in Victorian Britain', in *Science and Beliefs: From Natural Philosophy to Natural Science, 1700–1900*, ed. David M. Knight and Matthew Eddy (Aldershot, 2005), pp. 195–211.

49 BRHA, Voluntary Boarder Book, 1893–6 (CB/147–26).

50 George Savage, 'Marriage in Neurotic Subjects', *Journal of Mental Science*, XXIX (1883), p. 53.

51 Charles Darwin, *The Descent of Man, and Selection in Relation to Sex* (London, 1871), pp. 556–606.

52 Richard von Krafft-Ebing, *Psychopathia Sexualis: With Especial Reference to Antipathic Sexual Instinct, a Medico-forensic Study*, trans. F. Enke (London, 1899), p. 1.

53 After Krafft-Ebing's death, further revisions were produced by Alfred Fuchs and Albert Moll.

54 For more on the background of *Psychopathia Sexualis* see Renate Irene Hauser, 'Sexuality, Neurasthenia and the Law: Richard von Krafft-Ebing (1840–1902)', PhD thesis, University College London, 1992; Harry Oosterhuis, *Stepchildren of Nature: Krafft-Ebing, Psychiatry, and the Making of Sexual Identity* (Chicago, IL, and London, 2000).

55 Gert Hekma, *A History of Sexology: Social and Historical Aspects of Sexuality*, trans. Jan Bremmer (London and New York, 1989), p. 182.

56 H. R., 'Rev. of Psychopathia Sexualis: By Dr R. von. Krafft-Ebing', *Journal of Mental Science*, XXXVII/156 (1891), pp. 152–4.

57 Wilhelm Stekel, *Sadism and Masochism: The Psychology of Hatred and Cruelty*, trans. Louise Brink (London, 1953), vol. II.

58 Richard von Krafft-Ebing, *Psychopathia Sexualis, with Especial Reference to Contrary Sexual Instict: A Clinical-Forensic Study*, trans. Charles Gilbert Chaddock (Philadelphia, PA, and London, 1892), p. 138.

59 The first text that explicitly made the link was a psychoanalytic case study: L. E. Emerson, 'The Case of Miss A: A Preliminary Report of a Psychoanalytic Study and Treatment of a Case of Self-mutilation', *Psychoanalytic Review*, I (1913), pp. 41–54.

60 Richard von Krafft-Ebing, *Psychopathia Sexualis, with Especial Reference to Contrary Sexual Instinct: A Clinical-Forensic Study*, trans. Brian King (Burbank, CA, 1999), p. 181 (based on 12th German edition).

61 Connolly Norman, 'Sexual Perversion', in *Dictionary of Psychological Medicine*, ed. Daniel Hack Tuke (London, 1892), pp. 1156–7.

62 Havelock Ellis and John Addington Symonds, *Sexual Inversion: A Critical Edition*, ed. Ivan Crozier (Basingstoke, 2008), p. 39.

63 BRHA, Male Patient Casebook, 1892, CB/143–5.

64 BRHA, Male Patient Casebook, 1893, CB/145–50.

65 Cross-dressing and the adoption of traits considered female were both widely practised by male homosexuals in this era. It did not necessarily mean that they (or, indeed, Theodore B.) identified as women or were transsexual, although in some instances this may have been an impetus for castration, as later claimed by Havelock Ellis. Havelock Ellis, *Studies in the Psychology of Sex* (Philadelphia, PA, 1928), vol. VII, p. 94 n. 1.

66 For earlier examples, see Oosterhuis, *Stepchildren of Nature*, pp. 133–6. E. is case nine in both the seventh and tenth editions of *Psychopathia Sexualis*. Krafft-Ebing, *Psychopathia Sexualis* (1899), pp. 42–6.

67 Krafft-Ebing, *Psychopathia Sexualis* (1899), p. 45. Thomas Robert Malthus (1766–1834) wrote an influential theory of demography, suggesting that population growth would eventually outstrip food supply.

68 Krafft-Ebing, *Psychopathia Sexualis* (1899), p. 42.

69 Cases 96, 129 and 145 in the twelfth edition of *Psychopathia Sexualis* considered castration.

70 Richard von Krafft-Ebing, 'Zur Castratio virorum', *Arbeiten aus dem Gasammtgebiet der Psychiatrie und Neuropathologie*, vol. IV, pp. 189–92, cited in Oosterhuis, *Stepchildren of Nature*, p. 155.

71 Victor von Gyurkovechky, *Pathologie und Therapie der männlichen Impotenz* (Vienna, 1889), cited in Krafft-Ebing, *Psychopathia Sexualis* (1899), pp. 12–13.

72 The history of the sect has been ably traced by Laura Engelstein. Laura Engelstein, *Castration and the Heavenly Kingdom: A Russian Folktale* (Ithaca, NY, and London, 1999).

73 A. P. Cawadias, 'Male Eunuchism Considered in the Light of the Historical Method', *Proceedings of the Royal Society of Medicine*, XXXIX (1946), pp. 23–8; Jean D. Wilson and Claus Roehrborn, 'Long-term Consequences of Castration in Men: Lessons from the Skoptzy and the Eunuchs of the Chinese and Ottoman Courts', *Journal of Clinical Endocrinology and Metabolism*, LXXXIV/12 (1999), pp. 4324–31.

74 This connection was also made by Karl Menninger, who regarded mutilation 'willingly submitted to' for religious reasons as equivalent to self-inflicted injuries. Karl A. Menninger, *Man Against Himself* [1938] (San Diego, New York and London, 1985), p. 220.

75 'Self-mutilation by the Insane', *Medical Press and Circular*, II (1888), p. 260.

76 *Sheffield and Rotherham Independent*, 9 April 1869, issue 4910, p. 4; *Glasgow Herald*, 12 April 1869, issue 9134; *The Dundee Courier and Argus*, 15 April 1869, issue 4895.

77 Krafft-Ebing, *Psychopathia Sexualis* (1899), p. 5.

78 Charles Darwin, *The Descent of Man*, p. 585.

79 Henry Maudsley, 'The Genesis of Mind (II)', *Journal of Mental Science*, VIII (1862), p. 90.

80 For more on Pelikan, see Engelstein, *Castration and the Heavenly Kingdom*, pp. 60–68.

81 E. Teinturier, *Les Skoptzy* (Paris, 1877), pp. 28–36.

82 I. Kopernicky and J. B. Davis, 'On the Strange Peculiarities Observed by a Religious Sect of Moscovites Called Scoptsis', *Journal of the Anthropological Society of London*, VIII (1870), pp. 122–4.

83 Although Engelstein does note that male defendants were almost twice as likely as female to bear ritual scars: in most trials, 30–40 per cent of women, but around 60 per cent of men, were mutilated. Engelstein, *Castration and the Heavenly Kingdom*, p. 96.

84 James C. Howden, 'Notes of a Case – Mania Followed by Hyperaesthesia and Osteomalacia. Singular Family Tendency to Excessive Constipation and Self-mutilation', *Journal of Mental Science*, XXVIII/121 (1882), pp. 49–53. .

85 Krafft-Ebing, *Psychopathia Sexualis* (1899), p. 139.

86 Not to be confused with reproductive capacity, deemed of far greater physiological and psychological importance in women.

87 Pelikan quoted in Laura Engelstein, 'From Heresy to Harm: Self-castrators in the Civic Discourse of Late Tsarist Russia', in *Empire and Society: New Approaches to Russian History*, ed. Teruyuki Hara and Kimitaka Matsuzato (Sapporo, 1997), p. 12.

88 Engelstein, *Castration and the Heavenly Kingdom*, p. 36.

89 Adam, 'Self-mutilation', p. 1147. Adam was not alone in this declaration. See also 'On Moral and Criminal Epidemics', *Journal of Psychological Medicine and Mental Pathology*, IX/2 (1856), p. 249. Charles Arthur Mercier, 'A Classification of Feelings (part 3)', *Mind*, X/37 (1885), p. 3.

90 Cawadias, 'Male Eunuchism Considered in the Light of the Historical Method', p. 26.

91 Engelstein, *Castration and the Heavenly Kingdom*, p. 117.

92 Letter from Latyshev to Stalin (22 December 1938), translated in Engelstein, *Castration and the Heavenly Kingdom*, p. 229.

93 W. J. Bishop, 'Some Historical Cases of Auto-Surgery', *Proceedings of the Scottish Society for the History of Medicine, 1960–61* (1961), p. 23; Menninger, *Man Against Himself*, p. 248.

4   **Motiveless Malingerers:** Multiple Personality, Attention-seeking and Hysteria around 1900

1   Walter Channing, 'Case of Helen Miller – Self-mutilation – Tracheotomy', *American Journal of Insanity*, XXXIV (1878), p. 368.

2   Linda Gask, Mark Evans and David Kessler, 'Personality Disorder', *British Medical Journal*, CCCXXXXVII (2013), pp. 1–7. Conversely, in an interview Clare Shaw stated that she considered that this attitude towards BPD had got worse in recent years. Clare Shaw, interview by Sarah Chaney, 24 July 2015 (digital recording).

3   Mark S. Micale, *Approaching Hysteria: Disease and Its Interpretations* (Princeton, NJ, 1995), p. 19.

4   Helen King, 'Once Upon a Text: Hysteria from Hippocrates', in *Hysteria Beyond Freud*, ed. Sander L. Gilman et al. (Berkeley, Los Angeles and London, 1993), p. 7.

5   Hypochondriasis the disease was not the same as modern-day hypochondria – fear of non-existent illness – as it had both physical and mental symptoms. A fixation on bodily disease, it was long thought, could actually *produce* physical ailments. While hypochondriasis was viewed as a mental illness by the mid-Victorian period, it was sometimes considered serious enough to require asylum treatment.

6   Charles Chrétien Henri Marc, *De la folie, considérée dans ses rapports avec les questions médico-judiciaires* (Paris, 1840), vol. II, pp. 247–303. The Swiss doctor André Matthey described a similar propensity, which he called 'klopemanie' (mania for theft). André Matthey, *Nouvelles recherches sur les maladies de l'esprit* (Geneva, 1816), pp. 134–7.

7   J. Baker, 'Kleptomania', in *A Dictionary of Psychological Medicine*, ed. Daniel Hack Tuke (London, 1892), vol. II, pp. 726–9.

8   George Savage, 'An Address on the Borderland of Insanity', *British Medical Journal*, I/2357 (1906), p. 492.

9   Channing, 'Case of Helen Miller', p. 369.

10 Robert Saundby, 'Clinical Lecture on Toxic Hysteria', *The Lancet*, CXXXVII/3514 (January 1891), p. 2.

11 Elaine Showalter, *Hystories: Hysterical Epidemics and Modern Culture* (London, 1997).

12 Channing, 'Case of Helen Miller', p. 375.

13 Ibid., pp. 377–8.

14 Dr Budd, 'King's College Hospital (The Mania of Thrusting Needles into the Flesh)', *The Lancet*, LVI/1425 (1850), p. 676.

15 George M. Gould and Walter L. Pyle, *Anomalies and Curiosities of Medicine* (London and Philadelphia, PA, 1897), p. 735.

16 Ernest Hart, 'Hysteria: Wilful Self-infliction of Injury', *The Lancet*, LXXIX/2014 (1862), p. 355.

17 F. Bowreman Jessett, 'A Case of Faecal Fistula due to Self-mutilation Occurring Twice in the Same Patient', *The Lancet*, CXXXVIII/3818 (1896), p. 1214.

18 Mr Callender and Morrant Baker, 'St Bartholomew's Hospital (Hysteria)', *The Lancet*, C/2551 (1872), p. 78.

19 Micale, *Approaching Hysteria*, p. 24; Roy Porter, 'Body and Mind, the Doctor and the Patient: Negotiating Hysteria', in *Hysteria Beyond Freud*, pp. 261–5.

20 Beatrice A., Royal London Hospital Archive (RLHA) Microfilm Case Records (Surgical), TREVES F1898, pt. no. 901.

21 Beatrice A., RLHA Microfilm Case Records (Surgical), HUTCHINSON F1909, pt. no. 1154.

22 Beatrice A., RLHA, TREVES F1898.

23 Beatrice A., HUTCHINSON F1909. See also RLHA Microfilm Case Records (Surgical), FENWICK F1906, pt. no. 1695; OPENSHAW F1908, pt. no. 1814.

24 Ian Fraser, 'Foreign Bodies', *British Medical Journal*, 1/4088 (1939), p. 970.

25 Benjamin Collins Brodie, 'Extraction of Foreign Bodies', *The Lancet*, 1/1063, p. 500.

26 Maurice Craig, *Psychological Medicine: A Manual on Mental Diseases for Practitioners and Students* (London, 1905), pp. 267–8.

27 Sarah Chaney, 'Useful Members of Society or Motiveless Malingerers? Occupation and Malingering in British Asylum Psychiatry, 1870–1914', in *Work, Psychiatry and Society, c. 1750–2010*, ed. Waltraud Ernst (Manchester, 2016), pp. 284–7.

28 For more early examples of malingering, see Roger Cooter, 'Malingering in Modernity: Psychological Scripts and Adversarial Encounters During the First World War', in *War, Medicine and Modernity*, ed. Roger Cooter, Mark Harrison and Steve Sturdy (Stroud, 1999), pp. 125–48.

29 'Motiveless Malingerers', *British Medical Journal*, 1/470 (1870), p. 15.

30 Ibid., p. 16.

31 James Startin, 'Remarks on Feigned or Hysterical Diseases of the Skin', *British Medical Journal*, 1/471 (1870), pp. 25–7; Thomas Flower, 'Feigned or Hysterical Disease of Skin', *British Medical Journal*, 1/482 (1870), pp. 307–8; C. Hilton Fagge, 'Notes on Some Feigned Cutaneous Affections', *British Medical Journal*, 1/476 (1870), pp. 151–2.

32 Erasmus Wilson, *Lectures on Dermatology: Delivered in the Royal College of Surgeons of England in 1874–1875* (London, 1875), pp. 192–208; Henry Radcliffe Crocker, *Diseases of the Skin: Their Description, Pathology, Diagnosis and Treatment* (London, 1893), p. 288; James Galloway and Humphry Davy Rolleston, 'Feigned Diseases of the Skin', in *A System of Medicine*, ed. T. Clifford Allbutt (London, 1899), pp. 937–9.

33 Galloway and Rolleston, 'Feigned Diseases of the Skin', p. 937; Wilson, *Lectures on Dermatology*, p. 203.

34 Henry MacCormac, 'Autophytic Dermatitis', *British Medical Journal*, II/4014 (1937), p. 1153.

35 Neurasthenia was popularized by American neurologist George Miller Beard, who brought together a group of disorders found in 'brain-working households', all of which, he claimed, were 'diseases of civilization, and of modern civilization, and mainly of the nineteenth century, and of the United States'. George Miller Beard, *A Practical Treatise on Nervous Exhaustion (Neurasthenia)* (New York, 1889), pp. 23–5.

36 MacCormac, 'Autophytic Dermatitis', p. 1155.

37 Jean-Martin Charcot, *Clinical Lectures on the Diseases of the Nervous System*, ed. and trans. Ruth Harris (New York, 1991), pp. 14, 42, 94.

38 Pierre Janet, *The Major Symptoms of Hysteria: Fifteen Lectures Given in the Medical School of Harvard University* (New York and London, 1907), p. 273.

39 For more on Janet, see Henri F. Ellenberger, *The Discovery of the Unconscious: The History and Evolution of Dynamic Psychiatry* (New York, 1970), pp. 331–417; Henri F. Ellenberger, *Beyond the Unconscious: Essays of Henri F. Ellenberger in the History of Psychiatry*, ed. Mark S. Micale (Princeton, NJ, 1993), pp. 155–74; John I. Brooks, *The Eclectic Legacy: Academic Philosophy and the Human Sciences in Nineteenth-century France* (Cranbury, NJ, 1998), pp. 163–93.

40 Pierre Janet, 'On the Pathogenesis of Some Impulsions', *Journal of Abnormal Psychology* (1906), p. 8.

41 Pierre Janet, *Névroses et idées fixes* (Paris, 1898), pp. 388–90.

42 Psychasthenia was a term Janet used to describe lurid obsessions, compulsions and phobias. Pierre Janet, *Les Obsessions et la psychasthénie* (Paris, 1903), pp. 232–3.

43 Janet, 'On the Pathogenesis of Some Impulsions', p. 7.

44 Ibid., p. 13.

45 These promises appear in asylum case records. For example, Emily Kate T., Bethlem Royal Hospital Archives (BRHA), Female Patient Casebook 1888 (CB/135–347); Henry B., BRHA Male Patient Casebook 1895 (CB/151–97).

46 Georges Dieulafoy, 'Escarres multiples et récidivantes depuis deux ans deux bras et au pied. – Amputation du bras gauche. Discussion sur la nature de ces escarres. – Pathomimie', *La Presse Médicale* (1908), p. 371 (all translations my own).

47 'A Medical Puzzle Solved: Self-inflicted Injuries', *The Standard* (London), 11 June 1908.

48 Frederick Parkes Weber, 'Artificial "Erythrodoema" of Finger Tips' (Case Notes), 28 November 1936, in Wellcome Library, London (WLL), The Papers of Frederick Parkes Weber, PP/FPW/B163/1.

49 Henry MacCormac, 'Autophytic Dermatitis', *Proceedings of the Royal Society of Medicine (Dermatological Section)*, XXVIII (1935), p. 734; H. Haldin Davis, 'Dermatitis Artefacta', *Clinical Journal*, 53 (1924), p. 216.

50 Henry MacCormac, 'Self-inflicted Hysterical Lesions of the Skin, with Special Reference to the After-history', *British Journal of Dermatology and Syphilis*, XXXVIII (1926), p. 372.

51 This distinction is made very clearly in H. G. Adamson, 'Acne Urticata and Other Forms of "Neurotic Excoriations"', *British Journal of Dermatology*, XXVII/1 (1915), p. 11.

52 MacCormac, 'Self-inflicted Hysterical Lesions', pp. 372–5.

53 Pierre Janet, *L'Automatisme psychologique* (Paris, 1889). See Ian Hacking, *Rewriting the Soul: Multiple Personality and the Sciences of Memory* (Princeton, NJ, 1998); Showalter, *Hystories*.

54 William James, *The Principles of Psychology*, vol. 1 (London, 1890), pp. 390–93.

55 From 1895 until at least 1901, when his name disappeared from the published record. 'List of Members and Associates', *Proceedings of the Society for Psychical Research*, 10 (1895), p. 625. Calling card and letter from Pierre Janet to Theo Hyslop, 28 April (no year given but presumably around the time the book was published in 1895), pasted into WLL copy of Hyslop, *Mental Physiology*.

56 Theo Hyslop, 'On "Double Consciousness"', *British Medical Journal*, II/2021 (1899), p. 782.

57 BRHA, Voluntary Boarder Book, 1893–6 (CB/147–26).

58 Hyslop, 'On "Double Consciousness"', p. 782.

59 BRHA, Voluntary Boarder Book, 1893–6 (CB/147–26).

60 Hyslop, 'On "Double Consciousness"', p. 786.

61 F.W.H. Myers, *Human Personality and Its Survival of Bodily Death* (London, 1903), pp. 43–4.

62 Ibid., p. 355.

63 George Pernet, 'The Psychological Aspect of Dermatitis Factitia', *Transactions of the American Dermatological Association*, XXX (1909), pp. 21–5.

64 George Pernet, 'Two Cases of Dermatitis Factitia', *Proceedings of the Royal Society of Medicine (Dermatological Section)*, VIII (1915), p. 91.

65 It was actually Breuer, and not Freud, who wrote this section in *Studies on Hysteria*. Sigmund Freud and Josef Breuer, *Studies on Hysteria* [1895], trans. Angela Richards and James Strachey (Harmondsworth, 1991), pp. 279–92.

66 Pernet, 'Two Cases of Dermatitis Factitia', p. 89.

67 S. E. Dore, 'Report on a Case of Dermatitis Artefacta', *Proceedings of the Royal Society of Medicine (Dermatological Section)*, XIX (1926), pp. 47–8.

68 Weber, 'The Association of Hysteria with Malingering', p. 1542. For a similar suggestion, before the psychological view was applied, see 'Motiveless Malingerers', *BMJ*, p. 16.

69 Savage, 'An Address on the Borderland of Insanity', pp. 489–90. For more on the history of this idea as applied to rape, see Joanna Bourke, *Rape: A History from 1860 to the Present* (London, 2007), pp. 28–41.

70 MacCormac, 'Autophytic Dermatitis', p. 734.

5   **Focal Suicide:** Hypersexuality, Masochism and the Death Instinct
    in Psychoanalysis

  1 Elizabeth Ferrars was born in Burma in 1907, as Morna MacTaggart. Ferrars
     became well known in later decades as a writer of detective fiction, and was one
     of the founding members of the Crime Writers' Association. *Don't Monkey with
     Murder* was published early in her career, her fourth book. Elizabeth Ferrars,
     Don't Monkey with Murder (Harmondsworth, 1951).
  2 Ibid., p. 22.
  3 Ibid., p. 40.
  4 Ibid., p. 189.
  5 Armando R. Favazza, *Bodies Under Siege: Self-mutilation, Nonsuicidal Self-injury,
     and Body Modification in Culture and Psychiatry*, 2nd edn (Baltimore, MD, 1996),
     p. 232; Patricia A. Adler and Peter Adler, *The Tender Cut: Inside the Hidden
     World of Self-injury* (New York and London, 2011), p. 14.
  6 Martin Bauml Duberman, '"I Am Not Contented": Female Masochism and
     Lesbianism in Early Twentieth-century New England', *Signs: Journal of Women
     in Culture and Society*, V/4 (1980), p. 827.
  7 Louville Eugene Emerson, 'The Case of Miss A: A Preliminary Report of a
     Psychoanalytic Study and Treatment of a Case of Self-mutilation', *Psychoanalytic
     Review*, I (1913), p. 43.
  8 Louville Eugene Emerson, 'Emerson and Freud: A Study in Contrasts',
     Psychoanalytic Review, XX (1933), p. 44.
  9 Emerson, 'The Case of Miss A', p. 42.
 10 Louise J. Kaplan, *Female Perversions: The Temptations of Madame Bovary*
     (London, 1991), p. 553; Emerson, 'The Case of Miss A', p. 41. Delicate self-cutting
     is discussed in the next chapter.
 11 Stefan Collini, *Public Moralists: Political Thought and Intellectual Life in Britain,
     1850–1930* (Oxford, 1991), pp. 331–41. For the USA see Elizabeth Lunbeck,
     The Psychiatric Persuasion: Knowledge, Gender, and Power in Modern America
     (Princeton, NJ, 1994), pp. 72–3.
 12 Putnam (1846–1918) was one of the earliest supporters of psychoanalysis in
     the United States, and wrote one of the first articles in English on the topic
     in 1906, which he connected to his earlier interests in hypnosis and automatic
     writing. Sonu Shamdasani, 'Putnam, James Jackson', in *Dictionary of Medical
     Biography*, ed. William F. Bynum and Helen Bynum (Westport, CT, 2006),
     vol. IV, 1037–8.
 13 Burghölzli is the University of Zurich psychiatric hospital, founded by Wilhelm
     Griesinger and well known in psychiatric circles by the end of the nineteenth
     century. William McGuire, ed., *The Freud/Jung Letters: The Correspondence
     between Sigmund Freud and C. G. Jung*, trans. Ralph Manheim and R.F.C. Hull
     (Princeton, NJ, 1974).
 14 Francis Clark-Lowes, *Freud's Apostle: Wilhelm Stekel and the Early History
     of Psychoanalysis* (Sandy, 2010), p. 11. This followed the *Jahrbuch für*

psychoanalytische und psychopathologische Forschungen, established in 1908 and edited by Bleuler, Freud and Jung.

15 Karl A. Menninger, 'A Psychoanalytic Study of the Significance of Self-mutilations', *Psychoanalytic Quarterly*, IV (1935), p. 422.

16 Mikkel Borch-Jacobsen and Sonu Shamdasani, *The Freud Files: An Inquiry into the History of Psychoanalysis* (Cambridge, 2012), pp. 223–30.

17 Sigmund Freud, 'From the History of an Infantile Neurosis' [1918], in *The Standard Edition of the Complete Psychological Works of Sigmund Freud*, trans. James Strachey (London, 1974), vol. XVII, p. 7.

18 Ibid., pp. 99–100. Pankejeff consulted Freud, and later Brunswick, in 1926, on account of an obsession with a scar on his nose, caused by electrolysis. Brunswick countered that 'nothing whatsoever was visible on the small, snub, typically Russian nose of the patient' and interpreted this perceived injury as an ongoing neurotic obsession with the self-inflicted 'castration'. Ruth Mack Brunswick, 'A Supplement to Freud's "History of an Infantile Neurosis"', *International Journal of Psychoanalysis*, IX (1928), p. 439.

19 For more background on Meyer and his life and work from 1892 to 1917, see Susan D. Lamb, *Pathologist of the Mind: Adolf Meyer and the Origins of American Psychiatry* (Baltimore, MD, 2014). Lamb views Meyer as a key influence in the publication of the first *Diagnostic and Statistical Manual* (DSM) of the American Psychiatric Association in 1952, two years after his death.

20 Lunbeck, *The Psychiatric Persuasion*, pp. 22–3.

21 Nathan G. Hale, *The Rise and Crisis of Psychoanalysis in the United States: Freud and the Americans, 1917–1985* (Oxford, 1995), p. 4.

22 Louville Eugene Emerson, 'Psychoanalysis and Hospitals', *Psychoanalytic Review*, I (1914), pp. 286–7.

23 Lunbeck, *The Psychiatric Persuasion*, p. 3.

24 Emerson, 'Psychoanalysis and Hospitals', p. 285.

25 Both elements are clearly outlined in Lunbeck, *The Psychiatric Persuasion*, pp. 35–45. See also Hale, *Freud and the Americans*, pp. 94–5.

26 Lunbeck points out that 'it is impossible to reconstruct the mix of subtle suggestion and emotional incentives that in nearly every case yielded the information he sought.' Lunbeck, *The Psychiatric Persuasion*, p. 215.

27 In contrast, it took 292 sessions to delve into Rachel's unconscious memories.

28 Emerson, 'The Case of Miss A', pp. 43–50.

29 Duberman, '"I Am Not Contented"', p. 827; Emerson, 'The Case of Miss A', p. 44.

30 Emerson, 'The Case of Miss A', p. 44.

31 Duberman, '"I Am Not Contented"', p. 827.

32 Emerson, 'The Case of Miss A', p. 43.

33 Duberman, '"I Am Not Contented"', p. 827.

34 Lunbeck, *The Psychiatric Persuasion*, pp. 214, 219.

35 Duberman, '"I Am Not Contented"', pp. 826, 829.

36 Emerson, 'The Case of Miss A', pp. 51–2.

37 G. M. Jones, 'Extraordinary Self-mutilation', *The Lancet*, LXX/1769 (1857), p. 88.

38 George H. Monks, 'A Group of Unique and Unusual Surgical Cases', *Medical and Surgical Reports of the Boston City Hospital*, 11th series (1900), p. 143.

39 In 1907, the state of Indiana enacted the first sterilization law for those deemed 'unfit': this included people with learning disabilities and mental illness. In 1909, California and Washington passed similar laws and, in the next decade, 28 other states followed suit.

40 Louville Eugene Emerson, 'Some Psychoanalytic Studies of Character', *Journal of Abnormal Psychology*, XI/4 (1916), p. 265.

41 Sigmund Freud, 'Contributions to a Discussion on Masturbation' [1912], in *The Standard Edition of the Complete Psychological Works of Sigmund Freud*, trans. James Strachey, vol. XII, pp. 239–54.

42 Louville Eugene Emerson, 'The Psychoanalytic Treatment of Hystero-epilepsy', *Journal of Abnormal Psychology*, X/5 (1915), p. 316.

43 Wilhelm Stekel, *Auto-erotism: A Psychiatric Study of Masturbation and Neurosis*, trans. James S. Van Teslaar (New York, 1951), p. 80.

44 Wilhelm Stekel, *Sadism and Masochism: The Psychology of Hatred and Cruelty*, trans. Louise Brink (London, 1953), vol. II, p. 212.

45 Emerson, 'The Case of Miss A', pp. 51, 44.

46 Nathaniel Hawthorne, *The Scarlet Letter* [1850], ed. R. K. Gollin and Paul Lauter (Boston, MA, 2002), p. 350.

47 Stekel, *Sadism and Masochism*, vol. II, p. 161.

48 Emerson, 'The Case of Miss A', p. 41. Emphasis in original.

49 Richard von Krafft-Ebing, *Psychopathia Sexualis, with Especial Reference to Contrary Sexual Instinct: A Clinical-Forensic Study*, trans. Brian King (Burbank, CA, 1999), p. 170 (based on 12th German edition).

50 L. L. McArthur, 'Presentation of a Case of Mutilating Operations in a Hysterical Patient', *Journal of Nervous and Mental Diseases*, XXXVIII/7 (1911), p. 426.

51 Louville Eugene Emerson, 'The Psychopathology of the Family', *Journal of Abnormal Psychology*, IX/5 (1914), p. 337.

52 Duberman, '"I Am Not Contented"', p. 829.

53 Menninger, 'A Psychoanalytic Study', p. 418.

54 Karl A. Menninger, *Man Against Himself* [1938] (San Diego, New York and London, 1985), p. 211. Emphasis in original. In this later version, the Kansan auto-mechanic became a steamfitter's assistant from Chicago, a change indicating the popular readership Menninger hoped for, in that he made greater effort to protect patient confidentiality.

55 Menninger, 'A Psychoanalytic Study', p. 419.

56 Ibid., pp. 418–20.

57 Adler and Adler, *The Tender Cut*, p. 14.

58 Lawrence Jacob Friedman, *Menninger: The Family and the Clinic* (New York, 1990), p. xi. For more on Menninger, see Sonu Shamdasani, 'Menninger, Karl A.', in *Dictionary of Medical Biography*, ed. Bynum and Bynum, vol. IV, pp. 867–9.

59 Karl A. Menninger, *The Human Mind* (New York and London, 1930), p. 14.

60 Ibid., p. ix. Although Menninger cast himself as expressing the views of his era, Hale saw him as the most extreme example of an 'optimistic conservative interpretation' of psychoanalysis. Hale, *Freud and the Americans*, p. 82.

61 Karl A. Menninger, *The Selected Correspondence of Karl A. Menninger, 1919–1945*, ed. Howard J. Faulkner and Virginia D. Pruitt (Columbia, MO, 1995), p. 99.

62 Hale, *Freud and the Americans*, p. 7.

63 Friedman, *Menninger*, p. 110. Menninger's letters indicate that his rhetorical style was not limited to his published material; for example, Menninger to Franz Alexander, 15 March 1940, in *The Selected Correspondence of Karl A. Menninger*, pp. 330–31.

64 Sigmund Freud, 'Beyond the Pleasure Principle' [1920], in *The Standard Edition of the Complete Psychological Works of Sigmund Freud*, trans. James Strachey, vol. XVIII, pp. 7–64.

65 Menninger, *Man Against Himself*, p. 6.

66 'The Ubiquity of Suicide', *British Medical Journal*, 1/4075 (1939), p. 273.

67 Karl A. Menninger, *Sparks: Reflections from the Records of a Pioneer Psychiatrist*, ed. Lucy Freeman (New York, 1973), pp. 135–6.

68 Karl A. Menninger, 'Psychoanalytic Aspects of Suicide', *International Journal of Psychoanalysis*, XIV (1933), pp. 378–82.

69 Ibid., p. 388.

70 Ibid., pp. 378–9.

71 Menninger, *Man Against Himself*, pp. 249–50.

72 Ibid., pp. 254–5.

73 Ibid., p. 259.

74 Ibid., p. 55.

75 Karl A. Menninger, 'Purposive Accidents as an Expression of Self-destructive Tendencies', *International Journal of Psychoanalysis*, XVII (1936), p. 6.

76 Menninger, *Man Against Himself*, p. 279. The original passage is in Sigmund Freud, 'Fragment of an Analysis of a Case of Hysteria', in *The Standard Edition of the Complete Psychological Works of Sigmund Freud*, trans. James Strachey, vol. VII, p. 120.

77 Menninger, 'Purposive Accidents as an Expression of Self-destructive Tendencies', p. 9.

78 J. S. Baker, 'Do Traffic Accidents Happen by Chance?' *National Safety News*, 3, September 1929, pp. 12–14.

79 Menninger, *Man Against Himself*, p. 280.

80 Ibid., pp. 292–3.

81 Ibid., p. 293.

6 Delicate Self-cutting: Schizophrenia and the 'Borderline' in Post-war North America

1 Joanne Greenberg, 'Author's Notes on *I Never Promised You a Rose Garden*', www.mountaintopauthor.com, accessed 6 July 2015.

2 Joanne Greenberg, *I Never Promised You a Rose Garden* [1964] (New York, 2004), pp. 9–10.

3 Ping-Nie Pao, 'The Syndrome of Delicate Self-cutting', *British Journal of Medical Psychology*, XXXXII (1969), pp. 195–206.

4 Ibid., p. 195.

5 Neo-Kraepelinians followed a similar descriptive and biological approach to Emil Kraepelin (1856–1926), who emphasized heredity and associated biological factors in his classification of mental illness. Unlike other practitioners in his era, and psychoanalysts, Kraepelin drew a clear line between mental health and illness. See Hannah S. Decker, *The Making of DSM-III: A Diagnostic Manual's Conquest of American Psychiatry* (Oxford, 2013), pp. 35–51. .

6 Ronald Hayman, *The Death and Life of Sylvia Plath* (London, 1992), p. 55.

7 Sylvia Plath, *The Bell Jar* (London, 1963), p. 156.

8 Ibid., pp. 176–8.

9 Hayman, *The Death and Life of Sylvia Plath*, p. 56.

10 Al Alvarez, *The Savage God: A Study of Suicide* (Harmondsworth, 1974), p. 35.

11 Ibid., p. 53.

12 Erwin Stengel, *Suicide and Attempted Suicide* (Harmondsworth, 1967), p. 71.

13 Ibid., p. 97.

14 Alvarez, *The Savage God*, pp. 305–6; Chris Millard, *A History of Self-harm in Britain: A Genealogy of Cutting and Overdosing* (London, 2015), pp. 21–2.

15 Millard, *A History of Self-harm in Britain*, pp. 1–4.

16 Armando Favazza, interview by Sarah Chaney, 6 August 2015.

17 Plath, *The Bell Jar*, p. 154.

18 For example Myre Sim's *Guide to Psychiatry*, 4th edn (1981), quoted in Millard, *A History of Self-harm in Britain*, p. 17.

19 Greenberg, *I Never Promised You a Rose Garden*, p. 23.

20 Ibid., pp. 48–9.

21 Ibid., pp. 178–80.

22 Frieda Fromm-Reichmann, *Principles of Intensive Psychotherapy* (Edinburgh, 1953), p. 83.

23 Greenberg, *I Never Promised You a Rose Garden*, p. 37.

24 Ibid., p. 184.

25 Ibid., p. 169.

26 William Kurelek, *Someone With Me: An Autobiography* (Toronto, 1980), p. 17.

27 Ibid., pp. 17–18.

28 Pao, 'The Syndrome of Delicate Self-cutting', p. 195.

29 Harold Graff and Richard Mallin, 'The Syndrome of the Wrist Cutter', *American Journal of Psychiatry*, CXXIV (1967), pp. 36–42; Robert M. Goldwyn, John L.

Cahill and Henry Grunebaum, 'Self-inflicted Injury to the Wrist', *Plastic and Reconstructive Surgery*, XXXIX/6 (1967), pp. 583–9; Harold Graff, 'Outpatient Care: The Chronic Wrist-Slasher', *Hospital Topics*, XXXXV/11 (1967), pp. 61–5; Henry Grunebaum and Gerald Klerman, 'Wrist Slashing', *American Journal of Psychiatry*, CXXIV (1967), pp. 527–34.

30 Graff and Mallin, 'The Syndrome of the Wrist Cutter', p. 36.

31 Armando R. Favazza, *Bodies Under Siege: Self-mutilation, Nonsuicidal Self-injury, and Body Modification in Culture and Psychiatry*, 3rd edn (Baltimore, MD, 2011), p. 147. Favazza, interview by Chaney.

32 Chris Millard, 'Making the Cut: The Production of "Self-harm" in Post-1945 Anglo-Saxon Psychiatry', *History of the Human Sciences*, XXVI/2 (2013), p. 135.

33 Edward M. Podvoll, 'Self-mutilation Within a Hospital Setting: A Study of Identity and Social Compliance', *British Journal of Medical Psychology*, XXXXII (1969), p. 213.

34 In the volume itself, Strong phrased this more carefully: 'Although these people are sometimes called cutters – even in this book as a quick shorthand – they are more than their disorder, their lives infinitely richer, their stories more complex, than that single label might indicate.' Marilee Strong, *A Bright Red Scream: Self-mutilation and the Language of Pain* (London, 2000), p. xv.

35 Graff, 'Outpatient Care', p. 62 (my emphasis).

36 As Pao was based at Chestnut Lodge, it's probable he knew that *Rose Garden* was based on a real example, and it is not unlikely that others in this small circle did too. Pao, 'The Syndrome of Delicate Self-cutting', p. 200.

37 Chris Millard, 'Self-mutilation and a Psychiatric Syndrome: Emergence, Exclusions and Contexts (1967–76)', MA thesis, University of York, 2007, pp. 34–5.

38 Daniel Offer and Peter Barglow, 'Adolescent and Young Adult Self-mutilation Incidents in a General Psychiatric Hospital', *Archives of General Psychiatry*, III (1960), pp. 194–204.

39 The study published was based on 24 female 'cutters'. Richard J. Rosenthal, Carl Rinzler, Rita Walsh and Edmund Klausner, 'Wrist-cutting Syndrome: The Meaning of a Gesture', *American Journal of Psychiatry*, CXXVIII/11 (1972), p. 1363.

40 Millard, 'Making the Cut', p. 138.

41 Alfred H. Stanton and Morris S. Schwartz, *The Mental Hospital: A Study of Institutional Participation in Psychiatric Illness and Treatment* (New York, 1954), p. 461.

42 Pao, 'The Syndrome of Delicate Self-cutting', p. 195.

43 Millard, 'Self-mutilation and a Psychiatric Syndrome', pp. 10–11.

44 Scott H. Nelson and Henry Grunebaum, 'A Follow-up Study of Wrist Slashers', *American Journal of Psychiatry*, CXXVII (1971), p. 1348; Graff, 'Outpatient Care', pp. 61–2.

45 Robert C. Burnham, 'Symposium on Impulsive Self-mutilation: Discussion', *British Journal of Medical Psychology*, XXXXII (1969), p. 223; Richard von Krafft-Ebing, *Psychopathia Sexualis, with Especial Reference to Contrary Sexual Instinct:*

A Clinical-Forensic Study, trans. Brian King (Burbank, CA, 1999), p. 170 (based on 12th German edition).

46 Pao, 'The Syndrome of Delicate Self-cutting', p. 201.

47 Elaine L. Chao and Kathleen P. Utgoff, 'Women in the Labor Force: A Databook', *Bureau of Labor Statistics* (2005), p. 1.

48 Kurelek, *Someone With Me*, pp. 21–3.

49 Ibid., p. 29.

50 Susanna Kaysen, *Girl, Interrupted* (New York, 1993), pp. 71–2.

51 A deleted scene shows Lisa burning the image of a cat into her forearm with a cigarette. James Mangold, dir., *Girl, Interrupted* (Columbia Pictures, 1999).

52 *DSM-III-R: Diagnostic and Statistical Manual of Mental Disorders* (Washington, DC, 1987), pp. 346–7.

53 Kaysen, *Girl, Interrupted*, p. 152.

54 Charley Baker, interview by Sarah Chaney, 3 August 2015 (digital recording).

55 Elizabeth Lunbeck, 'Borderline Histories: Psychoanalysis Inside and Out', *Science in Context*, XIX (2006), p. 153.

56 Offer and Barglow, 'Adolescent and Young Adult Self-mutilation Incidents in a General Psychiatric Hospital', p. 109.

57 Graff and Mallin, 'The Syndrome of the Wrist Cutter', p. 36.

58 Pao, 'The Syndrome of Delicate Self-cutting', p. 196.

59 Grunebaum and Klerman, 'Wrist Slashing', pp. 530–31.

60 Pao, 'The Syndrome of Delicate Self-cutting', p. 196.

61 Robert P. Knight, 'Borderline States', in *Essential Papers on Borderline Disorders: One Hundred Years at the Border*, ed. Michael H. Stone (New York, 1986), pp. 159–61. Of course, it is possible that by 'self-mutilation' Knight meant extreme cases of permanent injury, such as amputation, castration or enucleation, often the way the term is used today. However, in this era self-mutilation was used interchangeably with 'self-harm' and 'self-injury', suggesting a broader interpretation.

62 Otto Kernberg, 'Borderline Personality Organization', *Journal of the American Psychoanalytic Association*, XV (1967), p. 641.

63 Otto Kernberg, *Borderline Conditions and Pathological Narcissism* (New York, 1975), p. 177.

64 Reuben Fine, ed., *Current and Historical Perspectives on the Borderline Patient* (New York, 1989), p. 2.

65 Lunbeck, 'Borderline Histories', p. 163.

66 Decker, *The Making of DSM-III*, p. 30.

67 John Edward Cooper, *Psychiatric Diagnosis in New York and London: A Comparative Study of Mental Hospital Admissions* (London, 1972), pp. 138–9.

68 Carol North and Remi Cadoret, 'Diagnostic Discrepancy in Personal Accounts of Patients with "Schizophrenia"', *Archives of General Psychiatry*, XXXVIII/2 (February 1981), p. 133.

69 Carol North, *Welcome, Silence: My Triumph Over Schizophrenia* (New York, 1987). See Gail A. Hornstein, *To Redeem One Person is to Redeem the World: The Life of Frieda Fromm-Reichmann* (London, 2000), pp. 370–71.

70 John G. Gunderson and Margaret T. Singer, 'Defining Borderline Patients:
    An Overview', *American Journal of Psychiatry*, CXXXII (1975), p. 1.
71 Decker, *The Making of DSM-III*, p. 168.
72 Robert L. Spitzer, Jean Endicott and Miriam Gibbon, 'Crossing the Border into
    Borderline Personality and Borderline Schizophrenia: The Development of
    Criteria', in *Essential Papers on Borderline Disorders: One Hundred Years at the
    Border*, ed. Michael H. Stone (New York, 1986), pp. 527–48.
73 Kernberg, *Borderline Conditions*, p. 125.
74 H. G. Morgan, *Death Wishes? The Understanding and Management of Deliberate
    Self-harm* (Chichester, 1979); Robert R. Ross and Hugh Bryan McKay,
    Self-mutilation (Lexington, MA, 1979).

7   **Trigger Happy:** Culture, Contagion and Trauma in the Internet Age

1 Natalie Ostroff and Jim Taylor, 'Tumblr To Ban Self-harm and Eating Disorder
    Blogs', BBC, www.bbc.co.uk (26 March 2012). Instagram and Pinterest took
    a similar approach.
2 'Community Standards', Facebook, www.facebook.com, accessed 26 August 2016.
3 Jamie Grierson, 'British Teenager's Attempt to Join Isis in Syria Foiled by
    Undercover Reporter', *The Guardian*, 22 May 2015, www.guardian.com; Imogen
    Calderwood, 'Teenage "Terror Twins" who Fled Britain to Join ISIS Tried to
    Recruit their Whole Family', *Mail Online*, 4 October 2015, www.dailymail.co.uk.
4 For a similar occurrence, a little earlier, in the understanding of eating disorders, see
    Joan Jacobs Brumberg, 'From Psychiatric Syndrome to "Communicable" Disease:
    The Case of Anorexia Nervosa', in *Framing Disease: Studies in Cultural History*, ed.
    Charles Rosenberg and Janet Golden (New Brunswick, NJ, 1992), pp. 134–54.
5 Although a surge in these reports occurred in early 2015, a more recent survey has
    claimed that trigger warnings are not widely used at American universities. Tyler
    Kingkade, 'The Prevailing Narrative on Trigger Warnings is Just Plain Wrong',
    Huffington Post, 1 December 2015, www.huffingtonpost.com.
6 Caroline Kettlewell, *Skin Game: A Memoir* (New York, 1999), p. 9.
7 Ibid., p. 68.
8 Ibid., p. 66.
9 One example of the cultural spread of this idea is Elizabeth Wurtzel, *Prozac
    Nation: Young and Depressed in America* (London, 1996). This attitude has
    shifted considerably in recent years, as described in Katherine Sharpe, 'The
    Silence of Prozac', *The Lancet Psychiatry*, II/10 (October 2015), pp. 871–3.
10 Kettlewell, *Skin Game*, p. 156.
11 For more detail on this, see Barbara J. Brickman, '"Delicate" Cutters: Gendered
    Self-mutilation and Attractive Flesh in Medical Discourse', *Body & Society*, X/4
    (2004), pp. 87–111.
12 Armando R. Favazza and Mary Oman, 'Overview: Foundations of Cultural
    Psychiatry', *American Journal of Psychiatry*, CXXXV/3 (1 March 1978),
    pp. 293–303.

13 Armando R. Favazza, *Bodies Under Siege: Self-mutilation, Nonsuicidal Self-injury, and Body Modification in Culture and Psychiatry*, 2nd edn (Baltimore, MD, 1996), pp. x–xi.

14 Armando Favazza, interview by Sarah Chaney, 6 August 2015.

15 Charles Darwin, *The Descent of Man*, ed. James H. Birx (Amherst, NY, 1998), pp. 596–7.

16 George M. Gould and Walter L. Pyle, *Anomalies and Curiosities of Medicine* (London and Philadelphia, PA, 1897), p. 749. Gould and Pyle also related the emergence of cosmetic surgery to the same impulses. For more on this idea, see Sander L. Gilman, *Making the Body Beautiful: A Cultural History of Aesthetic Surgery* (Princeton, NJ, 1999).

17 This is not to say that practices like tattooing had never previously been considered culturally acceptable in the West (before and outside the middle-class scientific view), nor to deny that some of the nineteenth-century connotations relating tattooing and body modification to crime or degeneracy retain currency in some circles. Matt Lodder, 'Stamping Out the Persistent Myths and Misconceptions about Tattoos', *The Guardian*, 1 October 2011, www.guardian.com.

18 's.a.f.e. Alternatives', www.selfinjury.com, accessed 24 October 2015.

19 Brickman, '"Delicate" Cutters', p. 88.

20 Janis Whitlock, Amanda Purington and Marina Gershkovich, 'Media, the Internet and Nonsuicidal Self-injury', in *Understanding Nonsuicidal Self-injury: Origins, Assessment, and Treatment*, ed. Matthew K. Nock (Arlington, VA, 2009), p. 148.

21 Adrian Lyne, dir., *Fatal Attraction* (Paramount Pictures, 1987).

22 David Cronenberg, dir., *Videodrome* (Universal Pictures, 1983).

23 In addition to the novel, Levenkron also wrote a self-help guide on the topic. Steven Levenkron, *Cutting: Understanding and Overcoming Self-mutilation* (New York and London, 1998).

24 Kettlewell, *Skin Game*, p. 26.

25 'Everybody Hurts', *Melody Maker*, 23/30 December 1995, p. 41.

26 'Manic Depression', *Melody Maker*, 20 August 1994, p. 12; 'From Despair to Where', *Melody Maker*, 8 April 1995, pp. 29–34.

27 Andrew Smith, 'Is This Music to Die For?', *The Guardian*, 31 March 1995, p. A2.

28 There is a list of celebrity self-injury revelations from 1993 to 2004 in Whitlock, Purington and Gershkovich, 'Media, the Internet and Nonsuicidal Self-injury', p. 140. This includes Hollywood stars Johnny Depp and Christina Ricci.

29 Steve Lamacq, 'Blood on the Tracks', *NME*, 25 May 1991, p. 48.

30 An edited version of the discussion was released as a B-side to the single 'Theme from M.A.S.H.' Manic Street Preachers, 'Theme From M.A.S.H. (Suicide is Painless)' [Side A], 'Sleeping with the N.M.E.' [Side B], 1992.

31 Stuart Bailie, 'Culture, Alienation, Boredom and Despair', *NME*, 29 January 2005, pp. 28–9.

32 Ibid.
33 'Everybody Hurts', *Melody Maker*, p. 41.
34 Manic Street Preachers, *Generation Terrorists* (Columbia Records, 1992).
35 Manic Street Preachers, *The Holy Bible* (Epic Records, 1994). Reviews tended to compare *The Holy Bible* to Nirvana's *In Utero* (1993), which was retrospectively regarded as being singer Kurt Cobain's 'suicide note'. The *NME* review began: 'Oh Christ. Remember "In Utero"? Remember the demands, the questions, the theorizing as an expectant world was plunged headfirst into Kurt's brutal abyss? Remember what happened next?' Simon Williams, 'Revelations Terrorists', *NME*, 27 August 1994, p. 37.
36 For example, Simon Price, 'Archives of Pain', *Melody Maker*, 3 December 1994, p. 15.
37 Stuart Bailie, 'Manic's Depressive', *NME*, 1 October 1994, pp. 32–4.
38 'Everybody Hurts', *Melody Maker*, p. 41.
39 Smith, 'Is This Music to Die For?', p. A2.
40 Lucy Bowes et al., 'Risk of Depression and Self-harm in Teenagers Identifying with Goth Subculture: A Longitudinal Cohort Study', *The Lancet Psychiatry*, II/9 (August 2015), p. 799.
41 Daniel Offer and Peter Barglow, 'Adolescent and Young Adult Self-mutilation Incidents in a General Psychiatric Hospital', *Archives of General Psychiatry*, III (1960), p. 204.
42 Edward M. Podvoll, 'Self-mutilation Within a Hospital Setting: A Study of Identity and Social Compliance', *British Journal of Medical Psychology*, XXXXII (1969), p. 213.
43 Robert R. Ross and Hugh Bryan McKay, *Self-mutilation* (Lexington, MA, 1979), p. 2.
44 Ibid., p. 3.
45 Ibid., pp. 62–3.
46 P. C. Matthews, 'Epidemic Self-injury in an Adolescent Unit', *International Journal of Social Psychiatry*, XIV/2 (April 1968), pp. 125–33.
47 Paul M. Rosen and Barent W. Walsh, 'Patterns of Contagion in Self-mutilation Epidemics', *American Journal of Psychiatry*, CXXXXVI/5 (1989), p. 657.
48 Barent W. Walsh and Paul M. Rosen, 'Self-mutilation and Contagion: An Empirical Test', *American Journal of Psychiatry*, CXXXXII/1 (1985), p. 120.
49 Ross and McKay, *Self-mutilation*, p. 64.
50 Jane Bunclark, interview by Sarah Chaney, 10 August 2015 (digital recording).
51 Louise Roxanne Pembroke, ed., *Self-harm: Perspectives from Personal Experience* (London, 2009), p. 28.
52 Bunclark, interview by Chaney.
53 Ian Hulatt, interview by Sarah Chaney, 30 July 2015 (digital recording). See Ben Leapman, 'Self-harmers "Should Get Clean Blades"', *Daily Telegraph*, 6 Feburary 2006, www.telegraph.co.uk; Sarah Kate Templeton, 'Self-harmers to Be Given Clean Blades', *The Times*, 6 February 2006, www.timesonline.co.uk.
54 Bunclark, interview by Chaney, 10 August 2015.

55 Janis Whitlock, Jane L. Powers and John Eckenrode, 'The Virtual Cutting Edge: The Internet and Adolescent Self-injury', *Developmental Psychology*, xxxxii/3 (2006), p. 415.

56 Seaneen Molloy-Vaughan, 'My Body Comes with a Trigger Warning', www.mind. org.uk (23 September 2015). Molloy-Vaughan has blogged since 2007 at www. thesecretlifeofamanicdepressive.wordpress.com.

57 This is not limited to self-injury scars. The same may apply to people with eating disorders, among other things.

58 Greg Lukianoff and Jonathan Haidt, 'The Coddling of the American Mind', *The Atlantic*, www.theatlantic.com (September 2015); Ali Vingiano, 'How the "Trigger Warning" Took over the Internet', *BuzzFeed News*, 5 May 2014, www. buzzfeed.com.

59 Lukianoff and Haidt, 'The Coddling of the American Mind'.

60 Laurie Penny, 'Laurie Penny on Trigger Warnings: What We're Really Talking About', *New Statesman*, 21 May 2014, www.newstatesman.com.

61 Vingiano, 'How the "Trigger Warning" Took over the Internet'; Jenny Jarvie, 'Trigger Happy', *New Republic*, 4 March 2014, www.newrepublic.com. Clare Shaw also located her first encounter with 'triggers' with engagement in peer support services in the 1990s, while Ian Hulatt first heard the term from mental health service users. Clare Shaw, interview by Sarah Chaney, 24 July 2015 (digital recording); Ian Hulatt, interview by Sarah Chaney, 30 July 2015 (digital recording).

62 Roxane Gay, 'The Illusion of Safety/The Safety of Illusion', *The Rumpus*, 28 August 2012, www.therumpus.net.

63 Tim Smith, 'On the Death of a Child and Trigger Warnings', www.gashead.net, 23 April 2015.

64 *DSM-5*, p. 275.

65 Ruth Leys, *Trauma: A Genealogy* (Chicago, IL, and London, 2000), p. 242.

66 Edgar Jones and Simon C. Wessely, 'Psychological Trauma: A Historical Perspective', *Psychiatry*, v/7 (2006), p. 219; Edgar Jones et al., 'Flashbacks and Post-Traumatic Stress Disorder: The Genesis of a 20th-century Diagnosis', *British Journal of Psychiatry*, CLXXXII/2 (February 2003), pp. 158–63.

67 Jones and Wessely, 'Psychological Trauma', p. 219.

68 Favazza puts the figure at 60 per cent. Armando R. Favazza, *Bodies Under Siege: Self-mutilation, Nonsuicidal Self-injury, and Body Modification in Culture and Psychiatry*, 3rd edn (Baltimore, MD, 2011), p. 277; Marilee Strong, *A Bright Red Scream: Self-mutilation and the Language of Pain* (London, 2000), pp. 64–85.

69 'Forum Terms' (last updated 11 July 2011), LifeSIGNs, www.lifesigns.org.uk.

70 Hulatt, interview by Chaney.

71 NSHN Admin, 'Forum Rules', *National Self-harm Network*, www.nshn.co.uk, 8 March 2007.

72 Shaw, interview by Chaney.

73 In an often problematic sociological review, Adler and Adler outlined several key purposes of online self-harm communities, including helping themselves by

helping others, defining the act of self-harm and the forging of identities as self-injurers. Patricia A. Adler and Peter Adler, *The Tender Cut: Inside the Hidden World of Self-injury* (New York and London, 2011), pp. 128–43.

74 Clare Shaw, interview by Sarah Chaney, 24 July 2015 (digital recording). Bunclark, however, argued the opposite.

75 Antonio Casilli, Fred Pailler and Paola Tubaro, 'Online Networks of Eating-Disorder Websites: Why Censoring Pro-Ana Might Be a Bad Idea', *Perspectives in Public Health*, CXXXIII/2 (2013), pp. 94–5. For more background on pro-ana discussions, see Daphna Yeshua-Katz and Nicole Martins, 'Communicating Stigma: The Pro-Ana Paradox', *Health Communication*, XXVIII/5 (2012), pp. 499–508.

76 Charley Baker, interview by Sarah Chaney, 3 August 2015 (digital recording).

77 Caitlin Dewey, 'Inside Tumblr's Teen Suicide Epidemic', *Washington Post*, 24 February 2015, www.washingtonpost.com. For the original article (which says nothing about the Internet), see Madelyn S. Gould, Marjorie H. Kleinman, Alison M. Lake, Judith Forman and Jennifer Bassett Midle, 'Newspaper Coverage of Suicide and Initiation of Suicide Clusters in Teenagers in the USA, 1988–96: A Retrospective, Population-based, Case-control Study', *The Lancet Psychiatry*, I/1 (6 June 2014), pp. 34–43.

78 Favazza, *Bodies Under Siege* (2011), p. 226.

79 Chris Hayward, 'Foreword', in Lori G. Plante, *Bleeding to Ease the Pain: Cutting, Self-injury, and the Adolescent Search for Self* (Westport, CT, 2007), p. ix; Nadja Slee et al., 'Cognitive-behavioural Intervention for Self-harm: Randomised Controlled Trial', *British Journal of Psychiatry*, CLXXXXII (2008), p. 202.

80 Nancy K. Bristow et al., 'Trauma and Trigger Warnings in the History Classroom: A Roundtable Discussion', *The American Historian*, www.tah.oah. org, May 2015.

81 Dinesh Bhugra, *Culture and Self-harm: Attempted Suicide in South Asians in London* (Hove and New York, 2004).

Conclusion: Three Narratives of Bodily Harm

1 Clare Shaw, interview by Sarah Chaney, 24 July 2015 (digital recording).

2 Charley Baker, Clare Shaw and Fran Biley, eds, *Our Encounters with Self-harm* (Ross-on-Wye, 2013), p. xiv.

3 Ibid., p. 99.

4 Liz Atkin, interview by Sarah Chaney, 29 June 2015 (digital recording).

5 Eleanor Longden, 'The Voices in my Head', TED Talk, www.ted.com/talks, February 2013.

6 A view strongly held by the peer network Recovery in the Bin, www. recoveryinthebin.org. A critical view of recovery is well articulated in the blog entry 'Jagged Little Pill: Has the Recovery Narrative Gone Too Far?' on www. purplepersuasion.wordpress.com (11 June 2014).

7   NICE, *Self-harm in Over 8s: Long-term Management (CG133)* (2011), www.nice. org.uk; Mind, 'What is Self-harm?', www.mind.org.uk (accessed 14 December 2015).

8   Armando Favazza, interview by Sarah Chaney, 6 August 2015. See also Lisa Bird and Alison Faulkner, *Suicide and Self-harm* (London, 2000), p. 16; Patricia A. Adler and Peter Adler, *The Tender Cut: Inside the Hidden World of Self-injury* (New York and London, 2011), p. 24.

9   Mind, 'What is Self-harm?'.

10 In their sociological study, Adler and Adler excluded from their survey those people who carried out acts which seemed to them to have alternative goals, such as body decoration or what they called 'deceptive' efforts to 'garner medical attention'. Adler and Adler, *The Tender Cut*, p. 24. See also Janis Whitlock, Wendy Lader and Karen Conterio, 'The Internet and Self-injury: What Psychotherapists Should Know', *Journal of Clinical Psychology*, LXIII/11 (2007), p. 1136.

11 Chris Millard, *A History of Self-harm in Britain: A Genealogy of Cutting and Overdosing* (London, 2015), pp. 1–4.

12 Ian Hacking, 'Kinds of People: Moving Targets', *Proceedings of the British Academy*, CLI (2007), p. 313.

13 George Savage, 'An Address on the Borderland of Insanity', *British Medical Journal*, 1/2357 (1906), p. 490.

14 The term was added to the *Oxford English Dictionary Online* in 2006, with its earliest use dated back to 1980.

15 Sarah Wheeler, aka Thomas Tobias, founder of 'Mental Fight Club', interview by Sarah Chaney, 2 August 2015 (digital recording).

BIBLIOGRAPHY

Abraham, P. S., 'Self-mutilation in a Lioness', *Journal of Mental Science*, XXXII/137 (1886), pp. 46–50

—, 'Self-mutilation of a Lioness', *Medical Press and Circular*, 1 (1885), pp. 211–12

Adam, James, 'Cases of Self-mutilation by the Insane', *Journal of Mental Science*, XXIX/126 (1883), pp. 213–19

—, 'Self-mutilation', in *Dictionary of Psychological Medicine*, vol. II, ed. Daniel Hack Tuke (London, 1892), pp. 1147–52

Adams, James Eli, *Dandies and Desert Saints: Styles of Victorian Masculinity* (Ithaca, NY, 1995)

Adamson, H. G. 'Acne Urticata and Other Forms of "Neurotic Excoriations"', *British Journal of Dermatology*, XXVII/1 (1915), 1–12

Adler, Patricia A. and Peter Adler, *The Tender Cut: Inside the Hidden World of Self-injury* (New York and London, 2011)

Alvar, Jaime, *Romanising Oriental Gods: Myth, Salvation and Ethics in the Cults of Cybele, Isis and Mithras*, trans. Richard Gordon (Leiden, 2008)

Alvarez, Al, *The Savage God: A Study of Suicide* (Harmondsworth, 1974)

American Psychiatric Association, *DSM-III: Diagnostic and Statistical Manual of Mental Disorders* (Washington, DC, 1980)

—, *DSM-III-R: Diagnostic and Statistical Manual of Mental Disorders* (Washington, DC, 1987)

—, *DSM-5: Diagnostic and Statistical Manual of Mental Disorders* (Arlington, VA, 2013)

Anderson, Olive, *Suicide in Victorian and Edwardian England* (Oxford and New York, 1987)

Andrews, Judson B., 'Case of Excessive Hypodermic Use of Morphia: Three Hundred Needles Removed from the Body of an Insane Woman', *American Journal of Insanity*, XXIX (1872), pp. 13–20

'Annotations', *The Lancet*, CXIX/3047 (1882), pp. 113–20

'Asylum Reports for 1871', *Journal of Mental Science*, XVIII/82 (1872), pp. 262–76

Baker, Charley, and Brian Brown, 'Suicide, Self-harm and Survival Strategies in Contemporary Heavy Metal Music: A Cultural and Literary Analysis', *Journal of Medical Humanities*, XXXVII/1, pp. 1–20

—, Clare Shaw and Fran Biley, eds, *Our Encounters with Self-harm* (Ross-on-Wye, 2013)

Barry, Jonathan, 'Piety and the Patient: Medicine and Religion in Eighteenth Century Bristol', in *Patients and Practitioners: Lay Perceptions of Medicine in Pre-Industrial Society*, ed. Roy Porter (Cambridge and New York, 1985)

Beard, George Miller, *A Practical Treatise on Nervous Exhaustion (Neurasthenia)* (New York, 1889)

Beeton, Isabella, *The Book of Household Management* (London, 1868)

Bentham, Jeremy, *An Introduction to the Principles of Morals and Legislation*, ed. Benjamin Giles King (London, 1823)

Bertram, James Glass, *Flagellation and the Flagellants: A History of the Rod in All Countries, from the Earliest Period to the Present Time* (London, 1877)

Bhugra, Dinesh, *Culture and Self-harm: Attempted Suicide in South Asians in London* (Hove and New York, 2004)

The Bible: Authorized King James Version, ed. Robert P. Carroll and Stephen Prickett (Oxford, 1998)

Bird, Lisa, and Alison Faulkner, *Suicide and Self-harm* (London, 2000)

Bishop, W. J., 'Some Historical Cases of Auto-surgery', *Proceedings of the Scottish Society of the History of Medicine, Session 1960–61* (1961), pp. 23–32

Blandford, G. Fielding, *Insanity and Its Treatment: Lectures on the Treatment, Medical and Legal, of Insane Patients* (Edinburgh and London, 1871)

Boileau, Jacques, *History of Flagellation among Different Nations: A Narrative of the Strange Customs and Cruelties of the Romans, Greeks, Egyptians, Etc. with an Account of Its Practice among the Early Christians as a Religious Stimulant and Corrector of Morals* (London, 1888)

Borch-Jacobsen, Mikkel, and Sonu Shamdasani, *The Freud Files: An Inquiry into the History of Psychoanalysis* (Cambridge, 2012)

Bourke, Joanna, *Dismembering the Male: Men's Bodies, Britain and the Great War* (London, 1996)

—, *Rape: A History from 1860 to the Present* (London, 2007)

—, *The Story of Pain: From Prayer to Painkillers* (New York, 2014)

Bowes, Lucy, Rebecca Carnegie, Rebecca Pearson, Becky Mars, Lucy Biddle, Barbara Maughan, Glyn Lewis, Charles Fernyhough and Jon Heron, 'Risk of Depression and Self-harm in Teenagers Identifying with Goth Subculture: A Longitudinal Cohort Study', *The Lancet Psychiatry*, II/9 (20 August 2015), pp. 793–800

Brain, Peter, *Galen on Bloodletting: A Study of the Origins, Development, and Validity of His Opinions, with a Translation of the Three Works* (Cambridge; New York, 1986)

Brickman, Barbara J., '"Delicate" Cutters: Gendered Self-mutilation and Attractive Flesh in Medical Discourse', *Body & Society*, X/4 (2004), pp. 87–111

Brisson, Luc, *Sexual Ambivalence: Androgyny and Hermaphroditism in Graeco-Roman Antiquity*, trans. Janet Lloyd (London, 2002)

Bristow, Nancy K., Angus Johnston, Edward T. Linenthal, Michael J. Pfeifer, Jacqui Shine and Kidada E Williams, 'Trauma and Trigger Warnings in the History Classroom: A Roundtable Discussion', *The American Historian*, http://tah.oah. org, May 2015

Brodie, Benjamin Collins, 'Extraction of Foreign Bodies', *The Lancet*, 1/1063 (1844), pp. 497–502

Brooks, John I., *The Eclectic Legacy: Academic Philosophy and the Human Sciences in Nineteenth-century France* (Cranbury, NJ, 1998)

Brown, Peter Robert Lamont, *The Body and Society: Men, Women, and Sexual Renunciation in Early Christianity* (New York, 2008)

Brown, William J., 'Notes of a Case of Monomania with Self-mutilation and a Suicidal Tendency', *Journal of Mental Science*, XXIII/102 (1877), pp. 242–8

Brumberg, Joan Jacobs, *Fasting Girls: The Emergence of Anorexia Nervosa as a Modern Disease* (Cambridge, MA, 1988)

—, 'From Psychiatric Syndrome to "Communicable" Disease: The Case of Anorexia Nervosa', in *Framing Disease: Studies in Cultural History*, ed. Charles Rosenberg and Janet Golden, pp. 134–54 (New Brunswick, NJ, 1992)

Brunswick, Ruth Mack, 'A Supplement to Freud's "History of an Infantile Neurosis"', *International Journal of Psycho-analysis*, IX (1928), pp. 439–76

Brushfield, Thomas N., 'On Medical Certificates of Insanity', *The Lancet*, CXV/2958 (1880), pp. 711–13

Bucknill, John Charles, and Daniel Hack Tuke, *A Manual of Psychological Medicine* (London, 1879)

Budd, Dr, 'King's College Hospital (The Mania of Thrusting Needles into the Flesh)', *The Lancet*, LVI/1425 (1850), p. 676

Burnham, Robert C., 'Symposium on Impulsive Self-mutilation: Discussion', *British Journal of Medical Psychology*, XXXXII (1969), pp. 223–9

Butler, Judith, *Gender Trouble: Feminism and the Subversion of Identity* (New York, 2006)

Bynum, Caroline Walker, 'Fast, Feast and Flesh: The Religious Significance of Food to Medieval Women', *Representations*, XI (1985), pp. 1–25

Bynum, William F., and Helen Bynum, eds, *Dictionary of Medical Biography* (Westport, CT, 2006)

Calderwood, Imogen, 'Teenage "Terror Twins" who Fled Britain to Join ISIS Tried to Recruit their Whole Family', *Mail Online*, 4 October 2015, www.dailymail.co.uk

Callender, Mr, and Morrant Baker, 'St Bartholomew's Hospital (Hysteria)', *The Lancet*, C/2551 (1872), pp. 78–9

Caplan, Paula J., *The Myth of Women's Masochism* (Lincoln, NE, 1993)

Cappello, Mary, *Swallow: Foreign Bodies, Their Ingestion, Inspiration, and the Curious Doctor Who Extracted Them* (New York and London, 2011)

Cardyn, Lisa, 'Construction of Female Sexual Trauma in Turn-of-the-Century American Mental Medicine', in *Traumatic Pasts: History, Psychiatry and Trauma in the Modern Age, 1870–1930*, ed. Mark S. Micale and Paul Frederick Lerner (Cambridge and New York, 2001), pp. 172–204

Carlson, Marla, *Performing Bodies in Pain: Medieval and Post-modern Martyrs, Mystics, and Artists* (New York, 2010)

Carter, Kay Codell, 'The Decline of Therapeutic Bloodletting and the Collapse of Traditional Medicine' (New Brunswick, NJ, 2012)

'The Case of the Farmer Brooks', *The Lancet*, CIX/3046 (1882), p. 73

'The Case of Isaac Brooks', *Journal of Mental Science*, XXVIII (1882), pp. 69–74

Casilli, Antonio, Fred Pailler and Paola Tubaro, 'Online Networks of Eating-disorder Websites: Why Censoring Pro-ana Might be a Bad Idea', *Perspectives in Public Health*, CXXXIII/2 (2013), pp. 94–5

Catullus, Gaius Valerius, *The Poems of Catullus: An Annotated Translation*, trans. Jeannine Diddle Uzzi (Cambridge, 2015)

Cawadias, A. P., 'Male Eunuchism Considered in the Light of the Historical Method', *Proceedings of the Royal Society of Medicine*, XXXIX (1946), pp. 23–8

Celsus, Aulus Cornelius, *De Medicina*, trans. W. G. Spencer (London, 1938)

Chandler, Amy, 'Narrating the Self-injured Body', *Medical Humanities*, XL (2014), pp. 111–16

Chaney, Sarah, 'Anaesthetic Bodies and the Absence of Feeling: Pain and Medical Concepts of Self-mutilation in Later Nineteenth-century Psychiatry', *19: Interdisciplinary Studies in the Long Nineteenth Century*, XV (2012)

—, '"A Hideous Torture on Himself": Madness and Self-mutilation in Victorian Literature', *Journal of Medical Humanities*, XXXII/4 (2011), pp. 279–89

—, '"No 'Sane' Person Would Have Any Idea": Patients' Involvement in Late Nineteenth-century British Asylum Psychiatry', *Medical History*, LX/1 (2015), pp. 37–53

—, 'Useful Members of Society or Motiveless Malingerers? Occupation and Malingering in British Asylum Psychiatry, 1870–1914', in *Work, Psychiatry and Society, c. 1750–2010*, ed. Waltraud Ernst (Manchester, 2016), pp. 277–97

Channing, Walter, 'Case of Helen Miller – Self-mutilation – Tracheotomy', *American Journal of Insanity*, 34 (1878), pp. 368–78

Chao, Elaine L., and Kathleen P. Utgoff, 'Women in the Labor Force: A Databook', www.bls.gov, 2005

Charcot, Jean-Martin, *Clinical Lectures on the Diseases of the Nervous System*, ed. and trans. Ruth Harris (New York, 1991)

Clark-Lowes, Francis, *Freud's Apostle: Wilhelm Stekel and the Early History of Psychoanalysis* (Sandy, 2010)

Collie, John, 'Fraud and Skin Eruptions', *The Lancet*, CLXXXVIII/4868 (1916), pp. 1008–10

Collini, Stefan, *Public Moralists: Political Thought and Intellectual Life in Britain, 1850–1930* (Oxford, 1991)

Conolly, John, *The Treatment of the Insane without Mechanical Restraint* (London, 1856)

Cooper, John Edward, *Psychiatric Diagnosis in New York and London: A Comparative Study of Mental Hospital Admissions* (London, 1972)

Cooter, Roger, 'Malingering in Modernity: Psychological Scripts and Adversarial Encounters during the First World War', in *War, Medicine and Modernity*, ed. Roger Cooter, Mark Harrison and Steve Sturdy (Stroud, 1999), pp. 125–48

Craig, Maurice, *Psychological Medicine: A Manual on Mental Diseases for Practitioners and Students* (London, 1905)

Cresswell, Mark, 'Self-harm "Survivors" and Psychiatry in England, 1988–1996', *Social Theory & Health*, III/4 (November 2005), pp. 259–85

Cresswell, Mark, and Zulfia Karimova, 'Self-harm and Medicine's Moral Code: A Historical Perspective, 1950–2000', *Ethical Human Psychology and Psychiatry*, XII/2 (August 2010), pp. 158–75

Crocker, Henry Radcliffe, *Diseases of the Skin: Their Description, Pathology, Diagnosis and Treatment* (London, 1893)

Cronenberg, David, dir., *Videodrome* (Universal Pictures, 1983)

Cunningham, Andrew, *The Anatomical Renaissance: The Resurrection of the Anatomical Projects of the Ancients* (Brookfield, VT, 1997)

Curious Cases of Flagellation in France: Considered from a Legal, Medical and Historical Standpoint with Reference to Analogous Cases in England, Germany, Italy, America, Australia and the Soudan (London, 1901)

Dale, Melissa S., 'Understanding Emasculation: Western Medical Perspectives on Chinese Eunuchs', *Social History of Medicine*, XXIII/1 (2010), pp. 38–55

Darby, Robert, 'The Masturbation Taboo and the Rise of Routine Male Circumcision: A Review of the Historiography', *Journal of Social History*, XXXVI/3 (2003), pp. 737–57

—, *A Surgical Temptation: The Demonization of the Foreskin and the Rise of Circumcision in Britain* (Chicago, IL, 2005)

Darwin, Charles, *The Descent of Man*, ed. H. James Birx (Amherst, NY, 1998)

—, *The Descent of Man, and Selection in Relation to Sex* (London, 1871)

Decker, Hannah S., *The Making of DSM-III: A Diagnostic Manual's Conquest of American Psychiatry* (Oxford, 2013)

Dewey, Caitlin, 'Inside Tumblr's Teen Suicide Epidemic', *Washington Post*, 24 February 2015, www.washingtonpost.com

Dieulafoy, Georges, 'Escarres multiples et récidivantes depuis deux ans deux bras et au pied. – Amputation du bras gauche. Discussion sur la nature de ces escarres. – Pathomimie', *La Presse Médicale*, 1908, pp. 369–73

Digby, Anne, *Madness, Morality, and Medicine: A Study of the York Retreat, 1796–1914* (Cambridge and New York, 1985)

Dixon, Thomas, 'The Invention of Altruism: Auguste Comte's Positive Polity and Respectable Unbelief in Victorian Britain', in *Science and Beliefs: From Natural Philosophy to Natural Science, 1700–1900*, ed. David M. Knight and Matthew Eddy (Aldershot, 2005), pp. 195–211

—, *The Invention of Altruism: Making Moral Meanings in Victorian Britain* (Oxford and New York, 2008)

Dixon, William Hepworth, *Spiritual Wives* (London, 1868)

'Domestic News', *The Cornwall Royal Gazette, Falmouth Packet and Plymouth Journal*, 10 January 1845

Dore, S. E., 'Report on a Case of Dermatitis Artefacta', *Proceedings of the Royal Society of Medicine (Dermatological Section)*, 19 (1926), pp. 47–8

Doyle, Arthur Conan, *The Adventures of Sherlock Holmes* (London, 1994)

Duberman, Martin Bauml, '"I Am Not Contented": Female Masochism and Lesbianism in Early Twentieth-century New England', *Signs: Journal of Women in Culture and Society*, V/4 (1980), pp. 825–41

Eghigian, Greg A., *Making Security Social: Disability, Insurance, and the Birth of the Social Entitlement State in Germany* (Ann Arbor, MI, 2000)

Ellenberger, Henri F., *Beyond the Unconscious: Essays of Henri F. Ellenberger in the History of Psychiatry*, ed. Mark S. Micale (Princeton, NJ, 1993)

—, *The Discovery of the Unconscious: The History and Evolution of Dynamic Psychiatry* (New York, 1970)

Ellis, Havelock, *Studies in the Psychology of Sex* (Philadelphia, PA, 1928)

Ellis, Havelock, and John Addington Symonds, *Sexual Inversion: A Critical Edition*, ed. Ivan Crozier (Basingstoke, 2008)

Ellis, William Charles, *A Treatise on the Nature, Symptoms, Causes and Treatment of Insanity* (London, 1838)

Emerson, Louville Eugene, 'The Case of Miss A: A Preliminary Report of a Psychoanalytic Study and Treatment of a Case of Self-mutilation', *Psychoanalytic Review*, I (1913), pp. 41–54

—, 'Emerson and Freud: A Study in Contrasts', *Psychoanalytic Review*, XX (1933), pp. 208–14

—, 'Psychoanalysis and Hospitals', *Psychoanalytic Review*, I (1914), pp. 285–94

—, 'A Psychoanalytic Study of a Severe Case of Hysteria (part 1)', *Journal of Abnormal Psychology*, VII/6 (1913), pp. 385–406

—, 'A Psychoanalytic Study of a Severe Case of Hysteria (part 2)', *Journal of Abnormal Psychology*, VIII/1 (1913), pp. 44–56

—, 'A Psychoanalytic Study of a Severe Case of Hysteria (part 3)', *Journal of Abnormal Psychology*, VIII/3 (1913), pp. 180–207

—, 'The Psychoanalytic Treatment of Hystero-epilepsy', *Journal of Abnormal Psychology*, X/5 (1915), pp. 315–28

—, 'The Psychopathology of the Family', *Journal of Abnormal Psychology*, IX/5 (1914), pp. 333–40

—, 'Some Psychoanalytic Studies of Character', *Journal of Abnormal Psychology*, XI/4 (1916), pp. 265–74

Engelstein, Laura, *Castration and the Heavenly Kingdom: A Russian Folktale* (Ithaca, NY, and London, 1999)

—, 'From Heresy to Harm: Self-castrators in the Civic Discourse of Late Tsarist Russia', in *Empire and Society: New Approaches to Russian History*, ed. Teruyuki Hara and Kimitaka Matsuzato (Sapporo, 1997), pp. 1–22

Eusebius, *The History of the Church from Christ to Constantine*, ed. G. A. Williamson and Andrew Louth (Harmondsworth and New York, 1989)

'The Extraordinary Confession at Leek', *Manchester Times*, 14 January 1882

'The Extraordinary Confession of Perjury Near Leek', *The Guardian*, 7 January 1882

'The Extraordinary Death-bed Confession', *Sheffield and Rotherham Independent*, 7 January 1882

Facebook, 'Community Standards', www.facebook.com, 2015, accessed 26 August 2016

Fagge, C. Hilton, 'Notes on Some Feigned Cutaneous Affections', *British Medical Journal*, I/476 (1870), pp. 151–2

Favazza, Armando R., *Bodies Under Siege: Self-mutilation and Body Modification in Culture and Psychiatry*, 2nd edn (Baltimore, MD, 1996)

—, *Bodies Under Siege: Self-mutilation, Nonsuicidal Self-injury, and Body Modification in Culture and Psychiatry*, 3rd edn (Baltimore, MD, 2011)

Favazza, Armando R., and Mary Oman, 'Overview: Foundations of Cultural Psychiatry', *American Journal of Psychiatry*, CXXXV/3 (1 March 1978), pp. 293–303

Ferrars, Elizabeth, *Don't Monkey with Murder* (Harmondsworth, 1951)

Figley, Charles R., ed., *Encyclopedia of Trauma: An Interdisciplinary Guide* (Thousand Oaks, CA, 2012)

Fine, Reuben, *Current and Historical Perspectives on the Borderline Patient* (New York, 1989)

Flower, Thomas, 'Feigned or Hysterical Disease of Skin', *British Medical Journal*, I/482 (1870), pp. 307–8

'Forum Terms', *LifeSIGNS*, www.lifesigns.org.uk, 2015

Foucault, Michel, *The History of Sexuality*, vol. I: *The Will to Knowledge*, trans. Robert Hurley (London, 1998)

—, *Madness and Civilization: A History of Insanity in the Age of Reason*, trans. Richard Howard (London, 1989)

Fraser, Ian, 'Foreign Bodies', *British Medical Journal*, I/4088 (1939), pp. 967–71

Frazer, James, *The Golden Bough: A Study of Magic and Religion* [1891] (London, 1993)

French, Roger Kenneth, *Dissection and Vivisection in the European Renaissance* (Aldershot, 1999)

Freud, Sigmund, *The Standard Edition of the Complete Psychological Works of Sigmund Freud*, ed. James Strachey (London, 1974)

Freud, Sigmund, and Josef Breuer, *Studies on Hysteria*, ed. Angela Richards, trans. James Strachey (Harmondsworth, 1991)

Freud, Sigmund, and Carl Gustav Jung, *The Freud/Jung Letters: The Correspondence between Sigmund Freud and C. G. Jung*, ed. William McGuire, trans. Ralph Manheim and R.F.C. Hull (London, 1994)

Friedman, Lawrence Jacob, *Menninger: The Family and the Clinic* (New York, 1990)

Fromm-Reichmann, Frieda, *Principles of Intensive Psychotherapy* (Edinburgh, 1953)

Fullerton, Ronald A., and Girish N. Punj, 'Kleptomania: A Brief Intellectual
    History', in *The Romance of Marketing History: Proceedings of the 11th Conference
    on Historical Analysis and Research in Marketing* (East Lansing, MI, 2003),
    pp. 201–9
Furst, Lilian R., *Before Freud: Hysteria and Hypnosis in Later Nineteenth-century
    Psychiatric Cases* (Lewisburg, PA, 2008)
Galen, *Galen on Anatomical Procedures*, trans. Charles Singer (London, 1956)
Galloway, James, and Humphry Davy Rolleston, 'Feigned Diseases of the Skin',
    in *A System of Medicine*, ed. T. Clifford Allbutt (London, 1899), pp. 937–9
Gask, Linda, Mark Evans and David Kessler, 'Personality Disorder', *British Medical
    Journal*, CCCXXXXVII (2013), pp. 1–7
Gates, Barbara T., 'Suicide and the Victorian Physicians', *Journal of the History of the
    Behavioral Sciences*, XVI (1980), pp. 164–74
—, *Victorian Suicide: Mad Crimes and Sad Histories* (Princeton, NJ, 1988)
Gay, Roxane, 'The Illusion of Safety/The Safety of Illusion', *The Rumpus*, 28 August
    2012, www.therumpus.net
Gijswijt-Hofstra, Marijke, and Roy Porter, eds, *Cultures of Neurasthenia from Beard
    to the First World War* (Amsterdam and New York, 2001)
Gilman, Sander L., 'From Psychiatric Symptom to Diagnostic Category: Self-harm
    from the Victorians to DSM-5', *History of Psychiatry*, XXIV/2 (2013), pp. 148–65
—, *Making the Body Beautiful: A Cultural History of Aesthetic Surgery* (Princeton,
    NJ, 1999)
Goffman, Erving, *Asylums: Essays on the Social Situation of Mental Patients and
    Other Inmates* (Harmondsworth and New York, 1975)
Goldstein, Jan, *Console and Classify: The French Psychiatric Profession in the
    Nineteenth Century* (Chicago, IL, and London, 2001)
Goldwyn, Robert M., John L. Cahill and Henry Grunebaum, 'Self-inflicted Injury
    to the Wrist', *Plastic and Reconstructive Surgery*, CCCIX/6 (1967), pp. 583–9
Gould, George M., and Walter L. Pyle, *Anomalies and Curiosities of Medicine*
    (London and Philadelphia, PA, 1897)
Gould, Madelyn S., Marjorie H. Kleinman, Alison M. Lake, Judith Forman and
    Jennifer Bassett Midle, 'Newspaper Coverage of Suicide and Initiation of Suicide
    Clusters in Teenagers in the USA, 1988–96: A Retrospective, Population-based,
    Case-control Study', *The Lancet Psychiatry*, I/1 (6 June 2014)
Graff, Harold, 'Outpatient Care: The Chronic Wrist-slasher', *Hospital Topics*,
    XXXXV/11 (1967), pp. 61–5
Graff, Harold, and Richard Mallin, 'The Syndrome of the Wrist Cutter', *American
    Journal of Psychiatry*, CXXIV (1967), pp. 36–42
Gratz, Kim L. 'Measurement of Deliberate Self-harm: Preliminary Data on the
    Deliberate Self-harm Inventory', *Journal of Psychopathology and Behavioral
    Assessment*, XXIII/4 (2001), pp. 253–63
Greenberg, Joanne, *I Never Promised You a Rose Garden* [1964] (New York, 2004)
Greg, William R., 'On the Failure of "Natural Selection" in the Case of Man', *Fraser's
    Magazine for Town and Country*, LXXVIII (July 1868), pp. 353–62

Gregory, Andrew, *Harvey's Heart: The Discovery of Blood Circulation* (Cambridge, 2001)

Grierson, Jamie, 'British Teenager's Attempt to Join Isis in Syria Foiled by Undercover Reporter', *The Guardian*, 22 May 2015

Griesinger, Wilhelm, 'German Psychiatrie; An Introductory Lecture, Read at the Opening of the Psychiatric Clinique, in Zürich', *Journal of Mental Science*, IX/48 (1864), pp. 531–47

Grob, Gerald N., *Mental Institutions in America: Social Policy to 1875* (New York, 1973)

Grunebaum, Henry, and Gerald Klerman, 'Wrist Slashing', *American Journal of Psychiatry*, CXXIV (1967), pp. 527–34

Gunderson, John G., and Margaret T. Singer, 'Defining Borderline Patients: An Overview', *American Journal of Psychiatry*, CXXXII (1975), pp. 1–10

Gyurkovechky, Victor von, *Pathologie und Therapie der Männlichen Impotenz* (Vienna, 1889)

Hacking, Ian, 'Kinds of People: Moving Targets', *Proceedings of the British Academy*, CLI (2007), pp. 285–318

—, *Rewriting the Soul: Multiple Personality and the Sciences of Memory* (Princeton, NJ, 1998)

Haldin Davis, H., 'Dermatitis Artefacta', *Clinical Journal*, LIII (1924), pp. 211–16

Hale, Nathan G., *Freud and the Americans: The Beginnings of Psychoanalysis in the United States, 1876–1917* (New York, 1971)

—, *The Rise and Crisis of Psychoanalysis in the United States: Freud and the Americans, 1917–1985* (Oxford, 1995)

Hall, Lesley, *Hidden Anxieties: Male Sexuality, 1900–1950* (Cambridge, 1991)

—, '"It Was Affecting the Medical Profession": The History of Masturbatory Insanity Revisited', *Paedagogica Historica*, XXXIX/6 (2003), pp. 685–99

Hart, Ernest, 'Hysteria: Wilful Self-infliction of Injury', *The Lancet*, LXXIX/2014 (1862), p. 355

Harvey, William, *The Works of William Harvey*, trans. Robert Willis (Philadelphia, PA, 1989)

Hauser, Renate Irene, 'Sexuality, Neurasthenia and the Law: Richard von Krafft-Ebing (1840–1902)', PhD thesis, University College London, 1992

Hawthorne, Nathaniel, *The Scarlet Letter* [1850], ed. R. K. Gollin and Paul Lauter (Boston, MA, 2002)

Hawton, K., S. Simkin, J. J. Deeks, S. O'Connor, A. Keen, D. G. Altman, G. Philo and C. Bulstrode, 'Effects of a Drug Overdose in a Television Drama on Presentations to Hospital for Self Poisoning: Time Series and Questionnaire Study', *BMJ* (*Clinical Research Edn*), CCCXVIII/7189 (10 April 1999), pp. 972–7

Hayman, Ronald, *The Death and Life of Sylvia Plath* (London, 1992)

Hayward, Rhodri, *Resisting History: Religious Transcendence and the Invention of the Unconscious* (Manchester, NY, 2007)

Hekma, Gert, *A History of Sexology: Social and Historical Aspects of Sexuality*, ed. Jan Bremmer (London and New York, 1989)

Herdt, Gilbert H., ed., *Third Sex, Third Gender: Beyond Sexual Dimorphism in Culture and History* (New York, 1994)

Hill, Robert Gardiner, *A Concise History of the Entire Abolition of Mechanical Restraint in the Treatment of the Insane* (London, 1857)

Hornstein, Gail A., *To Redeem One Person is to Redeem the World: The Life of Frieda Fromm-Reichmann* (London, 2000)

Horvitz, Lori, 'Life Doesn't Come with Trigger Warnings. Why Should Books?', *The Guardian*, 18 May 2015

Howden, James C., 'Notes of a Case – Mania Followed by Hyperaesthesia and Osteomalacia. Singular Family Tendency to Excessive Constipation and Self-mutilation', *Journal of Mental Science*, XXVIII/121 (1882), pp. 49–53

H. R., 'Rev. of Psychopathia Sexualis: By Dr R. Von. Krafft-Ebing. 5th Edition. Ferdinand Enke, Stuttgart, 1890', *Journal of Mental Science*, XXXVII/156 (1891), pp. 152–4

Hyslop, Theo, *Mental Physiology: Especially in its Relations to Mental Disorders* (London, 1895)

—, 'On "Double Consciousness"', *British Medical Journal*, II/2021 (1899), pp. 782–6

Icks, Martijn, *The Crimes of Elagabalus: The Life and Legacy of Rome's Decadent Boy Emperor* (Cambridge, MA, 2012)

'Index-catalogue of the Library of the Surgeon-General's Office, United States Army', 2nd series (Washington, DC, 1910)

'James Adam (Obituary)', *Journal of Mental Science*, LV (1909), pp. 208–9

James, William, *The Principles of Psychology* (London, 1890)

Janet, Pierre, *L'Automatisme psychologique* (Paris, 1889)

—, *Les Obsessions et la psychasthénie* (Paris, 1903)

—, *The Major Symptoms of Hysteria: Fifteen Lectures given in the Medical School of Harvard University* (New York and London, 1907)

—, *Névroses et idées fixes* (Paris, 1898)

—, 'On the Pathogenesis of Some Impulsions', *Journal of Abnormal Psychology*, I/1 (1906), pp. 1–17

Jansson, Åsa, 'From Statistics to Diagnostics: Medical Certificates, Melancholia, and "Suicidal Propensities" in Victorian Medicine', *Journal of Social History*, XXXXVI/3 (2013), pp. 716–31

Jarvie, Jenny, 'Trigger Happy', *New Republic*, 4 March 2014, www.newrepublic.com

Jessett, F. Bowreman, 'A Case of Faecal Fistula due to Self-mutilation Occurring Twice in the Same Patient', *The Lancet*, CXXXXVIII/3818 (1896), pp. 1213–15

Jones, Edgar, Robert Hodgins Vermaas, Helen McCartney, Charlotte Beech, Ian Palmer, Kenneth Hyams and Simon C. Wessely, 'Flashbacks and Post-traumatic Stress Disorder: The Genesis of a 20th-century Diagnosis', *British Journal of Psychiatry*, CLXXXII/2 (1 February 2003), pp. 158–63

Jones, Edgar, and Simon C. Wessely, 'Psychological Trauma: A Historical Perspective', *Psychiatry*, V/7 (2006), pp. 217–20

Jones, G. M., 'Extraordinary Self-mutilation', *The Lancet*, LXX/1769 (1857), pp. 88–9

Jung, Carl Gustav, *Jung Contra Freud: The 1912 New York Lectures on the Theory of Psychoanalysis*, trans. R.F.C. Hull (Oxford, 2012)

Justin, *Apologies*, ed. and trans. P. M. Minns (Oxford, 2009)

Kaplan, Louise J., *Female Perversions: The Temptations of Madame Bovary* (London, 1991)

Kaysen, Susanna, *Girl, Interrupted* (New York, 1993)

Kernberg, Otto, *Borderline Conditions and Pathological Narcissism* (New York, 1975)

—, 'Borderline Personality Organization', *Journal of the American Psychoanalytic Association*, XV (1967), pp. 641–85

Kettlewell, Caroline, *Skin Game: A Memoir* (New York, 1999)

Kevles, Daniel J., *In the Name of Eugenics: Genetics and the Uses of Human Heredity* (Cambridge, MA, 1995)

King, Helen, 'Once Upon a Text: Hysteria from Hippocrates', in *Hysteria Beyond Freud*, ed. Sander L. Gilman, Helen King, Roy Porter, G. S. Rousseau and Elaine Showalter (Berkeley, Los Angeles and London, 1993), pp. 3–90

Kingkade, Tyler, 'The Prevailing Narrative on Trigger Warnings is Just Plain Wrong', *The Huffington Post*, 1 December 2015, www.huffingtonpost.com

Kirk, Robert G. W., and Neil Pemberton, *Leech* (London, 2013)

Klonsky, E. David, 'The Functions of Deliberate Self-injury: A Review of the Evidence', *Clinical Psychology Review*, XXVII (2007), pp. 226–39

Knight, Robert P., 'Borderline States', in *Essential Papers on Borderline Disorders: One Hundred Years at the Border*, ed. Michael H. Stone (New York, 1986), pp. 159–73

Kopernicky, I., and J. B. Davis, 'On the Strange Peculiarities Observed by a Religious Sect of Moscovites Called Scoptsis', *Journal of the Anthropological Society of London*, VIII (1870), pp. 121–35

Krafft-Ebing, R. von, *Psychopathia Sexualis with Especial Reference to Contrary Sexual Instinct: A Clinical-Forensic Study*, trans. Charles Gilbert Chaddock, vol. VII (Philadelphia, PA, and London, 1894)

—, *Psychopathia Sexualis: With Especial Reference to Antipathic Sexual Instinct, a Medico-Forensic Study*, trans. J. Redman (London, 1899)

—, *Psychopathia Sexualis: With Especial Reference to Contrary Sexual Instinct: A Clinical-Forensic Study* (Burbank, CA, 1999)

—, *Text-book of Insanity: Based on Clinical Observations for Practitioners and Students of Medicine*, ed. Charles Gilbert Chaddock (Philadelphia, PA, 1904)

Kuefler, Mathew, *The Manly Eunuch: Masculinity, Gender Ambiguity, and Christian Ideology in Late Antiquity* (London, 2001)

Kurelek, William, *Someone With Me: An Autobiography* (Toronto, 1980)

Kuriyama, Shigehisa, 'Interpreting the History of Bloodletting', *Journal of the History of Medicine and Allied Sciences*, L (1995), pp. 11–46

Lacourse, Eric, Michel Claes and Martine Villeneuve, 'Heavy Metal Music and Adolescent Suicidal Risk', *Journal of Youth and Adolescence*, XXX/3 (2001), pp. 321–32

Lamb, Susan D., *Pathologist of the Mind: Adolf Meyer and the Origins of American Psychiatry* (Baltimore, MD, 2014)

Lancellotti, Maria Grazia, *Attis, Between Myth and History: King, Priest, and God* (Leiden, 2002)

Laqueur, Thomas, *Making Sex: Body and Gender from the Greeks to Freud* (Cambridge, MA, and London, 1990)

—, *Solitary Sex: A Cultural History of Masturbation* (New York, 2003)

Largier, Niklaus, *In Praise of the Whip: A Cultural History of Arousal*, trans. Graham Harman (New York, 2007)

Leapman, Ben, 'Self-harmers "Should Get Clean Blades"', *Daily Telegraph*, 6 February 2006

Lerner, Paul Frederick, *Hysterical Men: War, Psychiatry, and the Politics of Trauma in Germany, 1890–1930* (London, 2003)

Levenkron, Steven, *Cutting: Understanding and Overcoming Self-mutilation* (New York and London, 1998)

—, *The Luckiest Girl in the World* (New York, 1997)

Leys, Ruth, *Trauma: A Genealogy* (Chicago, IL, and London, 2000)

Lodder, Matt, 'Stamping out the Persistent Myths and Misconceptions about Tattoos', *The Guardian*, 1 October 2011

Lombardo, Paul A., ed., *A Century of Eugenics in America: From the Indiana Experiment to the Human Genome Era* (Bloomington, IN, 2010)

Lorber, Judith, 'Believing Is Seeing: Biology as Ideology', *Gender and Society*, VII/4 (1993), pp. 568–81

Loverin, Bailey, 'Trigger Warnings Encourage Free Thought and Debate', *New York Times*, 19 May 2014, www.nytimes.com

Lukianoff, Greg, and Jonathan Haidt, 'The Coddling of the American Mind', *The Atlantic*, September 2015, www.theatlantic.com

Lunbeck, Elizabeth, *The Americanization of Narcissism* (Cambridge, MA, and London, 2014)

—, 'Borderline Histories: Psychoanalysis Inside and Out', *Science in Context*, XIX/1 (2006), pp. 151–73

—, *The Psychiatric Persuasion: Knowledge, Gender, and Power in Modern America* (Princeton, NJ, 1994)

Lunbeck, Elizabeth, and Bennett Simon, *Family Romance, Family Secrets: Case Notes from an American Psychoanalysis, 1912* (New Haven, CT, and London, 2003)

Lyne, Adrian, dir., *Fatal Attraction* (Paramount Pictures, 1987)

MacCormac, Henry, 'Autophytic Dermatitis', *Proceedings of the Royal Society of Medicine (Dermatological Section)*, XXVIII (1935), 734

—, 'Autophytic Dermatitis', *British Medical Journal*, II/4014 (1937), pp. 1153–5

—, 'Self-inflicted Hysterical Lesions of the Skin, with Special Reference to the After-history', *British Journal of Dermatology and Syphilis*, XXXVIII (1926), pp. 371–5

MacDonald, Michael, 'The Medicalization of Suicide in England: Laymen, Physicians, and Cultural Change, 1500–1870', in *Framing Disease: Studies in Cultural History*, ed. Charles Rosenberg and Janet Golden (New Brunswick, NJ, 1992), pp. 85–103

MacDonald, Michael, and Terence R. Murphy, *Sleepless Souls: Suicide in Early Modern England* (Oxford and New York, 1990)

Mandeville, Bernard, *A Treatise of the Hypochondriack and Hysterick Passions* (London, 1711)

Mangold, James, dir., *Girl, Interrupted* (Columbia Pictures, 1999)

Marc, Charles Chrétien Henri, *De la folie, considérée dans ses rapports avec les questions médico-judiciaires* (Paris, 1840)

Marcus, Steven, *The Other Victorians: A Study of Sexuality and Pornography in Mid-Nineteenth-century England* (London, 1966)

Marten, John, *Onania, or the Heinous Sin of Self-pollution, and All Its Frightful Consequences in Both Sexes, Considered* (London, 1716)

Martin, Graham, Michael Clarke and Colby Pearce, 'Adolescent Suicide: Music Preference as an Indicator of Vulnerability', *Journal of the American Academy of Child and Adolescent Psychiatry*, XXXII/3 (1993), pp. 530–35

Mason, Michael, *The Making of Victorian Sexual Attitudes* (Oxford and New York, 1994)

Matthews, P. C., 'Epidemic Self-injury in an Adolescent Unit', *International Journal of Social Psychiatry*, XIV/2 (1 April 1968), pp. 125–33

Matthey, André, *Nouvelles recherches sur les maladies de l'esprit* (Geneva, 1816)

Maudsley, Henry, 'The Genesis of Mind', *Journal of Mental Science*, VII/40 (1862), pp. 461–94

—, 'The Genesis of Mind (II)', *Journal of Mental Science*, VIII (1862), pp. 61–102.

Maury Deas, P., 'The Uses and Limitations of Mechanical Restraint as a Means of Treatment of the Insane', *Journal of Mental Science*, XXXXII (1896), pp. 102–13

McAlinden, Anne-Marie, *'Grooming', and the Sexual Abuse of Children: Institutional, Internet and Familial Dimensions* (Oxford, 2013)

McArthur, L. L., 'Presentation of a Case of Mutilating Operations in a Hysterical Patient', *Journal of Nervous and Mental Disease*, XXXVIII/7 (1911), pp. 425–8

McIntosh, William Carmichael, 'On Morbid Impulse', *Medical Critic and Psychological Journal*, III (1863), pp. 101–23

—, 'On Some of the Varieties of Morbid Impulse and Perverted Instinct', *Journal of Mental Science*, XI/56 (1866), pp. 512–33

Menninger, Karl A., *Love Against Hate* (New York, 1942)

—, *Man Against Himself* (San Diego, New York and London, 1985)

—, 'Psychoanalytic Aspects of Suicide', *International Journal of Psycho-Analysis*, XIV (1933), pp. 376–90

—, 'A Psychoanalytic Study of the Significance of Self-mutilations', *Psychoanalysis Quarterly*, IV (1935), pp. 408–66

—, 'Purposive Accidents as an Expression of Self-destructive Tendencies', *International Journal of Psycho-Analysis*, XVII (1936), pp. 6–16

—, *Sparks: Reflections from the Records of a Pioneer Psychiatrist*, ed. Lucy Freeman (New York, 1973)

—, *The Human Mind* (New York and London, 1930)

he Selected Correspondence of Karl A. Menninger, 1919–1945, ed. Howard J.
Faulkner and Virginia D. Pruitt (Columbia, MO, 1995)

Mercier, Charles Arthur, 'A Classification of Feelings (part 3)', *Mind*, X/37 (1885),
pp. 1–26

Micale, Mark S., *Approaching Hysteria: Disease and Its Interpretations*
(Princeton, NJ, 1995)

Millard, Chris, *A History of Self-harm in Britain: A Genealogy of Cutting and
Overdosing* (London, 2015)

—, 'Making the Cut: The Production of "Self-harm" in Post-1945 Anglo-Saxon
Psychiatry', *History of the Human Sciences*, XXVI/2 (2013), pp. 126–50

—, 'Re-inventing the "Cry for Help": "Attempted Suicide" in Britain in the
Mid-twentieth Century *c.* 1937–1969', PhD thesis, Queen Mary University
of London, 2012

—, 'Self-mutilation and a Psychiatric Syndrome: Emergence, Exclusions and
Contexts (1967–1976)', MA thesis, University of York, 2007

Monks, George H., 'A Group of Unique and Unusual Surgical Cases', *Medical and
Surgical Reports of the Boston City Hospital*, 11th series (1900), pp. 143–57

Moore, Alison, 'Rethinking Gendered Perversion and Degeneration in Visions of
Sadism and Masochism, 1886–1930', *Journal of the History of Sexuality*, XVIII/1
(2009), pp. 138–57

Morgan, H. G., *Death Wishes? The Understanding and Management of Deliberate
Self-harm* (Chichester, 1979)

Moscucci, Ornella, *The Science of Woman: Gynaecology and Gender in England,
1800–1929* (Cambridge and New York, 1993)

'Motiveless Malingerers', *British Medical Journal*, I/470 (1870), pp. 15–16

Myers, F.W.H., *Human Personality and Its Survival of Bodily Death*
(London, 1903)

Nelson, Scott H., and Henry Grunebaum, 'A Follow-up Study of Wrist Slashers',
American Journal of Psychiatry, CXXVII (1971), pp. 1345–9

NICE (National Institute for Clinical Excellence), *Self-harm in Over 8s: Long-term
Management (CG133)*, www.nice.org.uk (November 2011)

Nicoll, Alexander, 'A Remarkable Case of Persistent Ingestion of Needles',
The Lancet, CLXXI/4411 (1908), pp. 772–8

Niebyl, Peter Heuer, 'Venesection and the Concept of the Foreign Body:
A Historical Study in the Therapeutic Consequences of Humoral and
Traumatic Concepts of Disease', PhD thesis, Yale University, 1970

Norman, Connolly, 'Sexual Perversion', in *Dictionary of Psychological Medicine*,
ed. Daniel Hack Tuke (London, 1892), pp. 1156–7

North, Carol, *Welcome, Silence: My Triumph Over Schizophrenia* (New York, 1987)

North, Carol, and Remi Cadoret, 'Diagnostic Discrepancy in Personal Accounts
of Patients with "Schizophrenia"', *Archives of General Psychiatry*, XXVIII/2
(1 February 1981), p. 133

Nutton, Vivian, *Ancient Medicine* (London and New York, 2005)

'Obituary: George Pernet', *British Medical Journal*, I (1940), p. 113

Offer, Daniel, and Peter Barglow, 'Adolescent and Young Adult Self-mutilation Incidents in a General Psychiatric Hospital', *Archives of General Psychiatry*, III (1960), pp. 194–204

Oldstone-Moore, Christopher, 'The Beard Movement in Victorian Britain', *Victorian Studies*, XXXXVIII/1 (2005), pp. 7–34

'On Moral and Criminal Epidemics', *Journal of Psychological Medicine and Mental Pathology*, IX/2 (1856), pp. 240–81

O'Neill, Timothy H., 'The Invisible Man? Problematising Gender and Male Medicine in Britain and America, 1800–1950', PhD thesis, University of Manchester, 2003

Oosterhuis, Harry, *Stepchildren of Nature: Krafft-Ebing, Psychiatry, and the Making of Sexual Indentity* (Chicago, IL, and London, 2000)

Oppenheim, Janet, *'Shattered Nerves': Doctors, Patients, and Depression in Victorian England* (New York, 1991)

Ostroff, Natalie, and Jim Taylor, 'Tumblr to Ban Self-harm and Eating Disorder Blogs', BBC, www.bbc.co.uk, 26 March 2012

Ovid, *Fasti*, ed. G. P. Goold, trans. James George Frazer (Cambridge, MA, 2014)

—, *Metamorphoses, Books IX–XII*, trans. D. E. Hill (Warminster, Wilts, 1999)

Pao, Ping-Nie, 'The Syndrome of Delicate Self-cutting', *British Journal of Medical Psychology*, XXXXII (1969), pp. 195–206

Parry-Jones, B., and W. L. Parry-Jones, 'Self-mutilation in 4 Historical Cases of Bulimia', *British Journal of Psychiatry*, CLXIII (1993), pp. 394–402

Parry-Jones, William Llywelyn, *The Trade in Lunacy: A Study of Private Madhouses in England in the Eighteenth and Nineteenth Centuries* (London, 1972)

Pembroke, Louise Roxanne, ed., *Self-harm: Perspectives from Personal Experience* (London, 2009)

Penny, Laurie, 'Laurie Penny on Trigger Warnings: What We're Really Talking about', *New Statesman*, 21 May 2014

Pernet, George, 'The Psychological Aspect of Dermatitis Factitia', *Transactions of the American Dermatological Association*, XXX (1909), pp. 20–26

—, 'Two Cases of Dermatitis Factitia', *Proceedings of the Royal Society of Medicine (Dermatological Section)*, VIII (1915), pp. 89–91

Pick, Daniel, *Faces of Degeneration: A European Disorder, c.1848–c.1918* (Cambridge and New York, 1989)

Plante, Lori G., *Bleeding to Ease the Pain: Cutting, Self-injury, and the Adolescent Search for Self* (Westport, CT, 2007)

Plath, Sylvia, *The Bell Jar* (London, 1963)

Platt, Stephen, 'The Aftermath of Angie's Overdose: Is Soap (Opera) Damaging to Your Health?', *British Medical Journal*, CCLXXXXIV (1987), pp. 954–7

Podvoll, Edward M., 'Self-mutilation Within a Hospital Setting: A Study of Identity and Social Compliance', *British Journal of Medical Psychology*, XXXXII (1969), pp. 213–21

Porter, Roy, 'Body and Mind, the Doctor and the Patient: Negotiating Hysteria', in *Hysteria Beyond Freud*, ed. Sander L. Gilman, Roy Porter, Helen King, G. S.

Rousseau and Elaine Showalter (Berkeley, Los Angeles and London, 1993), pp. 225–85

Preston, Laurence W., 'A Right to Exist: Eunuchs and the State in Nineteenth-century India', *Modern Asian Studies*, XXI/2 (1987), pp. 371–87

Prichard, James Cowles, *A Treatise on Insanity and Other Disorders Affecting the Mind* (London, 1835)

Pritchard Davies, Francis, 'Chemical Restraint and Alcohol', *Journal of Mental Science*, XXVI/116 (1881), pp. 526–30

Putnam, James Jackson, 'Recent Experiences in the Study and Treatment of Hysteria at the Massachusetts General Hospital; with Remarks on Freud's Method of Treatment by "Psycho-Analysis"', *Journal of Abnormal Psychology*, I/1 (1906), pp. 26–41

Rayner, Henry, 'Melancholia and Hypochondriasis', in *A System of Medicine*, ed. T. Clifford Allbutt (London, 1899), pp. 361–81

Reade, William Winwood, *The Martyrdom of Man* (London, 1884)

Reeves, Carol Anne, 'Insanity and Nervous Diseases amongst Jewish Immigrants to the East End of London, 1880–1920', PhD thesis, University of London, 2001

Renvoize, E., 'The Association of Medical Officers of Asylums and Hospitals for the Insane, the Medico-Psychological Association, and Their Presidents', in *150 Years of British Psychiatry, 1841–1991*, ed. G. E. Berrios and Hugh L. Freeman (London, 1991), pp. 29–78

Rey, Roselyne, *History of Pain*, trans. Louise Elliott Wallace, J. A. Cadden and S. W. Cadden (Paris, 1993)

Richardson, Henry Barber, *Patients Have Families* (New York, 1945)

Ringrose, Kathryn M., *The Perfect Servant: Eunuchs and the Social Construction of Gender in Byzantium* (London, 2003)

Risse, G. B., 'Renaissance of Bloodletting – Chapter in Modern Therapeutics', *Journal of the History of Medicine and Allied Sciences*, XXXIV (1979), pp. 3–22

Ritchie, Robert, 'An Inquiry into a Frequent Cause of Insanity in Young Men', *The Lancet*, LXXVII/1955–60 (1861), pp. 159–61 and 284–6

Roberts, Jane H., Rachel Pryke, Margaret Murphy and Lucie Russell, 'Young People who Self Harm by Cutting', *British Medical Journal*, CCCXXXXVII (2013), pp. 1–2

Rose, Diana, '"Having a Diagnosis is a Qualification for the Job"', *BMJ (Clinical Research Edition)*, CCCXXVI/7402 (14 June 2003), pp. 1331

Rose, Nikolas, *Inventing Our Selves: Psychology, Power and Personhood* (Cambridge and New York, 1996)

Rosen, Paul M., and Barent W. Walsh, 'Patterns of Contagion in Self-mutilation Epidemics', *American Journal of Psychiatry*, CXXXXVI/5 (1989), pp. 656–8

Rosenberg, Charles E., and Janet Golden, eds, *Framing Disease: Studies in Cultural History* (New Brunswick, NJ, 1992)

Rosenthal, Richard J., Carl Rinzler, Rita Walsh and Edmund Klausner, 'Wrist-cutting Syndrome: The Meaning of a Gesture', *American Journal of Psychiatry*, CXXVIII/11 (1972), pp. 1363–8

Ross, Robert R., and Hugh Bryan McKay, *Self-mutilation* (Lexington, MA, 1979)

Bibliography

Rousselle, Aline, *Porneia: On Desire and the Body in Antiquity*, trans. Felicia Pheasant (Oxford, 1988)

Rudnytsky, Peter L., 'Rescuing Psychoanalysis from Freud: The Common Project of Stekel, Jung and Ferenczi', *Psychoanalysis and History*, VIII/1 (2006), pp. 125–59

Samuel, Lawrence R., *Shrink: A Cultural History of Psychoanalysis in America* (Lincoln, NE, 2013)

Saundby, Robert, 'Clinical Lecture on Toxic Hysteria', *The Lancet*, CXXXVII/3514 (January 1891), pp. 2–4

Savage, George, 'An Address on the Borderland of Insanity', *British Medical Journal*, 1/2357 (1906), pp. 489–92

—, 'The Influence of Surroundings on the Production of Insanity', *Journal of Mental Science*, XXXVII/159 (1891), pp. 529–35

—, 'Marriage in Neurotic Subjects', *Journal of Mental Science*, XXIX (1883), pp. 49–54

—, 'The Mechanical Restraint of the Insane', *The Lancet*, CXXXII/3398 (1888), pp. 738–9

—, 'Moral Insanity', *Journal of Mental Science*, XXVII/118 (1881), pp. 147–55

—, 'Presidential Address, Delivered at the Annual Meeting of the Medico-Psychological Association', *Journal of Mental Science*, XXXII/139 (1886), pp. 313–31

Savage, George, and Charles Arthur Mercier, 'Insanity of Conduct', *Journal of Mental Science*, XXXXII/176 (1896), pp. 1–17

Schaffner, Wolfgang, 'Event, Series, Trauma: The Probabilistic Revolution of the Mind in the Late Nineteenth and Early Twentieth Centuries', in *Traumatic Pasts: History, Psychiatry and Trauma in the Modern Age, 1870–1930*, ed. Mark S. Micale and Paul Frederick Lerner (Cambridge and New York, 2001), pp. 81–91

Schroeder, Stephen R., Mary Lou Oster-Granite and Travis Thompson, eds, *Self-injurious Behavior: Gene–Brain–Behavior Relationship* (Washington, DC, 2002)

Scull, Andrew T., '"A Chance to Cut is a Chance to Cure": Sexual Surgery for Psychosis in Three Nineteenth-century Societies', in *The Insanity of Place / The Place of Insanity* (London and New York, 2006), pp. 151–71

—, *Museums of Madness: The Social Organization of Insanity in Nineteenth-century England* (London, 1979)

—, 'Psychiatry and Social Control in the Nineteenth and Twentieth Centuries', in *The Insanity of Place / The Place of Insanity* (London and New York, 2006), pp. 107–28

'Self-mutilation by the Insane', *Medical Press and Circular*, II (1888), pp. 260–61

Sengoopta, Chandak, *The Most Secret Quintessence of Life: Sex, Glands, and Hormones, 1850–1950* (Chicago, IL, and London, 2006)

Seymour, E. J., 'Thoughts on the Nature and Treatment of Several Severe Diseases of the Human Body', in *Three Hundred Years of Psychiatry, 1535–1860*, ed. Richard Alfred Hunter and Ida Macalpine (London and New York, 1847), pp. 960–62

Shamdasani, Sonu, 'Claire, Lise, Jean, Nadia and Gisele: Preliminary Notes towards a Characterisation of Pierre Janet's Psychasthenia', in *Cultures of Neurasthenia: From Beard to the First World War*, ed. Roy Porter and Marijke Gijswijt-Hofstra (Amsterdam, 2001), pp. 362–85

—, 'Psychotherapy: The Invention of a Word', *History of the Human Sciences*, XVIII/1 (2005), pp. 1–22

Sharpe, Katherine, 'The Silence of Prozac', *The Lancet Psychiatry*, II/10 (10 October 2015), pp. 871–3

Shaw, James, *Epitome of Mental Diseases: For Practitioners and Students* (Bristol and London, 1892)

Shorter, Edward, 'Paralysis: The Rise and Fall of a "Hysterical" Symptom', *Journal of Social History*, XIX/4 (1986), pp. 549–82

Shortt, John, 'The Kojahs of Southern India', *Journal of the Anthropological Institute of Great Britain and Ireland*, 2 (1873), pp. 402–7

Showalter, Elaine, *The Female Malady: Women, Madness, and English Culture, 1830–1980* (London, 1987)

—, *Hystories: Hysterical Epidemics and Modern Culture* (London, 1997)

Slee, Nadja, Nadia Garnefski, Rien van der Leeden, Ella Arensman and Philip Spinhoven, 'Cognitive-Behavioural Intervention for Self-harm: Randomised Controlled Trial', *British Journal of Psychiatry*, CLXXXXII (2008), pp. 202–11

Smith, Roger, *Being Human: Historical Knowledge and the Creation of Human Nature* (New York, 2007)

—, *Inhibition: History and Meaning in the Sciences of Mind and Brain* (London, 1992)

Smith, Tim, 'On the Death of a Child and Trigger Warnings', Gashead.net, www.gashead.net, 23 April 2015

Smith-Rosenberg, Carroll, *Disorderly Conduct: Visions of Gender in Victorian America* (New York and Oxford, 1986)

Spencer, Herbert, 'The Comparative Psychology of Man', *Mind*, I/1 (1876), pp. 7–20

Spitzer, Robert L., Jean Endicott and Miriam Gibbon, 'Crossing the Border into Borderline Personality and Borderline Schizophrenia: The Development of Criteria', in *Essential Papers on Borderline Disorders: One Hundred Years at the Border*, ed. Michael H. Stone (New York, 1986), pp. 527–48

Stanton, Alfred H., and Morris S. Schwartz, *The Mental Hospital: A Study of Institutional Participation in Psychiatric Illness and Treatment* (New York, 1954)

Starr, Douglas P., *Blood: An Epic History of Medicine and Commerce* (New York, 1998)

Startin, James, 'Remarks on Feigned or Hysterical Diseases of the Skin', *British Medical Journal*, I/471 (1870), pp. 25–7

Steggals, Peter, *Making Sense of Self-harm: the Cultural Meaning and Social Context of Nonsuicidal Self-injury* (Basingstoke, 2015)

Stekel, Wilhelm, *Auto-erotism: A Psychiatric Study of Masturbation and Neurosis*, trans. James A. Van Teslaar (New York, 1951)

—, *Sadism and Masochism: The Psychology of Hatred and Cruelty*, trans. Louise Brink (London, 1953)

Stengel, Erwin, *Suicide and Attempted Suicide* (Harmondsworth, 1967)

Stengel, Erwin, and Nancy Gwendolen Cook, *Attempted Suicide: Its Social Significance and Effects* (London, 1958)

Stone, Michael H., *Essential Papers on Borderline Disorders: One Hundred Years at the Border* (New York, 1986)

Strong, Marilee, *A Bright Red Scream: Self-mutilation and the Language of Pain* (London, 2000)

Tarr, Joel A., and Mark Tebeau, 'Housewives as Home Safety Managers: The Changing Perception of the Home as a Place of Hazard and Risk, 1870–1940', in *Accidents in History: Injuries, Fatalities and Social Relations*, ed. Roger Cooter and Bill Luckin (Atlanta, GA, 1997), pp. 196–233

Taylor, Gary, *Castration: An Abbreviated History of Western Manhood* (New York and London, 2000)

Teinturier, E., *Les Skoptzy* (Paris, 1877)

Templeton, Sarah Kate, 'Self-harmers to be Given Clean Blades', *The Times*, 5 February 2006

Thomson, George, *Galeno-pale; or, a Chymical Trial of the Galenists* (London, 1665)

Thomson, Mathew, 'Family, Community, and State: The Micro-politics of Mental Deficiency', in *From Idiocy to Mental Deficiency: Historical Perspectives on People with Learning Disabilities*, ed. David Wright and Anne Digby (New York, 1996), pp. 207–30

—, *Psychological Subjects: Identity, Culture, and Health in Twentieth-century Britain* (Oxford and New York, 2006)

Timms, Noel, *Psychiatric Social Work in Great Britain (1939–1962)* (New York, 1964)

Toch, Hans, *Men in Crisis: Human Breakdowns in Prison* (Chicago, IL, 1975)

Torok, Robyn, 'Developing an Explanatory Model for the Process of Online Radicalisation and Terrorism', *Security Informatics*, II/1 (12 February 2013), p. 6

Tosh, John, *A Man's Place: Masculinity and the Middle-class Home in Victorian England* (New Haven, CT, and London, 1999)

Tougher, Shaun, *The Eunuch in Byzantine History and Society* (Abingdon, Oxon, 2008)

Tuke, Daniel Hack, 'American Retrospect: The Insane in the United States', *Journal of Mental Science*, XXXI/133 (1 April 1885), pp. 89–116

—, 'Case of Moral Insanity or Congenital Moral Defect, with Commentary', *Journal of Mental Science*, XXXI/135 (1885), pp. 360–66

—, ed., *A Dictionary of Psychological Medicine* (London, 1892)

—, *Prichard and Symonds in Especial Relation to Mental Science, with Chapters on Moral Insanity* (London, 1891)

—, *Reform in the Treatment of the Insane: Early History of the Retreat, York: Its Objects and Influence, with a Report of the Celebrations of its Centenary* (London, 1892)

Tuke, Samuel, *Description of the Retreat, an Institution near York, for Insane Persons of the Society of Friends* (York, 1813)

Tylor, Edward B., 'Primitive Society (Part I)', *Contemporary Review*, XXI (1872), pp. 701–18

'The Ubiquity of Suicide', *British Medical Journal*, I/4075 (1939), pp. 273–4

Upchurch, Charles, 'Forgetting the Unthinkable: Cross-dressers and British Society in the Case of the Queen vs. Boulton and Others', *Gender & History*, XII/1 (2000), pp. 127–57

Vandermeersch, Patrick, 'Self-flagellation in the Early Modern Era', in *The Sense of Suffering: Constructions of Physical Pain in Early Modern Culture*, ed. Karl A. E. Dijkhuizen and Jan Frans van Enenkel (Boston, MA, 2009), pp. 253–65

Vesalius, Andreas, *On the Fabric of the Human Body (De Humani Corporis Fabrica), An Annotated Translation of the 1543 and 1555 Editions*, ed. Vivian Nutton (Evanston, IL, 2003)

Vingiano, Ali, 'How the "Trigger Warning" Took over the Internet', *BuzzFeed News*, 5 May 2014, www.buzzfeed.com

Walkowitz, Judith R., *City of Dreadful Delight: Narratives of Sexual Danger in Late-Victorian London* (London, 1992)

—, 'Jack the Ripper and the Myth of Male Violence', *Feminist Studies*, VIII/3 (1982), pp. 542–74

—, *Prostitution and Victorian Society: Women, Class and the State* (Cambridge, 1980)

Wallace, Alfred R., 'The Origin of Human Races and the Antiquity of Man Deduced from the Theory of "Natural Selection"', *Journal of the Anthropological Society of London*, II (1864), pp. clviii–clxxxvii

Walsh, Barent W., and Paul M. Rosen, 'Self-mutilation and Contagion: An Empirical Test', *American Journal of Psychiatry*, CXXXXII/1 (1985), pp. 119–20

—, *Self-mutilation: Theory, Research, and Treatment* (New York and London, 1988)

Weber, Frederick Parkes, 'The Association of Hysteria with Malingering', *The Lancet*, CLXXVIII/4605 (1911), pp. 1542–3

Weinstein, Deborah, *The Pathological Family: Postwar America and the Rise of Family Therapy* (London, 2013)

Wessely, Simon C., and Edgar Jones, *Shell Shock to PTSD: Military Psychiatry from 1900 to the Gulf War* (Hove and New York, 2005)

Whitlock, Janis, Wendy Lader and Karen Conterio, 'The Internet and Self-injury: What Psychotherapists Should Know', *Journal of Clinical Psychology*, LXIII/11 (2007), pp. 1135–43

Whitlock, Janis, Jane L. Powers and John Eckenrode, 'The Virtual Cutting Edge: The Internet and Adolescent Self-injury', *Developmental Psychology*, XXXXII/3 (2006), pp. 407–17

Whitlock, Janis, Amanda Purington and Marina Gershkovich, 'Media, the Internet and Nonsuicidal Self-injury', in *Understanding Nonsuicidal Self-injury: Origins, Assessment, and Treatment*, ed. Matthew Nock (Arlington, VA, 2009), pp. 139–55

Whittle, Helen, Catherine Hamilton-Giachritsis, Anthony Beech and Guy Collings, 'A Review of Online Grooming: Characteristics and Concerns', *Aggression and Violent Behavior*, XVIII/1 (January 2013)

Willis, Thomas, *The London Practice of Physick* (London, 1689)

Wilson, Erasmus, *Lectures on Dermatology: Delivered in the Royal College of Surgeons of England in 1874–1875* (London, 1875)

Wilson, Jean D., and Claus Roehrborn, 'Long-term Consequences of Castration in Men: Lessons from the Skoptzy and the Eunuchs of the Chinese and Ottoman Courts', *Journal of Clinical Endocrinology and Metabolism*, LXXXIV/12 (1999), pp. 4324–31

Winchester, Simon, *The Surgeon of Crowthorne: A Tale of Murder, Madness and the Love of Words* (London, 1998)

Winslow, Forbes, *The Anatomy of Suicide* (London, 1840)

Wootton, David, *Bad Medicine: Doctors Doing Harm since Hippocrates* (Oxford, 2006)

Wurtzel, Elizabeth, *Prozac Nation: Young and Depressed in America* (London, 1996)

Wynter, Andrew, *The Borderlands of Insanity* (London, 1877)

Yampolsky, Eva, 'La Perversion du suicide, entre la pathologie et la morale',
 Criminocorpus: Revue hypermédia (forthcoming, Autumn 2016)
Yellowlees, David, 'Masturbation', *Journal of Mental Science*, XXII/98 (1876), pp. 336–7
—, 'Masturbation', in *Dictionary of Psychological Medicine*, ed. Daniel Hack Tuke,
 (London, 1892), p. 785
Yeshua-Katz, Daphna, and Nicole Martins, 'Communicating Stigma: The Pro-Ana
 Paradox', *Health Communication*, XXVIII/5 (2012), pp. 499–508
Young, Robert, Helen Sweeting and Patrick West, 'Prevalence of Deliberate Self-harm
 and Attempted Suicide within Contemporary Goth Youth Subculture: Longitudinal
 Cohort Study', *British Medical Journal*, CCCXXXII/7549 (2006), pp. 1058–61

Archives and Unpublished Material

Bethlem Royal Hospital Archives (BRHA), Bethlem Royal Hospital, Monks
 Orchard Road, Beckenham, BR3 3BX (www.museumofthemind.org.uk)
 Annual Reports, 1880–1900 (BAR-18–BAR-38)
 Patient Casebooks, 1880–1900 (CB-116–164), includes Voluntary Boarders
 Casebooks, 1886–1900
 Resident Physician's Weekly Reports, 1885–1905 (BWR-01, BWR-02)
 Standing Rules and Orders (SRO series)
 Under the Dome (hospital magazine), 1892–1905 (UTD-01– UTD-14)
Kent County Archives (KCA), Kent History and Library Centre, James Whatman
 Way, Maidstone ME14 1LQ (www.kent.gov.uk)
 Records of Malling Place, Private Mental Nursing Home 1829–1977 (Ch84)
Oxford University Press Archive (OUPA), Oxford University Press, Great Clarendon
 Street, Oxford OX2 6DP (http://global.oup.com/uk/archives)
 Un-numbered discarded slips for *Oxford English Dictionary* editions
Queen Square Archives (QSA), National Hospital, Queen Square Library, UCL
 Institute of Neurology and the National Hospital, London WC1N 3BG
 (www.queensquare.org.uk/archives)
 Casebooks, 1878–1905
Royal London Hospital Archive (RLHA), 9 Prescot Street, London E1 8PR
 (www.bartshealth.nhs.uk)
 Inpatient Registers, 1885–1910 (LH/M/1/13–48)
 Case Notes, Surgical (Microfilm), 1893–1910 (LH/M/14, boxes 1–9)
 Case Notes, Medical (Microfilm), 1893–1910 (LH/M/14, boxes 50–65)
Wellcome Library, London (WLL), 183 Euston Road, London NW1 2BE
 (www.wellcomelibrary.org)
 James Adam, Diaries as Physician-Superintendent of Crichton Royal Institution,
 1880–1882 (MSS.5517-5519)
 Frederick Parkes Weber Collection, Self-mutilations for Various Purposes,
 1901–1954, PP/FPW/B.163 (box 84, 5 files)

HELP AND ADVICE

One of the aims of this book is to provide a critical perspective on the psychiatric model of self-harm. While this may help some people who injure themselves, many will still need to access other forms of support at times. If you or someone you know is looking for help and advice, here are some starting points.

Human Rights

The Bill of Rights for Those who Self-harm by Deb Martinson
www.fortrefuge.com/SelfInjuryBillOfRights.html
This is an American text outlining the basic human rights that someone who has injured themselves should expect in medical care, including Accident & Emergency.

Mind
www.mind.org.uk
The charity Mind provides advice and information on all aspects of mental health, including legal advice.

Telephone and Online Support

Samaritans
www.samaritans.org / Tel. 116 123
The Samaritans' (UK) phone lines are open 24/7, offering advice free of charge. They also offer drop-in, email and postal services.

SANEline
www.sane.org.uk / Tel. 0300 304 7000
SANEline offers emotional support and information from 6pm–11pm, every day of the year.

Harmless
www.harmless.org.uk
Harmless is a specialist self-harm support service, set up as a user-led charity. They have online advice and provide email and postal support.

Self-injury Support
www.selfinjurysupport.org.uk / Tel. 0808 800 8088
For women and girls; formerly Bristol Crisis Service for Women. This support group began as a user-led initiative. They run a Women's Self Injury Helpline, and their website also includes an extensive list of support groups and resources across the UK.

CALM
www.thecalmzone.net / 0800 58 58 58
For men. The Campaign Against Living Miserably provides support for men experiencing suicidal thoughts or distress. The telephone line is open 5pm–midnight every day. They also have a webchat service.

7 Cups of Tea
www.7cups.com
7 Cups of Tea offers online support from trained listeners at any time.

Mental Health Services

GP services and primary care are usually the first point of access to mental health services in the UK, including psychotherapy. Specialist self-harm support varies across NHS trusts. The Maudsley Hospital in London runs a national Self-harm Outpatient Service. You can be referred by a GP, consultant or community mental health team.

Non-clinical services available to those in need include The Maytree Suicide Respite Centre (www.maytree.org.uk) and Dial House in Leeds (www.lslcs.org.uk).

Arts and User-led Support Groups

Creative user-led groups exist in some parts of the UK. The way they are accessed and the services they offer vary considerably (some require a referral). A few of those that are open to everyone include:

Survivors Poetry, www.survivorspoetry.org. A mental health survivors poetry network, with local groups in various parts of England

The Dragon Café, London, www.dragoncafe.co.uk. A creative social space open to all every Monday

CoolTan Arts, London, www.cooltanarts.org.uk. Runs a variety of workshops and walks. Many activities are open to everyone

Creative Future, Brighton, www.creativefuture.org.uk. Courses, events and workshops for marginalized artists.

Outside In, Chichester, www.outsidein.org.uk. Set up by Pallant House Gallery, it provides a platform for marginalized artists

Creativity Works, Bristol, www.creativityworks.org.uk. Run arts and health projects in Bristol, Bath and North East Somerset

Online Peer Support Forums

National Self-harm Network, www.nshn.co.uk
Life Signs, www.lifesigns.org.uk/what
Recover Your Life, www.recoveryourlife.com
Self-injury.net, https://self-injury.net/forums

Other Peer Support or Service User Groups

These are just a few among many mental health support groups focused on specific symptoms or experiences:

Hearing Voices Network, www.hearing-voices.org. Many local chapters and support groups exist

Beat, www.b-eat.co.uk. Eating disorders charity that includes a help finder for local peer support groups

NSUN (formerly National Survivor User Network), www.nsun.org.uk. Provides peer-to-peer support, information and networking

Bipolar UK, www.bipolaruk.org. Local support groups and more

Emergence, www.emergenceplus.org.uk. Service-user led organization providing support and advice for people diagnosed with personality disorders

Survivors History, http://studymore.org.uk/mpu.htm. London-based history group, with an extremely comprehensive website of mental health history

ACKNOWLEDGEMENTS

This book would not have been possible without the support and assistance of a large number of people. During my research, I used various archives and libraries, and I am grateful to the staff at those institutions for their assistance: in particular, Colin Gale, archivist at Bethlem Museum of the Mind, and Jonathan Evans, archivist at the Royal London Hospital. I would also like to thank staff at the Oxford University Press, the Kent County Archives and the National Hospital for Neurology, Queen Square, London. Particular thanks are due to the friendly folk at the Wellcome Library, especially Ross, Phoebe, Jette and Danny, who have offered both support and an appropriately welcoming place to work. This book has been published with the help of a grant from the late Miss Isobel Thornley's Bequest to the University of London. I also gratefully acknowledge the financial support of the Wellcome Trust, in funding the PhD that began my research on the topic of self-harm.

I am extremely grateful for the time and interest of the interviewees who participated in the later chapters: Liz Atkin, Charley Baker, Jane Bunclark, Armando Favazza, Ian Hulatt, Clare Shaw and the late and very much missed Sarah Wheeler. Not only did they give generously of their time in interviews, they also offered comments on written material. Particular thanks are due to Liz and Clare for allowing me to use their personal stories in the conclusion. I would also like to thank Louise Pembroke for directing me to additional resources on survivor history, and for the use of her cartoons from *Self-Harm: Perspectives from Personal Experience*.

My friends and colleagues at University College London and Queen Mary University of London and beyond have provided invaluable criticism, advice and support. In particular, I would like to thank my PhD supervisor, Sonu Shamdasani, for his unfailing support for and interest in my project and his advice at every stage, and Roger Smith and Joanna Bourke, who examined my thesis and supported its adaptation into this book. I would also like to give especial thanks to the friends and colleagues who kindly read draft chapters of the book and offered useful suggestions and criticisms: Jenny Adlem, Mike Alexander, Niall Boyce, Sally Frampton, Åsa Jansson, Alice Leggatt, Chris Millard, Tom Quick, Mohammed Rashed, Danny Rees and Debbie Shipton. I am especially grateful to Chris and Åsa for helping me to think critically through some of the ideas raised in the introduction.

I would also like to thank all the other colleagues who have offered suggestions throughout my research project, in particular Gemma Angel, Peter Campbell, Lauren Cracknell, Roger Cooter, Ivan Crozier, Thomas Dixon, Corina Dobos, Lesley Hall, Rhodri Hayward, Matei Iagher, Sarah Marks, Joanne Ella Parsons, Carole Reeves, Steve Ridge, Andrew Roberts, Andreas Sommer, Emma Sutton, Jen Wallis and Andrew Wear. Thanks are also due to Jenny Walke and Max Reeves for keeping me going through the 'Mansions in the Orchard' project, to Jane Fradgley, whose *held* photography project led to countless stimulating discussions and friendship, and to Christine Bradbury, for the fortuitous present of a copy of *Don't Monkey With Murder*.

My thanks are due to everyone at Reaktion Books, in particular Ben Hayes for advice, suggestions, enthusiasm and coffee, and Aimee Selby for tireless editing.

Last but very much not least, thank you to all my other friends and loved ones. Above all to my parents, Brian and Kathy, and my little sister Alison, for never losing faith in me. To Sophia for being there during some of the worst times. And to Michelle and Gareth, Sadie and Willow for keeping me smiling.

And to Stewart, for late-night discussions, ideas, inspiration and love.

PHOTO ACKNOWLEDGEMENTS

The author and publishers wish to express their thanks to the following sources of illustrative material and/or permission to reproduce it:

© Bethlem Museum of the Mind: pp. 63, 73; © The British Library Board: p. 90; © The Trustees of the British Museum, London: p. 27; © Camera Press/Ed Sirrs: p. 215; courtesy The Freud Museum, London: p. 150; photo by Jeff Goode/Toronto Star via Getty Images: p. 187; © Maxwell Hamilton: p. 217; © Dominic Johnson. Used with permission: p. 13; The Estate of William Kurelek, courtesy of the Wynick/Tuck Gallery, Toronto (Adamson Collection/Wellcome Library): p. 194; © Library of Congress, Prints and Photographs Division/Frances Benjamin Johnston: p. 147; The Metropolitan Museum of Art, New York: p. 36; courtesy National Archives and Records Administration (USA): p. 170; © National Portrait Gallery, London: p. 137; courtesy of Peerless Rockville: p. 189; © Louise Roxanne Pembroke: pp. 16, 237; courtesy of The Pierpont Morgan Library, New York: p. 39; courtesy of H. W. Taylor: p. 160; reproduced with permission of Time Inc. (UK): p. 219; © UCL Pathology Collections: p. 122; courtesy of the United States National Library of Medicine: p. 55; © Tom Varco: p. 209; Victoria State Library, Australia: p. 125; © The Walters Art Museum, Baltimore, MD: p. 157; © Wellcome Library, London: pp. 43, 45, 49, 60, 70, 85, 87, 100, 105, 106, 115, 117, 126, 140, 146, 155, 211, 230; © Yale University Art Gallery, New Haven, CT: p. 23.

INDEX

Page numbers in italic refer to illustrations